Essentials of E-Learning for Nurse Educators

Essentials of E-Learning for Nurse Educators

Tim J. Bristol, PhD, RN, CNE
Owner
NurseTim, Inc.
Waconia, Minnesota
Consultant
Nursing Education Consultants
Ingram, Texas
Contributing Faculty
Walden University
Minneapolis, Minnesota

JoAnn Zerwekh, EdD, RN
Executive Director
Nursing Education Consultants
Ingram, Texas
Associate Faculty—Online Faculty
University of Phoenix
Phoenix, Arizona

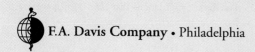 **F.A. Davis Company** • Philadelphia

F. A. Davis Company
1915 Arch Street
Philadelphia, PA 19103
www.fadavis.com

Printed in the United States of America

Last digit indicates print number: 10 9 8 7 6 5 4

Publisher, Nursing: Joanne P. DaCunha
Developmental Editor: Jennifer Schmidt
Director of Content Development: Darlene D. Pedersen
Project Editor: Tyler R. Baber
Design and Illustration Manager: Carolyn O'Brien

As new scientific information becomes available through basic and clinical research, recommended treatments and drug therapies undergo changes. The author(s) and publisher have done everything possible to make this book accurate, up to date, and in accord with accepted standards at the time of publication. The author(s), editors, and publisher are not responsible for errors or omissions or for consequences from application of the book, and make no warranty, expressed or implied, in regard to the contents of the book. Any practice described in this book should be applied by the reader in accordance with professional standards of care used in regard to the unique circumstances that may apply in each situation. The reader is advised always to check product information (package inserts) for changes and new information regarding dose and contraindications before administering any drug. Caution is especially urged when using new or infrequently ordered drugs.

Library of Congress Cataloging-in-Publication Data

Essentials of e-learning for nurse educators/[edited by] Tim J. Bristol, PhD, RN, CNE, Owner, Nurse Tim, Inc., Waconia, Minnesota; Contributing Faculty, Walden University, Minneapolis, Minnesota, JoAnn Zerwekh, EdD, RN Executive Director, Nursing Education Consultants, Ingram, Texas.
    p. ; cm.
  Includes bibliographical references and index.
  ISBN-13: 978-0-8036-2173-2
  ISBN-10: 0-8036-2173-6
1. Nursing—Study and teaching. 2. Internet in education. 3. Internet in medicine.
I. Bristol, Tim J., editor. II. Zerwekh, JoAnn, 1949- editor.
  [DNLM: 1. Education, Nursing—methods. 2. Computer-Assisted Instruction—methods.
3. Education, Distance—methods. 4. Internet. 5. Teaching—methods. WY 18]
  RT73.5.E87 2011
  610.73078'54678—dc22
                          2010047352

We want to thank Christina and John for their tireless support of all that has been involved in this great adventure. Their amazing friendship and encouragement has made it possible.

Foreword

As increasing numbers of the "net-generation" enter nursing schools and the nursing workforce, faculty and staff educators are challenged to provide educational experiences for learners who are savvy users of e-learning technologies. These learners may retrieve reading materials from electronic book readers and access information from smartphones, and often choose to enroll in online educational programs because they are accessible and convenient. These same learners relate to educators and each other through social networking Web sites and text messaging. To meet the needs of these learners, educational institutions have made significant investments in learning infrastructure such as classrooms equipped with videoconferencing and learner response systems, simulation centers with high-fidelity human patient simulators, as well as ubiquitous wireless access and online learning course management systems. Although today's nurse educators are likely to find themselves teaching in these "high-tech" classrooms and having clinical experiences in agencies where using e-learning is the norm, not all are prepared to do so.

Essentials of E-Learning for Nurse Educators addresses the needs of both new and experienced educators who must learn how to use e-leaning tools to facilitate learning and integrate them into courses and programs. Opening chapters of this book define e-learning, explain the theoretical underpinnings of learning with technology, and offer a design process to create an optimal learning environment. These chapters set the stage for subsequent in-depth discussions of how to teach in Web-supported courses, use technology in the curriculum, and develop and manage clinical simulations.

E-learning requires systems level planning for acquiring resources such as hardware and software, identifying stakeholders, developing the support team, and orienting learners and educators. The chapter on strategic planning will be useful to administrators and e-learning coordinators charged with leading the planning, implementing, and evaluating of the e-learning enterprise.

Learning is no longer scheduled for or measured by "seat time." Throughout the book, the chapter authors urge educators to be mindful of evaluating student learning outcomes and assessing the impact of e-learning. Concepts of continuous quality improvement are threaded throughout the book.

Nurse educators will find this book easy to use. There is a judicious balance of technical information and pedagogical principles. Each chapter includes, where relevant, teaching tips, examples of computer screen shots, checklists, and Web links to key resources and online learning activities. Tables, charts, and a glossary highlight key information.

Essentials of E-Learning for Nurse Educators adds to the increasing evidence for best practice in using e-learning for nursing education. This book is an essential addition to the nurse educator's library.

Diane M. Billings, EdD, RN, FAAN
Chancellor's Professor of Nursing Emeritus
Indiana University School of Nursing
Indianapolis, Indiana

Nurse educators of today have an amazing challenge ahead of them. They seek to serve a society that still needs the touch of the nurse at all stages in life. Yet educators must be attuned to the myriad of technology that is being infused into health care. Can these two challenges be met by today's educators? Can nursing students truly be prepared for the wave of the future?

We believe that the answer to these questions is a resounding "Yes." As you will see in the pages of this book, there are many ways to engage learners and prepare them for the future. One of the most important ways is to invoke the power of collaboration. Partner with colleagues in your department, in your college, and in your profession. Partner with learners. They bring such varied perspectives and they need to see you role modeling this crucial behavior (collaboration). Partner with vendors. Many offer excellent tools that are little or no cost. Others offer superior support for the tools in your school. Partner with industry. Your colleagues in other organizations, hospitals, and schools can help you obtain funding and succeed in your venture.

Finally partner with our team. We have put together a great collection of talent, perspective, and experience. From the young nurse to the seasoned educator, you will hear from a various professionals. You will look at concrete examples that you can take to practice right away.

This tool is packed full of features that will assist you in achieving your goals of creating innovative yet realistic learning experiences.

Innovative Experts: An author team that works in the same settings as you do.

Vignettes: Stories from the authors that highlight realistic examples.

Tech Tips: Practical and instantly applicable information.

Evidence-Based Practice Boxes: A solid foundation for the concepts being explored.

Tables/Figures: Visuals that clearly illustrate what you need to know for quick reference.

Sample Activities: From learning to assessment, many tools that have been used in multiple settings.

eNurse the Tour Guide: Will help emphasize key points on this important journey.

Appendixes: Crucial tools that apply to multiple settings.

Glossary: Addresses key terms so you can quickly find what you are looking for.

DavisPlus: Web site with links, samples, activities, and more.

Case Studies: Explore direct application of the concepts from each chapter; found in DavisPlus.

Contributors

Julia W. Aucoin, DNS, RN-BC, CNE
Nurse Research Scientist
Duke University Hospital
Durham, North Carolina

Margaret C. Blodgett, PhD, EdS, OTR
Associate Professor and Instructional Designer
Concordia University Wisconsin
Mequon, Wisconsin

Linda Caputi, MSN, EdD, RN, ANEF, CNE
Nursing Education Consultant
Linda Caputi, Inc.
Saint Charles, Illinois

Ellen Cummings, MSN, RN, CNRN, CNE
Nursing Faculty
Gateway Community College
Phoenix, Arizona

**Sharon Decker,
PhD, MSN, CCRN, ACNS-BC, ANEF**
Director of Clinical Simulation in the Anita
    Thigpen Perry SON
Texas Tech University Health Sciences Center
Lubbock, Texas

Cheryl Feken, RN, MS
Assistant Professor of Nursing
Clinical Simulation Coordinator
Tulsa Community College
Tulsa, Oklahoma

Ebony S. Fisher, MSN, PhD(c), RN
Online RN to BSN Program Chair
National American University
Rapid City, South Dakota

Teresa N. Gore, DNP, FNP-BC, NP-C
Assistant Clinical Professor and Simulation
    Learning Coordinator
Auburn University School of Nursing
Auburn, Alabama

Barbara A. Ihrke, PhD, RN
Dean, School of Nursing
Indiana Wesleyan University
Marion, Indiana

**Maria Lauer,
MSN, PhD(c) ,RN, APN-C, CNE**
Moorestown, New Jersey

John Miller, MN, ADN, BSN, CNE
3D Virtual Nursing and Medical Education
    Consulting
Tacoma Community College Nursing
MuveMarket and MUVErs
Tacoma, Washington

Patricia A.Z. (PZ) Nielsen MS, RN, NP
Assistant Professor of Nursing
College of Saint Scholastica
Duluth, Minnesota

Joann M. Oliver, MNEd, BSN, RN, CNE
Associate Professor of Nursing
Anne Arundel Community College
Arnold, Maryland

Marie E. Oliver, AS, AA
Millersville, Maryland

Cheryl D. Parker, MSN, PhD, RN
Senior Clinical Informatics Specialist—Motion
    Computing
Contributing Faculty—Walden University MSN-
    Nursing Informatics Track
Dallas, Texas

**Barbara Schreiner,
PhD, RN, CDE, BC-ADM**
Core Faculty, Nursing Programs
Capella University
Minneapolis, MN

Margi J. Schultz, PhD, RN, CNE
Director, Nursing Division
GateWay Community College
Phoenix, Arizona

**Charlene M. Smith,
DNS, MSEd, WHNP, RN, BC**
Associate Professor
Wegmans School of Nursing, St. John Fisher
    College
Rochester, New York

Beth A. Starnes-Vottero, PhD, RN, CNE
Assistant Professor of Nursing
Purdue University Calumet
Hammond, Indiana

Erich Widemark, PhD, RN, FNP-BC
FNP Program Manager
University of Phoenix
Phoenix, Arizona

Reviewers

Elizabeth Amos, PhD, RN, C, CS
Associate Professor
Graduate Coordinator
University of Nevada Reno
Reno, Nevada

Ronald Wade Ayers, MSN, RN, CNE
Instructor
Winston-Salem State University
Winston-Salem, North Carolina

Bridget Bailey, RN, MSN
Associate Professor
Iowa Lakes Community College
Emmetsburg, Iowa

**Cynthia Francis Bechtel,
PhD, RN, CNE, CEN**
Assistant Professor
Coordinator, MSN Program
Framingham State College
Framingham, Massachusetts

Mary Benham-Hutchins, RN, PhD
Assistant Professor
Northeastern University
Boston, Massachusetts

Wanda Bonnel, PhD, ARNP, ANEF
Associate Professor
University of Kansas
Kansas City, Kansas

Michelle Byrne, RN, PhD, CNOR
Professor
Program Coordinator MS Nursing Education
North Georgia College and State University
Dahlonega, Georgia

Kelly Dupuy, RN, BScN
Clinical Instructor
Staff Nurse
Mohawk College
Sick Kids Hospital
Hamilton, Ontario, Canada

Sally E. Erdel, MS, RN, CNE
Assistant Professor of Nursing
Bethel College
Mishawaka, Indiana

Alayne Fitzpatrick, APRN, BC, EdD
Associate Professor
Coordinator of Nursing Education Program
Fairleigh Dickinson University
Teaneck, New Jersey

Kathleen Flaherty, EdD, RN, CRRN, CNE
Nursing Professor
College of Mount Saint Vincent
Riverdale, New York

**Margaret M. Governo,
EdD, EdM, BC-CNS, FNP, PNP**
Professor
Wagner College
Staten Island, New York

Linda Grimsley, RN, DSN
Chair and Associate Professor
Albany State University
Albany, Georgia

Aprille Haynie, MSN, RN
Faculty
Huron School of Nursing
East Cleveland, Ohio

Patricia L. Hutchinson, EdD
Assistant Professor
Angelo State University
San Angelo, Texas

Zena Hyman, DNS, ANP-BC
Assistant Professor
Daemen College
Amherst, New York

Diane S. Keasler, BS, MS
Instructor/Instructional Designer
University of South Alabama College of Nursing
Mobile, Alabama

Debora E. Kirsch, RN, CNS, PhDc
Clinical Assistant Professor
Director of Undergraduate Nursing Studies
SUNY Upstate Medical University
Syracuse, New York

Joanne C. Langan, BS-Edu, BSN, PhD, RN
Assistant Dean, Community & Clinical Affairs
Saint Louis University School of Nursing
St. Louis, Missouri

Ramona Browder Lazenby,
  EdD, RN, FNP-BC, CNE
Professor
Associate Dean of Nursing
Auburn Montgomery School of Nursing
Montgomery, Alabama

S. Elena MacLachlan, RN, MS
Teaching Assistant
University of California at San Francisco
San Francisco, California

Betsy S. Mann, MSN, RN, CNE
Dean of Healthcare Education
East Central Community College
Decatur, Mississippi

Susan A. Moore, RN, PhD
Assistant Professor
University of Memphis
Memphis, Tennessee

Brenda Morris, EdD, MS, RN, CNE
Senior Director, Baccalaureate Programs
Clinical Associate Professor
Arizona State College of Nursing and Health
  Innovation
Phoenix, Arizona

Mary Carol G. Pomatto, EdD, ARNP-CNS
University Professor
Chair, Department of Nursing
Pittsburg State University
Pittsburg, Kansas

Carla E. Randall, Rn, PhD
Assistant Professor
University of Southern Maine
Lewiston, Maine

Debra L. Renna, MSN, CCRN
Nursing Instructor
Keiser University
Fort Lauderdale, Florida

Kristynia M. Robinson, PhD, FNPbc, RN
Associate Professor
Director of APN Programs
Assistant Dean of Graduate Nursing
University of Texas at El Paso
El Paso, Texas

Susan Parnell Scholtz, RN, PhD
Associate Professor of Nursing
St Luke's School of Nursing
Moravian College
Nazareth, Pennsylvania

Rosalee J. Seymour
Retired, Professor Emeritus
Johnson City, Tennessee

Pat Shannon, MS, MA, PNP-BC, CNE
Associate Professor
Grand Canyon University
Phoenix, Arizona

Thelma A. Stich, PhD, RN LC
Nurse Entrepreneur
www.Student NurseTutor.com, PLLC
Staten Island, New York

John Stone, RN, BScN, BA, MA, CPMHN
Professor
University of New Brunswick at Humber ITAL
Toronto, Ontario, Canada

Linda A. Streit, RN, DSN
Dean
Professor
Associate Dean for Graduate Programs
Georgia Baptist College of Nursing of Mercer
  University
Mercer University
Atlanta, Georgia

Joyce E. Thompson,
  DrPH, RN, CNM, FAAN, FACNM
Professor
Western Michigan University
Kalamazoo, Michigan

Margo L. Thompson, RN, MSN, EdD, CNE
Nursing Faculty Coordinator
Academic Advisor
Webster University
Kansas City, Missouri

Lois Tschetter, RN, EdD, CNE
Associate Professor
South Dakota State University
Brookings, South Dakota

Laura J. Wallace, RN, CNM, PhD
Associate Professor of Nursing
Brenau University
Gainesville, Georgia

Carol Winters-Moorhead, PhD, RN, CNE
Professor of Nursing
Director of MSN Nursing Education
    Concentration
East Carolina University
Greenville, North Carolina

Table of Contents

UNIT 1

Understanding E-Learning

Chapter 1

E-Learning Defined

JoAnn Zerwekh, MSN, EdD, RN

E-learning is about as vast a concept as nursing. To ask what e-learning is could be compared with asking what is the essence of nursing. The diversity within this concept is so great, no book can fully offer an accurate picture.

When considering the various areas of Web-based, Web-supported, and hybrid education, one begins to understand the diversity that is in the domain of e-learning. As we explore the possibilities of e-learning in nursing education, remember that the limits lay within you, the educator. You decide where the boundaries should be.

CLASSROOM

We can look at the common classroom. For a period of time, a group of learners and a faculty member come together to explore concepts of interest. E-learning comes into the picture when the learners text the instructor their thoughts. E-learning is seen again when the faculty offers a PowerPoint presentation on how best to manage certain challenges. Students then can open their laptops and work in small groups on simulated electronic medical records.

After these students go home, they finish writing their clinical reasoning challenges and upload the documents to the online course dropbox. Next, students log into facebook to add to the study guide that is being developed by their peers (Fig. 1.1).

CYBERSPACE

Now let's visit the online critical care course. This course is a continuing education experience for nurses in the Intensive Care Unit (ICU). Simultaneously, it serves as a three-credit course for fourth-semester nursing students. This concept is based on a principle discussed by Diane Billings (2003) and is called Online Communities of Professional Practice. *The two groups work together in a case-study based online learning environment. Each week the learning teams or groups are presented with a new case study. In the middle of the week, they are offered additional information to assist with the completion of the case study. The course work is completed through group discussions in an asynchronous discussion board. Every other week, each group presents its case to the larger class.*

Because this is a distance education course, the learners never physically meet. Three times throughout the semester, the faculty member holds a webinar or Web-conference (Fig. 1.2). They meet online with telephone audio conferencing. Participants take turns offering a mini-tutorial on a particular issue in critical care.

DavisPlus | For additional resources please visit
http://davisplus.fadavis.com

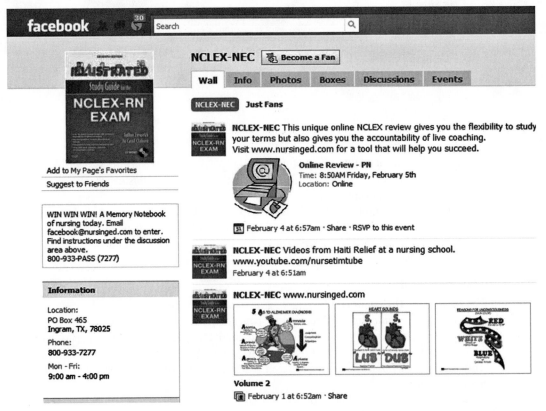

Figure 1.1   Facebook (screenshot). *Used with permission, Nursing Education Consultants, Inc., www.nursinged.com*

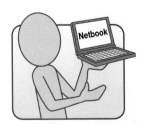

CLINICAL LABORATORY

Before laboratory, students log into their online resources and watch four videos that are assigned. They take a 10-item quiz on the videos. In the nursing laboratory, they grab a Netbook and take it to the bedside. In groups of three, they watch a 3-minute video from the Web and practice the nursing procedure on one another.

After laboratory, students log into their online course management system and create a DAR (data/action/response) note in the online journaling tool. The note is based on the activities that took place in laboratory.

CLINICAL EXPERIENCE

The day before a clinical experience, students receive an e-mail from the instructor. Each student obtains a brief scenario. They are directed to open the free concept map creator that comes with

TECHNOLOGY TIP 1.1

Check your student and instructor textbook online and CD resources for concept map creator tools, such as the one illustrated in Figure 1.4.

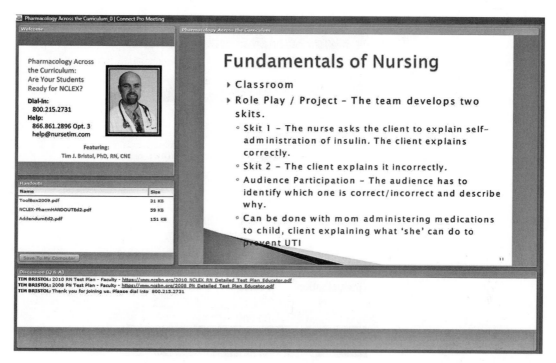

Figure 1.2 Webinar (screenshot).

their textbook and create a concept map on the scenario and then print it. Upon arrival to clinical, they give a paper copy of the concept map to the instructor. While students prepare for patient care, the instructor reviews the concept maps. In report, the instructor offers brief feedback on the concept maps. The students will find more detailed feedback in the online gradebook in the next few days.

During clinical, the students are using PDAs (handheld computers) for clinical decision support tools (resource guides/books, concept maps) and for tracking clinical events and activities (Fig. 1.3). The clinical decision tools allow the students to take notes directly in their e-books and share the notes over the Internet with the instructor and other students. With the clinical tracking tool, the data is synchronized to the Internet. The faculty login at a later time and approve or disapprove of the student's data. Once approved, the data is loaded into a portfolio that the student compiles throughout their academic career.

The opening scenarios show how pervasive the use of the computer, the Internet, and technology are in nursing education. This chapter provides a brief historical sketch of the history of distance education, e-learning, m-learning, along with definitions of Web-supported, hybrid (blended), and Web-based (online) education. Today's educators have probably come across many of these terms and how they have been used interchangeably. For purposes of consistency, this first chapter will provide the reader with an understanding of how these terms will be used in the chapters that follow.

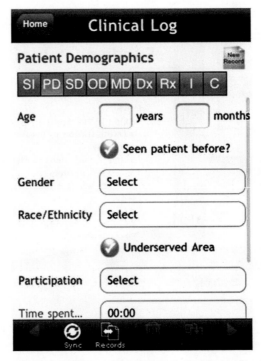

Figure 1.3   Clinical log with patient demographics. *Used with permission from nTrack from Skyscape, Inc.*

HISTORY

The literature about distance education is vast. Historically, it began more than 150 years ago in correspondence or home study courses with humble beginnings in the mid-1800s in Europe. The pioneers of distance education realized a need to provide education to a growing audience and used correspondence courses delivered via the technology available at the time (e.g., the postal system), as a means of meeting that need. In Bath, England about 1840, an Englishman, Sir Isaac Pittman, taught shorthand by correspondence course (Hinkle, 2009a).

As technology flourished with the development of radio and television, the complexion of distance education changed. It was about 1971 when the first e-mails were sent, providing an early milestone of major developments that were on the horizon as computer technology emerged as a significant player in distance education. According to *Baker's Guide to Distance Education* (2010), notable events such as cable and satellite television came into use in the 1970s and early 1980s and further enhanced distance-learning opportunities. Interestingly, in 1983 *Time Magazine* named the computer as its "Machine of the Year." In less than 20 years, by 2000, the term "e-learning" was being used, as the updated version for distance education or rather to include any type of learning activity that encompassed technology and the computer. Smart phones and other mobile devices for Internet usage also arrived in the 2000s. This added another layer of learning—mobile learning or "m-learning." "According to the United States Distance Learning Association, the number of Internet users worldwide surpassed 1 billion in 2005 and is expected to reach 2 billion in 2011" (Hinkle, 2009b, para 3).

Georgiev, Georgieva, and Smrikarov (2004) provided a visual model of distance learning (d-learning), e-learning, and m-learning (Fig. 1.4), in which m-learning is a new stage or part of e-learning. They added a new dimension to defining m-learning and that is to include the ability to learn everywhere at any time without permanent physical connection to a cable network. This is readily achieved by the use of mobile or smart phones, PDAs, digital cameras, portable computers, tablet PCs, voice recorders, pen scanners, and Kindle wireless reading devices.

DEFINITIONS

Following are definitions of commonly used terms that will be found in this book.

A traditional course is a course with no online technology used. The instructional material and content is delivered in person in either written or oral format. This is often referred to as face-to-face instruction (f-2-f) or instruction at a brick-and-mortar institution.

Distance learning takes place when the instructor and the students are separated by geographical or physical distance. The use of media and technology (i.e., voice, video, data, and/or print) is used to bridge the geographical gap. The instruction can be delivered to learners in a synchronous (at the same time or real-time) or asynchronous (not at the same time) manner.

A *Web-supported* course uses technology to facilitate what is essentially a face-to-face course. The instructor may use a learning or course management system (LMS or CMS) or Web pages to post the course syllabus and assignments.

A course that blends online and face-to-face delivery is called *hybrid* or *blended*. Hybrid courses have a considerable amount of the content delivered online and often use online discussion. The number of f-2-f encounters between instructor and student is reduced, but not of sufficient quantity to reduce the actual amount of seat time (amount of time the student is in the classroom seat). Hybrid courses incorporate online or Web-based learning activities, such as case studies, tutorials, self-testing exercises, simulations, and online group collaborations.

A *Web-based* course (**online**) is where all of the content is delivered online via a computer network. There is no f-2-f component. Physically, the computer network could be a local area network (LAN), an intranet within a particular organization, a wide area network (WAN), or it could be the Internet (worldwide Web). In a Web-based course, the instructor and students share a common technological link via the previously listed communication lines. Many refer to this type of course as e-learning, as more and more of the essential

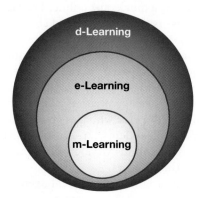

Figure 1.4 d-learning, e-learning, m-learning. *Source: Georgiev, T., Georgieva, E., & Smrikarov, A. (2004). M-learning: A new stage of e-learning. Retrieved from http://ecet.ecs.ru.acad.bg/cst04/Docs/sIV/428.pdf*

teaching activities use the Internet, helping to free learning from the constraints of time and space (McArthur, 2002).

The following section provides brief examples of Web-supported, hybrid, and Web-based e-learning. A more thorough discussion of each of these e-learning formats can be found in chapters 6, 7, and 8, respectively.

WEB-SUPPORTED

Web-supported e-learning (sometimes referred to as Web-enhanced) involves a f-2-f learning environment that is still fully onsite (sometimes referred to as ground-based). The course then uses Internet-based tools or a course management system to support the activities of the course.

Activities include in-class/out-of-class engagement, assessment, and organization. The engagement can come through many different tools. One tool used is the online audience response system such as i>clicker or LiveClassTech. These tools allow students to chat with the instructor, take notes on PowerPoint slides, and answer live quizzing questions all on the Internet during class (Fig. 1.5). Another tool includes social networking media. Twitter and Facebook can be used in the classroom to allow students to be a part of the discussion instead of just recipients of knowledge. Faculty also may wish to activate online case studies. Students work in small groups on their laptops. While logged onto the Internet, they interact with digital case studies and then answer questions electronically. Faculty walk around the room and interact with students while they are working. After a period of time, the faculty turns on the case study in the front of the room and reveals the answers to the questions.

Out-of-class engagement also includes various tools that allow faculty and students to collaborate. For example, after a pediatric lecture, students must log into an asynchronous discussion board to "synthesize" three key concepts from the day's lecture. Or, for instance, in a community health course, the faculty wants all of the class time to be project focused. So the instructor decides to create audio MP3 files (using a free audio recording and editing program, e.g., Audacity) of lecture content and upload them to the Web to either a URL (Web page) or the course management system. Students are required to listen to lecture before they come to class to be prepared for the projects that are assigned.

Assessment in a Web-supported class can vary greatly. Some faculty have students use their laptops in class and take a quick quiz online. The faculty displays the item analysis on the LCD projector and they discuss the outcome and content of the quiz. One group of faculty decided that they wanted more class time so they chose to create what they called an examination center. All examinations happened in the computer lab outside of class time. The faculty proctor examinations during their office hours. Because the examinations were in the online course management system, students can view their examination results right away.

Another assessment strategy involves online standardized examinations. Take, for example, a nursing program director who was concerned about attrition and, therefore, wanted to be able to identify at-risk students earlier. Students took online examinations that are nationally normed. The examinations were given in five different nursing courses. The results are closely analyzed by the advisors.

One rural nursing program had clinical agencies in three different counties. They noted that some students had to drive an extra 2 hours each week just to turn in post-clinical paperwork. They decided to put the paperwork online (documents and spreadsheets) and

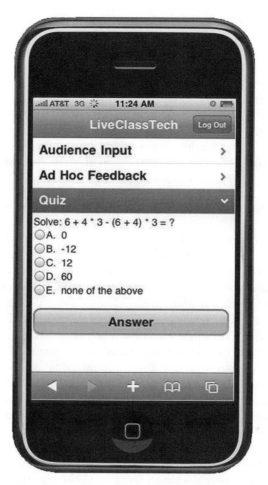

Figure 1.5 Audience response systems. *Used with permission, Liveclasstech.com*

have students digitally submit their material. The dropbox was used in the online course management system to collect these items.

Additional examples and management strategies for Web-supported courses are presented in Chapter 6.

HYBRID

The course that replaces partial "seat-time" with online or virtual activities may be considered a hybrid course, also described as blended or mixed-learning environments. These formats are probably the most popular online course formats. They offer great flexibility in programming and tend to demonstrate the "best" of both face-to-face education and online innovation.

In one program, the first-semester students meet in the nursing laboratory for 8 hours every other Saturday. The rest of the time is spent engaged in online discussion, case study, and video activities.

The fourth-semester students in another program are very busy with clinicals and projects. So, the faculty developed a strategy in which half of the seat-time in their leadership course would be completed online. They still meet once a week to work on Web-based projects and online learning modules.

In an accelerated post baccalaureate program, the students meet for 3 days at the beginning of the semester and for 3 days at the end of the semester. The rest of the semester they meet via webinar or Web-conference (each student has a Web cam on their personal computer at home and calls into the webinar on their phone) each week. The courses take on a seminar format so each week a different student is presenting content directed by the faculty.

Additional examples and management strategies for hybrid courses are presented in Chapter 7.

WEB-BASED

Web-based courses are distance education courses in which the faculty and students never meet physically as part of the course. These courses are sometimes referred to as online courses or e-learning courses. Web-based courses also can be facilitated through live technology such as telephone or webinar (Web-conference). Some examples of successful implementation of Web-based courses follow.

An Allied Health Division decided to make Medical Terminology their first completely online course. They knew there was a big demand in multiple disciplines but students were struggling with time constraints from other courses. The faculty adopted a predeveloped medical terminology course from a publishing company and adjusted it to meet their students' needs.

A liberal arts college felt its nursing department was ready to take the next steps in growth. This led them to explore the development of a fully online MSN educator program. The students would do all courses through the facilitation of asynchronous discussions. Each course would also have a synthesis project. A number of the courses used a facebook group for journal clubs. While in the teaching practicums, students were required to use Twitter for logging key events. The tweets were all tagged so others in the class could easily identify peers and follow each other. The tweets were then archived as part of the student's portfolio.

In a clinical teaching practicum, the students all learned to run a simple simulation on a high-fidelity simulator. They also learned how to stock a computerized medication dispenser and used an IV simulator in a learning event. For each of these areas, the students had to develop learning objectives, a simple lesson plan, and an assessment activity with scoring guide.

Additional examples and management strategies for Web-based courses are presented in Chapter 8.

CONCLUSION

In a recent study by the Alfred P. Sloan Foundation, it was noted that approximately 22% of U.S. college students, or 3.94 million students, were enrolled in at least one Web-based class in the fall 2007 semester. This was an increase of 12.9% from the previous fall 2006 semester as a result of the steady increase in the number of Web-based classes being offered. This study surveyed more than 2500 colleges and universities and found during the same period that overall higher education enrollment increased by only 1.2%. In fall 2002, the first year in

TECHNOLOGY TIP 1.2

Diigo is a free social bookmarking service. Social bookmarking allows students and educators to share their favorites on the Internet. In addition, it allows learners and educators to highlight and annotate Web pages—put sticky notes, archive, and annotate your favorite Web pages. See http://www.diigo.com/

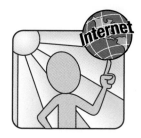

conducting and reporting the research, the Sloan Foundation found that 1.6 million students were taking at least one online class, meaning 9% of college students were taking online classes. That number eclipsed the 2 million in 2004 and topped the 3 million in 2005 (Allen & Seaman, 2008, p. 1). E-learning is here to stay and it is having a significant impact on nursing education. Paradigm shifts are already occurring requiring faculty to make fundamental changes to their teaching strategies. More than a third of public university faculty have taught an online course and more than half have recommended an online course to students, according to an unprecedented study of administrative and faculty views toward online learning released by the Association of Public and Land-grant Universities-Sloan National Commission on Online Learning (Seaman, 2009). It is an exciting time for all! As Ed Hoff, Chief Learning Officer for IBM, stated in 2008, "In this global, networked world, several technologies including search engines, blogs, podcasts, Web 2.0 applications and virtual worlds such as Second Life will be used for learning." We are already there!

REFERENCES

Allen, I. E., & Seaman, J. (2008). Staying the course: Online education in the United States, 2008. Retrieved from http://www.sloan-c.org/sites/default/files/staying_the_course-2.pdf

Baker's Guide to Christian Distance Education. (2010). Distance education timeline. Retrieved from http://www.bakersguide.com/Distance_Education_Timeline/

Billings, D. M. (2003). Online communities of professional practice. *Journal of Nursing Education, 42*(8), 335.

Diigo. (2010). Diigo. Research, share, collaborate. Retrieved from http://www.diigo.com/

Georgiev, T., Georgieva, E., & Smrikarov, A. (2004). M-learning: A new stage of e-learning. International Conference on Computer Systems and Technologies. Retrieved from http://ecet.ecs.ru.acad.bg/cst04/Docs/sIV/428.pdf

Hinkle, L. (2009a). Distance education history: The early years of distance learning. Retrieved from http://www.brighthub.com/education/online-learning/articles/24404.aspx

Hinkle, L. (2009b). The future of distance learning. Retrieved from http://www.brighthub.com/education/online-learning/articles/27955.aspx#ixzz0eJQq36x3

Kala, S., Isaramalai, S., & Pohthong, A. (2010). Electronic learning and constructivism: A model for nursing education. *Nurse Education Today, 30*, 61–66. doi:10.1016/j.nedt.2009.06.002

McArthur, D. (2002). Investing in digital resources. *New Directions for Higher Education, 119*, 77–84.

Seaman, J. (2009). Online learning as a strategic asset. Volume II: The Paradox of faculty voices: Views and experiences with online learning. Retrieved from http://www.aplu.org/NetCommunity/Document.Doc?id=1879

Time Magazine. (1983). The computer moves in. Retrieved from http://www.time.com/time/covers/0,16641,19830103,00.html

Chapter 2

Theoretical Basis of E-Learning

Julia Aucoin, DNS, RN-BC, CNE

Many nurses and faculty will describe their experience with theory as painful, useless, and misguided. Their experience may be limited by the theory or philosophy with which they were taught or exposed. Especially in this era of connectivity, when one carries a mobile device that pushes several e-mail accounts and phone numbers to one handheld, faculty often are concerned about exactly how student-centered (i.e., connected) each educator must be. Being connected 24/7 suggests to some that we should be available 24/7 to respond. But, looking at student-centered learning theory would suggest something different.

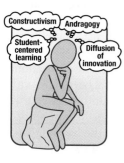

The term *theory* generally refers to a set of ideas, but also can reflect models and philosophies. This chapter will introduce you to types of theories that influence how we construct and practice e-learning, how we create a learning environment suitable to the learner, and how we can explain our practices to others. It is important to note that any theory of education is open to subjectivity based upon the individual perspective of the educator and the learner. In addition, while one theory emphasizes focused aspects of education it is not intended to neglect the other aspects. Therefore, being student-centered does not mean we are not supportive of self-actualizing or classical theory. In this chapter, we will discuss only four theoretical frameworks—student-centered learning, constructivism, andragogy, and diffusion of innovations.

STUDENT-CENTERED LEARNING

In 1997, Hannafin and Land wrote that recent focus on student-centeredness has spurred interest in new teaching and learning perspectives. Direct teaching methods had been criticized for lacking critical thinking and practical problem-solving skills. They saw the logistics of implementing student-centered learning as difficult, yet recognized that advances in technology systems would allow for more feasible approaches to engage, challenge, and stimulate the learner, by the nature of the activities that could be generated. Fast forward to 2011—would Hannafin and Land's ideas be equally provocative?

We have evolved from the simplicity and elegance of problem-based learning to Second Life (where users come to life in a virtual world), which places the learner truly in the center of the learning environment. Along the way, we have included synchronous and asynchronous discussion, Web field trips, viewing and posting on YouTube, and project management on document sharing sites. We know that some thought of schools as the setting for life-apprenticeships and

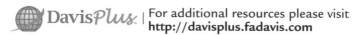

Davis*Plus* | For additional resources please visit **http://davisplus.fadavis.com**

TECHNOLOGY TIP 2.1

Use Google Scholar at http://scholar.google.com to find more details about education theory.

learning occurs through interactions in the environment. Hannafin and Land suggest that student-centered learning environments emphasize finding the personal meaning when relating new knowledge to existing thoughts. You will often find theories in this category referred to as student-centered learning. In this section, we will further explore the concept of student-centeredness and its relationship to the learning environment.

Much of what we consider in learner environment theory begins with the learning community. I would think all would agree that the current delivery of most academic online courses requires collaboration, openness to multiple perspectives, and a different tolerance for the words our students use to express their thinking, especially in light of the lack of non-verbal expression for validation of feelings or meaning. In 1997, Panitz wrote that "Collaboration is a philosophy of interaction and personal lifestyle where individuals are responsible for their own actions, including learning and respect for the abilities and contributions of their peers; cooperation is a structure of interaction designed to facilitate the accomplishment of a specific end product or goal through people working together in groups." (para 4) Although these references that I have included may seem old to you when e-learning is relatively new in the lifecycle of education, it is interesting to note the foresight with which many have approached the design of our current learning environments.

Cook-Sather (2002) suggests that the student who is most directly affected by educational policy and practice is often the least consulted. She chides that the system has been built without consulting those it is intended to serve. Cook-Sather further remarks that this is the result of the power base, and that the basic premise upon which different approaches depend, is trust. Therefore, student-centeredness should reflect a shared authority for the learning environment, a dynamic that is difficult to attain because the formal education of students is historically rooted in domination and teacher-centered pedagogies.

Freinet initiated cooperative pedagogy into French educational theory in the 1920s (Bertrand, 2003). He had returned from World War I with an injury that prevented him from projecting his voice to a group. Thus, he worked to develop a pedagogy that emphasized cooperation among the students as its premise. Freinet was successful in implementing his ideas, which are in use today in many French communities. His elements for education included: learning is an inductive process, the learner must take charge of oneself and charge of the group, and learning is a critical analysis of reality. Thus was born the idea that children learn by doing (keep in mind that doing is not always a psychomotor function) (Bertrand, 2003). Freinet patterned his work off Montessori, a much maligned model for the education of children.

The application of learning theory is as individual as the teacher and the learner. However, the creation of a learning environment that is respectful of what the learner brings has proven to be successful. In e-learning, not engaging the learner, not acknowledging the ideas of those you cannot see, and not building upon previous experiences creates a two-dimensional approach to learning. Yet student-centeredness creates a matrix approach in which there are multiple interactions occurring simultaneously, among the teacher, the learners, the materials, and the activities. It is this theoretical structure that can exponentially increase an individual's knowledge in a short period of time.

Strategies for Implementation

In 1990, Beaudoin wrote that distance education (which began in the 1920s) is a learner-centered system, where the teacher augments traditional tools by reinforcing learning through explanations, references, and thoughtful questioning. We have seen through the growth of Web-based tools, the power of directing a student to a new resource and the excitement of students when they discover the riches of that URL. In addition, the "passing of notes" in class to share resources among learners that support their individual projects is one of the least disruptive and most productive classroom activities we can promote.

Beaudoin (1990) suggests that we avoid syllabism, the tendency for students to be bound by the syllabus, and only produce what is requested without exploration or adaptation to their personal/professional needs. He further suggests that we focus on dialogue and not question and answer. In my experience, I'll offer that promoting dialogue among the learners rather than a volley of comments between the student and the teacher is only one of our challenges. The learners need to learn to value each others' thoughts and because we cannot see the "rolling of eyes" then we should facilitate an open and respectful exchange of ideas. Too often, comments are directed only at the professor and not to all or to the peer. Setting the tone for this early in the asynchronous discussion experience (for each course and each faculty) is important (Hanna, Conceicao-Runlee, & Glowacki-Dudka, 2000).

Bertrand (2003) offers that difficulty in creating a student-centered environment can be resolved by addressing these problems: student passivity generated by traditional teaching, absence of direct contact among students, weaknesses in implementing active methods, and low tolerance by faculty for student diversity. Thus, the strategies to implement would include: interactivity generated by what is still termed nontraditional techniques, encouraging student-to-student conversation, practicing active methods until they are comfortable and productive, and embracing the experience and worldview of our learners to enhance the experience for the student and the faculty.

This is why it is so important to create an introduction discussion for a long-term course with multiple learners. The student's introduction is an opportunity for the faculty to create a connection, whether that be professional or personal. This can make the relationship seem more tangible to the learner and open up the lines of communication. Remembering the student's expertise or employment then provides an anchor for comments, resources, and questions. Creating a private discussion in which students can share their personal developments also is helpful, like a hallway chat. Anything that simulates meaningful experiences in the online environment is useful. Although all universities will seek student input through a formal feedback tool, if it is your practice to use formative evaluation strategies while in person, then you'll want to see "How are we doing?" periodically online.

Facilitating rather than assigning group projects is critical to using learning environment theory. However, this is not feasible until the group has learned to be a group. Strategies that help members to teach each other, respect each other's contributions, and work well together can be employed before using an actual group assignment to meet course objectives. An example of this is to ask course members to choose a favorite color from a list of red, blue, and yellow. By doing so, teams are assigned and members then work together to promote their color to others. This is a simple, nonthreatening exercise that can help identify the strengths of each team member and recognize work contributions of each. Following this brief exercise (only 1 week), the teams can be retained, but the actual assignment distributed.

Many group projects initially fail in the online environment because learners try to apply face-to-face concepts to their work rather than learn new techniques for working together.

Cooperative testing is often used in a student-centered environment; however, in the online environment, we tend to be more concerned about cheating than in face-to-face (f-2-f). We can use the concept of cooperative testing by providing a list of questions to a pair of students and asking them to work together to complete the list. Students then divide the work into half for each and then give feedback to the other's half or each takes an approach to all the questions and then they incorporate both learner's information into the responses. The key is integration and discussion rather than copy and paste with duplication.

Interactive discussions require building upon each other's ideas. Often I see repetitive responses because the learners read the prompt, leave the site, and return with their unique response, not realizing that it has been posted several times in a similar manner by colleagues. When responding to discussion prompts, suggest to the learners that they read the prompt, then complete the readings to support one's thinking to respond. Before actually responding to the prompt, go into the site to read what others have written. Then it is easy to respond to the prompt, given what the learner knows from reading, reflecting, and considering what others have said. The discussion then feels more like a conversation just like in a ground class. No one would tolerate six people stating nearly identical ideas in a live classroom; there would be an expectation that we were respectful of what others have said. The asynchronous nature of discussion does not mean that we ignore what has happened while we were out thinking; it means that we create a dialogue for reflection of what everyone brings to the discussion.

CONSTRUCTIVISM

Constructivism is based on "continual and sympathetic observation" of students' interests (Dewey, 1964, p. 436). Thus, we should develop pedagogies that give students the opportunity to explore their ideas. The current intent of constructivism is to attend to learning processes and feedback with the student to change the pedagogical practice to better facilitate learning. Dewey also shared with us that intelligence is the result of social interactions.

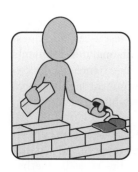

Constructivism relies upon three elements—cognitive styles, transfer of learning, and social construction of knowledge. Cognitive styles can be likened to mental models: conceptual thinking versus linear thinking. Educators are often challenged by those who differ from themselves. Conceptual thinkers see their ideas in balloons or clouds floating above their heads; the educator's responsibility is to draw the threads together to help the learner organize the thoughts. The linear thinker sees outlines, tables, and charts to illustrate the relationship between ideas. Transfer of learning can be likened to learning styles: multiple intelligences, personality temperament, and preferred delivery systems. The third element, the social construction of knowledge, is both social and cultural.

Most commonly known to nursing is Bandura's social cognitive theory. Many nurses have been educated using similar strategies, work within similar environments,

TECHNOLOGY TIP 2.2

The Center for Dewey Studies is located on the Internet at http://www.siuc.edu/~deweyctr/index.html

and interpret what they learn from a similar context, until you get into a continental or international classroom where perspectives can be quite different. It is this enriching component of e-learning that makes it enticing to so many learners. The appreciation for how we are geographically dissimilar and socially alike is what contributes most to the growth of learners learning online. Bandura suggested that we learn from each other and the media's influence. He explained his expression of social-cognitive as social because thought and action are fundamentally social and cognitive because thought processes influence motivation, emotions, and action (Bandura, 2001). A characteristic worthy of discussion is self-regulation. In learning, this refers to the learner's proactive efforts to mobilize emotional, cognitive, and environmental resources during learning as well as observe, judge, and react to the learner's own progress. Individuals can think over what is going on in addition to building upon interactions to construct knowledge.

Strategies for Implementation

Although there are many strategies we could consider, we will take this discussion from simple to complex. Listening (or reading) closely to what students say about their learning is key in the e-learning realm. Key to understanding constructivism is the educator's awareness of his or her own learning style. Many inventories are available online at no cost (without a detailed report) or low cost with a downloadable report. After the educator appreciates his or her own style, then it is important to study the styles that students bring to the course. The beauty of e-learning is that the course design can address all learning styles in some way so that there is something there for every learner. Those new to e-learning are often challenged by their own frame of reference (self-identified teaching style that mirrors their own learning style) rather than openly approaching the learning style of everyone who may be encountered. A quick search of learning style instruments will yield multiple choices to use for self-assessment. Equally important is to ask learners to assess their own styles to recognize self-contributions and respect those of others. Thus, the one learner who always must respond early and often is not ridiculed by others but recognized as an extrovert and achiever and perhaps the one who always responds last is not thought of as a laggard benefitting from the thinking of others, but an assimilator and consensus builder. From here it is easy to take a look at www.mindmap.com for ideas about conceptual thinking and traditional tables and charts, such as Anderson and Krathwohl's cognitive taxonomy, to determine your cognitive style (Forehand, 2005).

Self-regulation can be aided by providing feedback and sufficient information to be able to change behaviors or attitudes. For example, a healthy discussion presents new ideas that often differ from those of others; yet these ideas must be presented respectfully (students may need coaching in respectful communication). The learner can take this feedback to change how the next interaction might be read, with or without acknowledging how others perceived it. It is up to the learner to take your offline feedback and internalize it in his or her own way. However, if the behavior/attitude does not change, then you can respond to all in a summary note about respect to each other, the difficulties of only interpreting from the written word, and the ability of everyone to change the perceptions of those who receive the message. This can change the dynamic for the discussion again without directing any learner how the behavior or participation must be specifically altered.

By suggesting that no one repeat the response of another in an asynchronous discussion and only build, the construction of knowledge occurs with the addition of new resources and new ideas. The concept of a progressive dinner was popular in the 1980s, where a group of neighbors went to one home for appetizers, another for the main course, and a final for dessert, allowing for a different dining opportunity in each home and the construction of a dining experience, rather than the consumption of a meal. Making learning progressive, by using discussion questions to promote the ability to respond to a later assignment, is an example of successful implementation of constructivism.

ANDRAGOGY

It is important that we refer to the work of Knowles as andragogy rather than adult learning theory. This theory focuses on valuing the learner's experience and participation in learning as a way to facilitate motivation. Let me offer you some perspective. Knowles' publications began in the early 1940s with his first book on adult education being published in 1950. So consider the times—consider the influences of K–12 education during the 1920s to 1940s

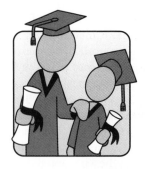

and the context in which Knowles wrote. When we refer to Knowles today and continue to believe that the andragogical principles only apply to adults, we are missing his points (Knowles, Holton, & Swanson, 2011).

Merriam (2001) offers us perspective on this, by stating that there is no one theory of adult learning that explains the process of learning in adults. My thoughts are that this is because we have significantly changed how we educate our students since the 1920s. Early research into the differences between adult and younger learners was a result of research; often, timed tests were given that concluded that younger meant better (Merriam, 2001). Studies conducted in the 1950s did not differentiate adults from children on problem solving or cognitive development. Many of the early conclusions were extrapolated from research that placed adults under the same conditions as children.

In 1968, Knowles first proposed the need to differentiate adult from preadult teaching. He adopted the concept of andragogy from the work of Kapp, who had adapted the elements of Plato's education theory. The original intent was to contrast *andr* (man) from *paid* (child), while *agogos* means leading (Thorpe, Edwards, & Hanson, 1993). Although Plato was instrumental in the concept, Kapp coined the term andragogy in 1833. There was an attempt to reintroduce it in 1920s; however, it was not until Knowles' repeated efforts that the term caught on. Knowles built on the concept of andragogy as the art and science of helping adults learn and thus, the term caught on as a rallying point to differentiate educators into specialties, adult or child.

Many of you could list multiple principles of adult learning but the concepts were originally limited to five assumptions. The adult learner:

• Has an independent self-concept and can direct own learning.
• Has accumulated a reservoir of life experiences as a rich resource for learning.
• Has learning needs closely related to changing social roles.
• Is problem-centered and interested in immediate application of knowledge.
• Is motivated to learn by internal rather than external factors.

The sense was that adults manage other aspects of their lives and, therefore, are capable of some assistance in planning their own learning (Merriam, 2001).

It is also interesting to note that andragogy is often referred to as adult learning principles. This may be a result of Knowles' admonition that andragogy is less of a theory and more of a model of assumptions that could serve to build theory (Knowles, 1989). Further questions arise regarding today's learners; this is due to the dependence upon structure for some adults and the independence of some children as learners. This same thought applies to the range of experience and functioning in a learning situation. Knowles revised his thinking to shift from a position of andragogy versus pedagogy to one of student-directed versus teacher-directed. Knowles' sense was that andragogy is defined more by the learning situation than by the age of the learner.

Strategies for Implementation

To build upon self-concept, it is important for the educator to support the learners in their identification of their self-concept. This is often managed by asking learners why they are enrolled in the learning experience and what their personal goals are for participation. Terms like voluntary versus mandatory, growth versus competence, and solve versus explore often are used when learners are given the opportunity to express why they are participating in the learning activity. After we have a sense of the learners' orientations to their learning, the educator can focus on building upon their self-concepts.

Through the introduction phase, when learners describe their personal or professional backgrounds, the educator can make notes. When the opportunity presents itself, the learners' experiences can be introduced into the discussion so that their next contributions are personally relevant. Prompts, such as "Tell us about how this applies to your practice setting," will allow for the learner to build upon the rich resources from their lives. Another prompt that you may find helpful when asked a question by a learner, is to ask all the learners, "Who has had a similar experience and can help with this question?"

Although the nurse really does not have a changing social role, the learning may change function or abilities to respond to the environment. The relevance of the learning should be made evident regarding how it will change the learner's perspective in the workplace. Too often, organizations are using two-dimensional (noninteractive) e-learning to deliver instruction to staff. Rather than frame how and why the information is useful, the learning is viewing slides and responding to multiple-choice questions. The educator's role in design or delivery is to provide context for learning so that the relevance is obvious and the learning can be anchored to a purpose.

To add to that relevance, it is important to highlight when immediate application of knowledge is a possibility. Not all learning, however, will have an immediate application and it is equally important to share that information with the learner. Nevertheless, the applicability of the knowledge should be made obvious to the learner for now and for the future. For example, when teaching rhythm strip interpretation, it is necessary to share the intent: daily use, new patient population, management of medications in response to the rhythm or basic introduction of information. Then the learner knows where and how to store the information so that it can be applied when called upon for practice.

The learner's motivation can be internal or external. The instructor can influence an external motivator to become more internal by providing relevance and playing upon the desire of the learner to provide the best patient care possible, often by having the learner imagine the patient is a family member. The educator should clarify the learner's motivation to determine if it makes any difference in the learner's willingness to participate and thereby actively learn. In the e-learning environment, asking for the motivation in advance and then following up with an action plan written by the learner for how the information will be applied, can demonstrate the shift in motivation caused by the education.

Applying any learner-focused activities such as small group work, buzz sessions, share-pairs, and case studies also will involve the learner actively, placing the focus where it can make the most difference in the learners' practices. Andragogy is evident when the outcomes are focused on learning more than on teaching.

ROGER'S THEORY OF DIFFUSION OF INNOVATIONS

Roger's Theory of Diffusion explains the process by which individuals adopt new innovations (Rogers, 2003). Making the case that Roger's Theory of Diffusion of Innovations is an education theory may be a stretch. However, if we think about education as the ultimate in diffusion of knowledge, then we can make a case for including it here. Similarly, the explosion of the Internet and learning management systems has allowed for broader diffusion of knowledge. Many of you may not have studied Roger's theory as a part of your discussions in graduate school, unless you took a course in implementation science or discovered it while learning about evidence-based practice principles. So we will begin with an orientation to the elements in the Diffusion of Innovations.

Diffusion is the process by which an innovation is communicated through certain channels over time among the members of a social system (Rogers, 2003); thus, the four elements are: innovation, communication, time, and social system. Further defining these elements may shed some light on how this fits into education theory. An innovation is an idea, practice, or object that is perceived as new by an individual or other unit of adoption. This seems quite subjective if you take a moment to think about it; innovation is not only in the eye of the beholder but all who view it. Yet there is little difference between awareness of an innovation and oblivion. The innovation becomes important as soon as awareness suggests it should be. Interestingly the novelty of the innovation could result from knowledge, persuasion, or the readiness to adopt. In thinking about innovation and e-learning, we can point to technologies, both hardware and software, that have made access to and usability of education delivery worthy of adoption. We also can think about a concept such as evidence-based practice, which differs from research utilization, and the advent of translational research and implementation science, none of which were included in nursing program curricula before the 1980s and for some programs is still sorely lacking. There are many similarities between innovation and discovery of new theories, concepts, and principles. Additional principles to consider when regarding the innovation are relative advantage, compatibility, complexity, trialability, and observability. The greater the presence of these five principles (less for complexity) the more rapid the innovation will be adopted. With teaching strategy, as with concept mapping, the adoption has depended on pilot testing, observable results, recognition of the advantage over linear models, compatibility with the faculty's perspective, and the simplicity with which it is delivered. If one considers e-learning to be an innovation, then its proliferation would be a result of the same principles. We often refer to using all the bells and whistles in a software program, which may either enhance or delay the use of an innovation. Software engineers are often more aggressively creative than user readiness warrants.

Diffusion is a type of communication in which the message is regarding the innovation. This second element of the theory is known as the communication channel, which depicts the means by which an innovation is presented by one who has knowledge of it to another who does not use the innovation. Interpersonal (f-2-f) and mass media are primary channels. More effective communication occurs between homophilous parties, that is, those with similar interests. With e-learning, nurses often pass on to others their strategies for continuing their formal academic education or required continuing education units. Communication is often rewarding to both participants when homophily is present. Diffusion of innovation is often slowed when the parties are more heterophilous. For example, the engineer cannot teach the faculty member to use the learning management system, but a superuser surely can. One nurse can offer to another nurse advice about how to maneuver in the learning management system, and as you might guess, word of mouth is an excellent way to make a positive or negative recommendation about a continuing education Website or delivery strategy.

The third element in the diffusion process is time, which is often an ignored concept in behavioral science research. The time element takes on many dimensions—passing on first knowledge of the innovation, the innovativeness of the party considering the innovation, and the number of parties who adopt the innovation in a period of time. Consider the advent of e-learning in the 1990s, the introduction of experts in e-learning by the beginning of the 2000s, and in 2011 the ubiquitous nature of hybrid models, which blend live and electronic teaching strategies to achieve a single outcome. The initial time element is dependent on knowledge of the innovation, persuasion to form an attitude about the innovation, decision to adopt or reject the innovation, implementation or application of the innovation, and confirmation to adopt or reject the innovation. The sequence of these elements is time-ordered and the innovation decision period can be quantified as the length of time required to move through all five elements. The second dimension, innovativeness, is the degree to which the party is early in adopting new ideas in comparison to their system. Rogers defined adopter categories as: innovators, early adopters, early majority, late majority, and laggards. In education, the innovator is often thought of as renegade or naïve, but if successful can influence an early majority; laggards are often ignored or given other assignments. Although many learners may want the freedom of e-learning, some recognize that they lack the discipline to conform to standards required for asynchronous discus-

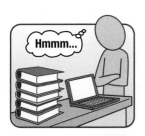

sions. These individuals may have several false or failed starts before they find an innovative approach that supports their individual needs. There are even some members of society who purposefully reject the idea that any learning could occur using a strategy other than face-to-face. Finally, the rate of adoption is the relative speed with which an innovation is adopted by the members of a social system. Most frequently the distribution is an S-shaped curve. The early adopters rising slowly, followed by the majority that adopts quickly, and finally the curve slows with the laggards. If you consider that distance learning has been available since the 1920s, but documentation of teaching has been in place since Aristotle and Plato, then e-learning has been adopted rather quickly as a strategy for distance learning.

The final element of the diffusion process is the social system, a set of interrelated units engaged in solutions to achieve a common goal. We can think of all 3.1 million nurses as a social system and, therefore, expect that all diffusion will be similar. However nurses operate in different settings and organizational cultures and live within different social systems. It could be that e-learning is valued in system A more than in system B and, thus, adoption of use of the e-learning strategies would be faster and easier in system A. The use of MP3 technology for streaming audio was adopted slowly as people converted from "traditional" CDs to MP3 players; the advent of the IPod changed the adoption cycle and the use of audio as a means to convey information to learners.

Strategies for Implementation

For application of Roger's theory, the four elements must all be present—innovation, communication, time, and social system. Projects in the e-learning environment focused on real-life solutions are the best way to use Roger's theory in the learning situation. Case studies in which any solution is possible to reach a patient outcome will support innovation. Managing vignettes using timers also can support innovation and critical thinking. Considering how to communicate ideas to an interprofessional team is an exercise to demonstrate another element of Roger's work.

One strategy to teach educators to use e-learning is to enroll them in the e-learning environment so that they can experience what their learners will feel. They can experience the innovation, discuss how it works for themselves as learners, gain confidence and skill in using the components, and choose how to use these new skills in their own practice. Rather than start off teaching strategies, changing the learning experience through using these strategies demonstrates the use of Roger's theory and changes the educators' practice.

CONCLUSION

Critics of e-learning are often fearful or inexperienced in the environment and unfamiliar with how to apply educational theory to their practice. These critics often come from those who have neither been a learner nor a facilitator in the "classroom." There is no better environment than e-learning to be sure that the voices of learners are heard in word and deed, because their voices are all we have. Given that I have taught a ventilator dependent student, a chronic pain student, and several on rigorous chemotherapeutic protocols, the e-learning environment is the only one in which their individual voices can be heard above the din of their lives and their faculty's power.

REFERENCES

Bandura, A. (2001). Social cognitive theory: An agentic perspective. *Annual Review of Psychology, 52,* 1–26.

Beaudoin, M. (1990). The instructor's changing role in distance education. *The American Journal of Distance Education, 4,* 2.

Bertrand, Y. (2003). *Contemporary theories and practice in education.* Madison, WI: Atwood.

Cook-Sather, A. (2002). Authorizing students' perspectives: Toward trust, dialogue, and change in education. *Educational Researcher, 31*(4), 3–14.

Dewey, J. (1964). My pedagogic creed. In R. D. Archambault (Ed.), *Dewey on education.* Chicago, IL: The University of Chicago Press.

Forehand, M. (2005). Bloom's taxonomy: Original and revised. In M. Orey (Ed.), *Emerging perspectives on learning, teaching, and technology.* Retrieved from http://projects.coe.uga.edu/epltt/

Hanna, D. E., Conceicao-Runlee, S., & Glowacki-Dudka, M. (2000). *147 Practical tips for teaching online groups: essentials of web-based education.* Madison, WI: Atwood.

Hannafin, M. J., & Land, S. M. (1997). The foundations and assumptions of technology-enhanced student-centered learning environments. *Instructional Science, 25,* 167–202.

Knowles, M. S. (1989). *The making of an adult educator.* San Francisco: Jossey-Bass.

Knowles, M. S., Holton, E. F., & Swanson, R. A. (Eds.). (2011). *The adult learner: The definitive classic in adult education and human resource development* (7th ed.). Woburn, MA: Butterworth-Heinemann.

Merriam, S. (2001). Andragogy and self-directed learning: Pillars of adult learning theory. *New Directions for Adult and Continuing Education, 89,* 3–13.

Panitz, T. (1997). *Ted's cooperative e-book.* Retrieved from http://home.capecod.net/~tpanitz/tedsarticles/coopdefinition.htm

Piaget, J. (1952). *The origins of intelligence in children.* New York, NY: International University Press.

Rogers, E. (2003). *Diffusion of innovations* (3rd ed.). New York, NY: Free Press.

Thorpe, M., Edwards, R., & Hanson, A. (1993). Culture and processes of adult learning. New York, NY: Routledge.

Chapter 3

Instructional Design for E-learning in Nursing Education

Patricia A. Z. (PZ) Nielsen, MS, RN, FNP

Sara has been teaching several nursing classes for a few years and has been longing to put them online. She has often thought about posting the syllabus, readings and assignments, and monitoring the class from her cabin porch. Now, it is Sara's turn to put her course online and it doesn't seem as easy as it once did. Sara has taken several online courses and realizes that what works in person doesn't work online. It is not a simple transfer. She wonders where to start and realizes that there are several things to take into consideration as she begins the journey of online course development.

Instructional design (ID) is the product of optimizing conditions for learners to achieve the cognitive, behavioral, and affective objectives ascribed to the learning activity, which, in this case, is assumed to be a course in a degree generating program, but could just as easily apply to a single learning event or a whole program. It may be easier to think of ID as a process instead of an outcome. Course designers and faculty usually are doing instructional designing to create an environment in which conditions are optimized for successful learning rather than looking at the final instructional design in and of itself. Either way, in working with instructional design the intent is to make the learning environment effective, efficient, and as engaging as possible.

HISTORY OF INSTRUCTIONAL DESIGN

Socrates is said to have developed the Socratic Method of instruction, which is based in debate, argument, contradiction, agreement, and, as we would say today, deep critical thinking that stems from dialogue. The apprenticeship-to-master model can be traced back to medieval times when boys went off to the homes of friends or allies to serve as pages to learn the arts of war and chivalry, and eventually become knights. This tradition still exists in formal nursing education as precepted clinical instruction, summer nurse internships, and in societies where promising youngsters learn the healing arts for the community from the current healer. In generations past, it was taught that wisdom was evil in that it tried to replace the only true wisdom of the church and God. As a result, teaching was often subjected to strict censorship to keep minds innocent and in a state of grace. Before the renaissance, formal

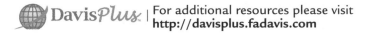

Davis*Plus* | For additional resources please visit
http://davisplus.fadavis.com

schooling was often limited to boys who were being trained for the priesthood. Indoctrination came to the forefront as the instructional design for instilling obedience, faith, and ritual (Reiser, 2001). In more recent times, the roots of instructional design are traceable to World War II (WWII). The military needed to train troops very rapidly in specific skill sets to carry out every aspect of combat from building ships and planes to cleaning, assembling, loading, aiming, and firing weapons. This required a strategy for rapid, precise task completion at a very high performance level. The behavioral theory of operant condition, proposed by B. F. Skinner, propelled this form of instructional design into action. Skinner's theory implied that anyone could learn anything with enough repetition and remediation. During the 1950s and 1960s, post-war classrooms were where children sat silently, wrote spelling words ten times each, repeated their times tables ten times each, and obeyed. High performance was rewarded, the best spelling paper was taped to the board, and low performance was remediated, a misspelled word was rewritten 50 times. Middle American students were prepared for life in the factory. They were quiet, task-oriented, with high performance expectations, and were able to apply themselves to repetitive activities without complaining or getting antsy. Ah, the good old days. This type of learning is still used in various situations in which precise performance is required including cardiopulmonary resuscitation training (CPR) and keyboarding.

After WWII and well into the 1950s, Benjamin Bloom studied how troop training had occurred in WWII and presented *Bloom's Taxonomy*, which identified the cognitive, behavioral, and affective domains of learning, and presented progressive levels of cognitive learning labeled as knowledge, understanding, application, analysis, synthesis, and evaluation. These levels of cognition have more recently been revamped into action verbs to more closely align with the activity of learning resulting in remembering, understanding, applying, analyzing, evaluating, and creating. *Bloom's Taxonomy* is still used in instructional design today.

Today, learning is moving away from both the teacher and the material as the center of the learning universe and toward student-centered learning. For this reason, we need to graduate learners who are equipped to manage themselves effectively in ill-defined situations immediately upon graduation. In nursing education, we want our undergraduates to be room ready for entry-level practice and our graduate students to be prepared to take on case loads immediately and quite independently.

Before getting into where one needs to go with online instructional design, what is it that is important to remember from this extremely brief history of instructional design? First, it is important to note that instructional design has been going on in one form or another for as long as people have participated in formal learning environments. Second, instructional design is valued for the purpose of creating space or environments that optimize the conditions for achieving predetermined learning objectives and goals. Goals vary. Some are quite large, for example, surviving on a battle field, and some are smaller and less easily identified. Others goals have nothing to do with content or material and everything to do with something entirely different such as developing the ability to deliver a cogent argument about one side of an issue without getting bowled over by an opponent. In addition, some learning objectives for classes will be behavioral, some cognitive, and others affective so the instructional design needs to facilitate learning in all three domains. Finally, we know from history that instructional design is fluid. It changes to accommodate outcomes that are desired in areas where those who are educated will practice. This means that as the world changes and new jobs are created, educational requirements will change and instructional design will change to create environments where what is needed can be learned.

INSTRUCTIONAL DESIGN MODELS

Instructor design models (IDMs) are methods used to provide a systematic thorough process of getting together all that is needed in the design of a course. There are many such models and all have more similarities than differences. Three IDMs are presented here to give instructional designers a sense of what various models have to offer and to provide some choice for instructional designers who care to use one or more of the models.

Gagne's Nine Events of Instruction

Robert Gagne, a behaviorist and contributor to instructional design, first wrote about the condition and processes necessary for learning in 1965. Although being primarily concerned with the behavioral changes that occur as a result of learning, Gagne realized that there are mental events that occur when an adult learner is presented with a stimulus to learning. He developed a nine-step process of instructional activities that correlate with the nine-step process of learning suggesting that, if the instruction process correlates with the learning process, learning outcomes will be more readily achieved. The nine steps include (Gagne, Briggs, & Wager, 1992):

1. Gain the learner's attention.
2. Inform learners of unit learning objectives.
3. Stimulate recall of prior learning.
4. Present the content, (or stimulus material).
5. Provide learner guidance.
6. Elicit performance.
7. Provide feedback.
8. Assess performance.
9. Enhance retention and transfer (Table 3.1).

TABLE 3.1	
Gagne's Nine Steps for Instructional Design	
Gagne's Instructional Event	**Learner's Corresponding Mental Process**
1. Gain the learner's attention	Pose a question, present a case, or find an interesting or controversial issue in the class reading. The point is to stimulate learner curiosity.
2. Inform learners of unit learning objectives	Learners want to be made aware of what they are to glean through their learning efforts. Be sure to include cognitive, behavioral, and affective objectives if this is what you intend, then later be sure to evaluate learning according to the domain and level of the unit objectives.

Continued

TABLE 3.1—cont'd	
Gagne's Nine Steps for Instructional Design	
Gagne's Instructional Event	**Learner's Corresponding Mental Process**
3. Stimulate recall of prior learning	Help the learner to recall that they know something and that new learning will build on what is already known. In addition, recalling previous learning stimulates short-term and long-term memory.
4. Present the content (or stimulus material)	Use various tactics to present content so that it feeds curiosity and motivates participation.
5. Provide learner guidance	Assist the learner with strategies and resources for learning at the intended level.
6. Elicit performance	Provide opportunities for learner elaboration, for learners to build on learning by drawing them out, or through seeking learning transference to a similar but not identical situation.
7. Provide feedback	Use the 2+2 method to identify what is going well and where there are concerns or areas for improvement.
8. Assess performance	Instructors need to know if learners reached the intended learning objectives and if course instruction helped or hindered this process; therefore, summative and formative assessment techniques should be built into each learning activity, unit, and course.
9. Enhance retention and transfer	Sequence instruction and learning outcomes so that learners can build from a solid base; encourage socialization into the practice world through integrating real-life problems; assess at a level appropriate to moving the learner forward in the program.

Adapted from Gagne, R.M., Briggs, L.J., & Wagner, W.W. (1992). *Principles of Instructional Design* (4th ed.). Fort Worth, TX: Harcourt Brace Jovanovich College Publishers.

The steps are used like a checklist to make sure that a course or learning moves through a series of steps or stages that, when completed, provide a well-rounded learning experience. An excellent resource for the Nine Steps that includes course illustrations for each step can be found at (http://ide.ed.psu.edu/idde/9events.htm).

TECHNOLOGY TIP 3.1

In every faculty meeting pull up The Nine Events of Instruction at http://ide.ed.psu.edu/idde/9events.htm. As a group, discuss one of the events and how it can apply to your classes.

The Dick and Carey Model

The Dick and Carey model of instructional design was first developed in 1978 as a general systems approach to instructional design. The model was considered to be unique at the time because it incorporated elements of general systems theory with behaviorist, constructivist, reductionist, and cognitivist schools of thought (Dick, 1996). This far-reaching integration across philosophical and theoretical boundaries was rare for its time. The Dick and Carey model breaks down learning activities into subunits, an instructivist tendency, predicting that mastery of the subunits will support further learning, the principle of scaffolding, which is a constructivist phenomena (Dick, Carey, & Carey, 2006). The Dick and Carey model itself reduces learning to a group of traits but links the traits together into a whole systems model that is embedded in a contextual environment important to learning success, both constructivist principles. Dick and Carey espoused the belief that every part of their system is connected to each other and that the entire instructional system works together with learners, course designers, and instructors to meet the objectives and goals of a course. Elements of the Dick and Carey model include: identify the instructional goals of the course; conduct instructional analysis; analyze learners and contexts; write performance objectives; develop assessment instruments; develop instructional strategies; develop and select instructional materials; design and conduct formative evaluation of instruction; revise instruction; and design and conduct summative evaluation. This model is used in the same way as the Gagne model. The instructor uses it to make sure every element of the instructional design that is needed to optimize the learning environment is accounted for (Table 3.2).

TABLE 3.2

The Dick and Carey Model of Instructional System Design

Steps in the Systems Design	Instructor and Designer Roles
Identify the Instructional Goals of the Course	The first job for the instructor is deciding what learners should be able to do at the end of each learning module and the entire course. Instructional goals are developed based on the assessment of learners' needs.
Conduct Instructional Analysis	The instructor considers instructional steps that will be most valuable in the achievement of learning goals. During this analysis, the instructor determines the knowledge, skills, and attitudes that learners must have before admittance to the class, which are known as entry behaviors and should be stipulated before the student's course starts.
Analyze Learners and Contexts	Here both learners and the contextual milieu, where they will learn and the setting in which they will practice their learning, are analyzed. Information from these analyses are integrated with information about the learners' previous knowledge, skill sets, and attitudes and then an instructional strategy is established.
Write Performance Objectives	Performance objectives are listed based on the instructional and learner analyses and the criteria for successful performance.

Continued

TABLE 3.2—cont'd	
The Dick and Carey Model of Instructional System Design	
Steps in the Systems Design	**Instructor and Designer Roles**
Develop Assessment Instruments	Instructional designers plan unit and course assessment strategies before the course, not as it goes along. Assessment strategies are developed for cognitive and behavioral learning and are to be directly related to the expectations identified in the performance objectives.
Develop Instructional Strategies	Instructional strategies need to be addressed for four time periods in a course: (1) preinstructional activities; (2) presentation of information; (3) practice and feedback; and (4) testing and follow-through activities and assessments. Instructional strategies should be based on current teaching/learning theories, evidence-based practice, course content, learner characteristics, and the medium of instructional delivery.
Develop and Select Instructional Materials	Instructional materials include all the devices and strategies used to produce instruction. These include the syllabus, Web pages, text books, hyperlinked materials, video streaming, computer-based multimedia, and so forth. In the ideal world, resource selection is based on course criteria. In reality, we often use what we have and add as we go.
Design and Conduct Formative Evaluation of Instruction	Frequent use of formative evaluation strategies helps instructors improve instruction and course quality both during a course and at the end of a course, or before it is offered the next time. There are many strategies to choose from including Brookfield's Critical Incident Questionnaire, asking learners about "the muddiest point," and the 1-minute essay on what was learned or not learned.
Revise Instruction	This may be triggered by formative assessment data and/or formal and informal evaluation of any other part of the cycle.
Design and Conduct Summative Evaluation	At the end of learning units and the end of a course, summative evaluations are done to measure achievement. In addition, formative evaluations are done to discover more about the value or worth of the course including the instructional design.

Adapted from Dick, W. (1996). The Dick & Carey Model: Will it survive the decade? *Educational Technology Research and Development,* 44(3), 55-63; Dick, W., Carey, L., & Carey, J.O. (2006). *The systematic design of instruction.* (6th ed.). San Francisco, CA: Berett-Koehler Publishers, Inc.

The ADDIE Model of Instruction

The ADDIE model is interesting in that it is well represented on the World Wide Web (WWW) and has a very common-sense approach to instructional design, but it is also odd in that it does not have a cited author or validation stream. Molenda, Pershing, and Reigeluth (1996) indicate that ADDIE is a model that has grown out of an oral tradition and exemplifies many models with similar characteristics. Even without a defined history, the ADDIE model seems to be the most popular of the instructional design models. According to this model:

- **A** stands for analyze, which directs the instructor to analyze learner characteristics and tasks to be learned.
- **D** stands for design the learning objectives and instructional approaches.
- The second **D** stands for develop instructional materials.
- **I** directs the instructor to deliver or distribute instructional materials that, in this case, will be online.
- **E** stands for evaluate.

Employing this model allows the user to come in at any point and go through the remaining steps then start all over again in an iterative fashion. This model is presented for two reasons. First, it is very simple and will get an instructor through the basics of instructional design without adding work or being intimidating, and second, because it looks so much like the Nursing Process that nursing faculty might have a natural affinity for it.

PEDAGOGIES FOR LEARNING

A Word About Pedagogy

Pedagogy refers to the study of being a teacher, which includes strategies for instruction and the style chosen by the teacher, in general or in a particular situation, to impart material to students or to create a space in which students might learn. Pedagogy has become part of several phrases that incorporate philosophical or epistemological antecedents. One example is critical pedagogy, which was championed by Paulo Freire as a method of teaching adults through dialogic interaction.

Andragogy, on the other hand, refers to the art of teaching adults. The androgogical model was developed by Malcolm Knowles. Some of his original principles relating to all adult education include (1) letting learners know why something is important; (2) showing learners how to direct themselves through information; and (3) relating the topic to the learners' experiences. In addition, (4) people will not learn until they are ready and motivated to learn. Often this (5) requires helping them overcome inhibitions, behaviors, and beliefs about learning (Knowles, Holton, & Swanson, 2005). All of these principles influence instructional design. Getting learners to engage is tremendously important in the online environment. Each of the androgogical principles increases the chance of getting and keeping learners engaged.

Constructivist versus instructivist pedagogy is something every instructional designer is likely to hear about. The constructivist viewpoint is, in many ways, reactionary to the more traditional instructivist view. Epistemologically, the instructivist view finds the world to be concrete and knowable to all in exactly the same way, whereas in the constructivist view reality is in the mind of the beholder, or is constructed from the interaction of experience, behavior, cognition, culture and so forth, by the learner or person of concern. When taken to the extreme, radical constructivism, means that reality is in the mind of the beholder and every reality is different. We will leave that to philosophers and epistemologists to debate. Instructivists break down information to the smallest units of analysis possible, which is called reductionism, finding that if one understands each little piece then adds the pieces together the whole will be knowable and make sense. Constructivists take a more holistic, fully assembled view of subject matter looking at it by itself and within its contextual framework.

In the instructivist view, learning is rigidly controlled and highly structured and no accommodation is made for individual differences, cultural sensitivity, or collaborative learning. The opposite is true for the constructivist pedagogy in which accommodation is made for individual differences, cultural sensitivity, and collaborative learning. The role of the teacher in the instructivist pedagogy is that of an authoritative-didactic imparter of knowledge. This person is the expert with a sharply focused vision of how instruction will be delivered and pointed expectations of how learners are to respond. On the other hand, the constructivist instructor acts as a facilitator, modifies instruction based on the course climate, and encourages learner control.

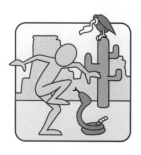

Before committing exclusively to one or the other of these pedagogies, there are a few things to remember. In nursing education, the instructor is indeed likely to be an expert and often that expertise is highly desirable. There may be points at which learners can self-determine learning goals and processes to meet their goals but in a highly regulated field such as nursing, there are many places where learning will be directed to fulfill accreditation requirements, meet state standards and, in the long run, create the best possibility for safe, quality patient care. It is a great idea in instructional design to work a course through a transition from a more directed perspective view to less directed perspective view intentionally. This is suggested for several reasons. If students feel as though faculty are not involved in assignments or discussions, they often feel abandoned. An ideal instructional design gives the student the perception that the faculty role could easily be eliminated.

Another point of consideration is that some students are unaccustomed to self-directed learning and such an environment could lead to failure if implemented too early in the term. On the other hand, an online course will hopefully mimic the real world and encourage independent learning, self-reflection, decision making, and self-evaluation as time goes on. As a side note, please also remember that no course resides in a vacuum. It is important for every faculty member to work with colleagues to determine the level of cognitive thinking and the level of independence learners in each course should have in the overall curriculum schema for the nursing program.

Narrative Pedagogy

Narrative pedagogy has its roots in post-modern interpretive philosophy. It's focus is on creating learning environments in which learners are encouraged to become self-directed, collaborative, co-creators of their educational experiences. The instructor may set the course in motion but then step back and becomes a facilitator of learning rather than the keeper and distributor of information. According to Freire (1993), the teacher is no longer the banker, making deposits of knowledge into students' flip-top heads. Instead, the teacher works in community with students to devise understanding through study, observation, and reflection that can be used to make the world a better place, so to speak, for all members of the learning community. Adopting narrative pedagogy requires that students and instructors examine not just information and skills but individual emotional reactions to learning situations. The reasoning that underpins the usefulness of this strategy for nursing educators is that nursing is as much about relationships, contextually based realities, and understanding diversity caused by a host of factors including culture, ethnicity, race, gender, socio-economic status, and life circumstances, as it is about understanding illness or injury progression. In addition, nursing is about managing and coping with problems that are not neat and tidy, do not follow the rules, are not fair, and do not evolve in a predictable manner. Educators using narrative pedagogy understand, accept, and celebrate this.

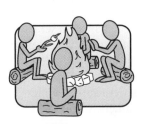

Narrative pedagogy does not suggest that conventional teaching strategies are no longer valid, it respectfully requests admittance into the educational arena to broaden learners horizons in learning through real-life and representations of real-life including art, poetry, music, literature, and movies. To learn from real-life events through narrative pedagogy, learners and instructors take time for reflective thinking and give voice to what they have learned through the intersection of experience and reflection by doing written work and openly expressing meaning through verbalization. Learning communities will only feel safe doing this if learning environments are designed and held to a standard of "collaboration, understanding, mutual trust, respect, equality, and acceptance of differences" (National League for Nursing, 2005). Using narrative pedagogy in online instruction requires that the instructional design supports a trusting environment. Further, it assumes a commitment by the faculty to making sure that learners really know how to think critically and express themselves reflectively through writing and dialogue.

Universal Design for Learning

The National Center on Universal Design for Learning (2009) reminds educators that "the goal of education is not simply the mastery of knowledge, it is the mastery of *learning*." Universal Design for Learning (UDL) is a pedagogy that recognizes that there is diversity in the classroom that is so ubiquitous that learning needs cannot be met by the traditional middle of the road one-size-fits-all curriculum. In addition, learning cannot be individualized to meet all different situations presented in each classroom. Types of diversity that UDL seeks to address through inclusivity rather than individuation of learning are variations on or multiple intelligences, differences in learning styles, abilities and disabilities, cultural and racial diversity, gender diversity, and socio-economic diversity (and any other diversity that can be named). Diversity is the norm not the exception and traditional instructional design that lacks depth and dimension for including all participants creates barriers to learning. UDL fills the gap in traditional pedagogy by creating learning environments and conditions for all learners. No small task to be sure, but thought by many to be the most impressive advance in learning theory and practice since movable print (Meyers & Rose, 2005). How can UDL be of use in instructional design? The list is long and the work for the designer is increased but front-loading the work will save on rework during a course. A simple overview of how to use UDL in the online environment learning units includes:

- Provide Multiple Means of Representation: Some students do very well with reading, but others do not. Much of online course is read-and-repeat, but there are more ways to present material than through the exclusive use of visual/auditory means. For example, while learning, mental health nursing students could be encouraged to watch a number of movies including *A Beautiful Mind* to understand schizophrenia and *On Golden Pond* to learn about aging, family conflict, and early dementia.

- Provide Multiple Means of Expression: Learners have varying degrees of success with writing, speaking, test taking, and so forth. Engagement in online learning will be a more satisfying experience leading to more engaged learners if there are multiple paths to expressing what has been learned.
- Provide Multiple Means of Engagement: Some learners thrive on a strict routine while others wilt away having to follow the same routine and prefer spontaneity. Instead of engaging all of the learners in one way, see if it is possible to find several ways to approach learning content. For example, one student might thrive on writing a discussion response but another might get far more out of photo-journaling the same material. The instructional design sets up the environment for optimizing conditions for learning, but the designer cannot control learning itself. It is in the best interest of the learner to provide avenues within optimizing conditions to allow for flexible possibilities in all of the three mentioned areas.

CONCEPTS TO INCLUDE IN INSTRUCTIONAL DESIGN

Leveled Learning

Bloom's Taxonomy has been mentioned often in this and other chapters. Why is it important in instructional design? Nursing is a *doing* profession. It is a clinical practice profession and although much of what professional nurses do is in their heads, so much of nursing is *thinking*, there are psychomotor behaviors and affective strategies that clearly have an effect on successful practice. Lower levels of learning in any domain are fairly easy to assess, but they do not reflect the reality of the practice environment, which is what nursing education prepares students to enter. Instruction within and across nursing programs needs to address a progression of learning throughout the levels of learning in all domains from simple to complex. This is conceptually easy to understand but difficult to address in the concrete structure of instructional design (Table 3.2). Bloom's Taxonomy helps the instructor and/or course designer develop leveled learning from simple to complex information, concepts, and procedures through cognitive function, psychomotor skills, behaviors, and affective or emotional development (Anderson & Krathwohl, 2001). Using Bloom's Taxonomy to assist with developing learning objectives and evaluation strategies—addressed later in the chapter—can be seen in Table 3.3. First, consider the level at which the entire course will be taught and then identify the optimal learning level for each course objective and subobjective and list all of these in the left-hand column. In the first row, label general levels of desirable learning outcomes according to Bloom's Taxonomy, remembering, understanding, applying, analyzing, and so forth. In the boxes created by the grid, write assessment ideas, discussion plans, test questions, and assignments that match the desired learning-level. Finally, calculate the percent of the course that is accounted for by each level of learning and review it according to the initial plan. This gives the instructor the opportunity to adjust the level of learning taught and/or assessed before the start of the class.

				Affective Domain—	
TABLE 3.3					
Revisiting Bloom's Taxonomy					
Cognitive Domain	Conceptual Framework	Psychomotor Domain	Conceptual Framework	Feelings and Attitudes	Conceptual Framework
Remembering	Learners recall information and recognize what has been distributed without information assimilation.	**Observe and Imitate**	Mimic, see what others are doing and replicate.	**Receiving**	Learners become aware of the learning experience not just the material; they listen, tune in, and realize that there are emotions, attitudes, and behaviors in play.
Understanding	Learners demonstrate an understanding and comprehension of information, concepts, and processes and are able to interpret and explain the meaning of material provided.	**Model and Manipulate**	Reproduce or replicate activity from precious success, memory, or instruction.	**Responding**	Learners react to material and the learning environment demonstrating changes associated with the emotions, attitudes, and behaviors in play.

Continued

TABLE 3.3—cont'd

Revisiting Bloom's Taxonomy

Cognitive Domain	Conceptual Framework	Psychomotor Domain	Conceptual Framework	Affective Domain—Feelings and Attitudes	Conceptual Framework
Applying	Learners are able to apply knowledge to real-life situations such as putting lessons into practice, solving problems, and/or managing activities.	Recognize Standards and Proceed with Precision	The learner recognizes the importance of performing skills according to standards that have been purposefully developed and respond to this independently with precision and with the ability to consistently demonstrate mastery of the skill.	Valuing	Learners attribute value to what is being learned and respond by expressing opinions, committing, or withdrawing their involvement.
Analyzing	Learners scrutinize received material looking for evidence to support assumptions. Knowledge is deconstructed to identify relationships and compare to standards in practice.	Correct	Learners use standards against which to evaluate their performance and make adjustments in performance.	Organizing and Conceptualizing Values	Learners qualify values associated with learning through resolving internal conflicts.

		Apply / Coach	Internalizing Values Characterizing the Individual
Evaluating	Learners attempt to appraise or assess information based on standards, values, criteria, and opinion to establish a sense of the correctness and worthiness of information.	Learners apply new-found skills to real-world situations.	Learners change, internalizing new values and transforming previously held patterns of beliefs that become part of the learner's character.
Creating	Learners integrate information gained through classroom knowledge, reflection, cultural and social underpinnings, and create meaning for themselves and nuances for transference to ill-define situations not directly addressed in a learning unit or course.	Skills become unconscious and automated and the learner is able to teach others this skill and/or transfer this learning to other ill-defined situations.	

Time and Space for Reflection Utilizing Technology as a Medium

It has long been considered valuable for teachers to create learning situations in which part of the input in thinking about experiences includes considering and reflecting on personal values, past experiences, feelings, and attitudes in order to create new meaning, better choices, and improved performance in the future as an output of learning. Often this does not happen because learners have not become skilled in the practice of reflection in learning. Strampel and Oliver (2007) site the importance of reflective learning in instructional design in their statement:

> [Reflective learning is a] complex process that strongly influences learning by increasing understanding, inducing conceptual change, and promoting critical evaluation and knowledge transfer. When instructors do not generate reflective learning opportunities in the classroom, prospects are lost for better learning outcomes. Much research has been devoted to conditions that must necessarily be present when fostering reflection. With the increase of technology-mediated learning in today's classroom, it is imperative that instructors understand how to ensure that these conditions are present when using technologies to create optimal reflective learning environments (p. 973).

As can be seen by integrating the previous discussion of constructivist and narrative pedagogy with a deeper understanding caused by stimulating reflective thinking, the instructional designer will realize the importance of intentionality in including strategies for reflective thinking in online instructional design. In this way, reflective learning is not just expected, it is planned for by building in situations that will create conditions for it to happen.

While planning for reflective learning it is important to remember that it too is leveled. It will probably not be surprising to find that Bloom's work is evident in reflective learning leveling and runs a parallel course. As a learner comes in contact with new information through an experience, cognitive excitation occurs. The learner becomes self-aware of the newness of what is being presented, and begins a process of wrestling with the material, falling into a pattern of cognitive dissonance (Gregoire, 2003, p. 156), deciding how she or he feels about it, deciphering how the information or experience will help or hinder his or her class work and/or nursing practice, and finally assimilates and accommodates the new information. Awareness followed by cognitive excitation and reflective thinking can be encouraged by the instructor asking questions, setting up problems to solve or tasks to accomplish so that the learner goes through cognitive disequilibrium (dissonance), which helps the learner come to an understanding or comprehension of the material rather than just memorizing it (Graessner, McNamara, and VanLehn, 2005).

As learners continue to engage with material, they move through phases of deeper understanding by looking at new material through the lens of past experiences. In this stage the learner returns to previous experiences, recalling what has happened in the past in terms of experiences and reactions, blends new thinking with old pictures and "tries out" newly formed ideas mentally to get a cerebral picture of what might have been or what might be. At this point, learners are able to describe the event in a nonjudgmental way, discussing in detail what they are thinking and feeling about new information. This stage of *descriptive reflection* can be promoted through written dialogue within a course. If the instructor asks each student to absorb material through reading or watching a movie, then asks each learner to reflect on how the information gained in the assignment is valuable to them in a explicit contextual example of their own choosing, the student will have both the opportunity for self-descriptive reflection and for reading and assimilating the reflections of others. This will not necessarily lead to changes in behavior or practice, but it is a step in the reflective process that will eventually lead to learning as change.

In the next stage—*dialogical reflection*—learners visit the question, "What does this material mean to me?" Learners associate with the information, integrate information into a previous knowledge base or skill-set, seek connections between the new information and the old, and appropriate what has been learned from both as one's own, internalizing it so that it becomes part of the learner who might then have difficulty identifying where "that" came from. For example, after a while a new nurse cannot easily explicate the stages of learning that have gone into understanding the value of precisely measured vital signs as they relate to patient management, she or he knows this. The dialogical phase of reflection can be encouraged in the online environment by having learners reconceptualize information they have been given for similar yet different scenarios, synthesize new material with additional material, and solve a more sophisticated problem than has been previously considered.

The final stage of reflective thinking is *critical reflection*. Here the learner moves beyond dialogical reflection by transferring knowledge to other situations, making associations between what has been learned in the given experience and other learning or life experiences, or synthesizes current learning with distant learning to create a new idea, process, or use for the thinking. In addition, the learner consciously evaluates what has been learned and places a value on the knowledge and potentially makes the transition from values and beliefs that were held before the learning event to values and beliefs inspired by the learning event. Instructional design will assist in drawing out this level of reflection by asking the learner questions that stimulate thinking about metacognition, that is, thinking about their thinking. For example, what did you think about some aspect of a learning unit before studying the unit and what do you think about the subject now that you have completed the unit. One example might be, what did you think about the self-care abilities of Haitian families before you watched the TV coverage of the 2010 earthquake disaster and studied nursing in environmental disasters, and what do you think about Haitian self-care abilities now? Why is this important to you in your personal and professional life? Why is it important that nurses concern themselves with global health and the health of complete strangers who have survived a natural disaster? How has your understanding of the role of disaster nursing changed through this learning exercise? Compare and contrast what you have learned in this exercise to what you think would be important for a nurse to know about self-care in the event of a sudden acute respiratory syndrome (SARS) epidemic?

Scaffolding

Scaffolding is loosely defined as any support that assists learners to achieve desired cognitive, behavioral, and affective learning goals. In the f2f environment the teacher-as-expert tends to be the main scaffold system providing information, practice situations, re-wording and re-teaching, providing study guides, and participating in selective tutoring. The online environment requires that technology be used by itself or as an interface between the teacher and learner to provide supports for learning. Instructional designers who are engaged in creating an environment for learning processes integrate *supportive situations* or scaffolding into the learning environment and plan so that learners can increase their knowledge or skill to a desired level. In a study done by Cagiltay (2006), there are four types of scaffolding appropriate to the online environment. These include conceptual scaffolding, procedural or process scaffolding, strategic scaffolding, and metacognition scaffolding. In addition, functional support for learning is provided directly through the CMS (course management system).

Functional scaffolding is usually built into the CMS and is related to helping the student store and retrieve information, send and receive messages, communicate with fellow learners and faculty, and get help with the CMS itself. Most of these are built into the system so the instructional designer will not have to develop them but will have to orient first-time users to them. Lack of success with functional scaffolds can cause the loss of a student from a course or program, so it is best for the instructional designer to plan carefully for a good orientation to the functional aspects of online learning and the CMS so that they can in turn support the learner.

Conceptual scaffolding is built into learning units to assist the learner in deciding what to consider, how or where to begin, and, in essence, help learners reason through complex problems. Some conceptual scaffolding can be built into the software that supports a course and some of it is created for learners within assignments and course room activities. An example of conceptual scaffolding is the glossary function apparent in many content modules in which words that may be unfamiliar to the user appear to be highlighted, indicating to the user that a click on the word will take the user rapidly to a definition of the term. The advantage of this is obvious. Many learners do not take the time to look up a word with which they are not familiar because it is a pain in the neck to get a dictionary and look up the word. Conceptual scaffolding that can be built into a learning module might include cueing or hinting at what a learner should do next or look for, grading rubrics that guide learners to exactly what must appear in an assignment to receive a certain grade, coaching comments that keep students going, and timely and specific feedback and performance advice.

Process or *procedural scaffolding* supports learning by guiding users through processes in a step-by-step manner (Cagiltay, 2006). When an instructional designer is considering scaffolding supports for help with learning processes and procedures, hyperlinks are often built into content modules. For example, if you happen to be teaching electrocardiogram interpretation or arrhythmias online, have your students click into http://www.youtube.com/watch?v=asR2-sb27Vw for a laugh and some seriously good learning inspiration. If you are looking for something that will take your students outside the box, try The Pink Glove Dance at http://www.youtube.com/watch?v=OEdVfyt-mLw. There are an enormous number of possibilities for supporting learning that stimulate learning outside the reading and repeating method. So much of online learning relies on reading that it is always a good idea to look for active learning scaffolding solutions and nonreading solutions to help maintain interest and engagement in the course.

Metacognitive (reflective) scaffolding is built in to foster reflection, which has been covered quite extensively. The role of the instructional designer is to build in time and space for metacognitive activities. This is done through prompting with questions designed to elicit reflective thinking. One of the most rewarding things for faculty to read occurs when a student who would normally answer the question "what did you learn?" with "nothing" instead can really see what they did, where further work is needed, and what might be done differently the next time.

Cognitive Load

For several years, educators have been encouraged to move from the traditional lecture-and-test format of the received or instructivist school of teaching and learning and move toward problem-based learning that provides the opportunity for learners to become engaged in solving real-life problems like the ones that they may be faced with after graduating and entering the professional world. One of the concepts that has evolved with the transition to problem-based learning, is the tendency to go hog wild and develop the richest most complex and diverse cases that can be dreamed up from a compilation of past patients, major disasters, and modern technology. The problem with these cases is that they are too rich for novice learners. Each case in problem-based learning or case-based learning and/or the sheer volume of content in a traditional case can be quantified as *cognitive load* (van Merriënboer & Sluijsmans, 2009). Cognitive load has three components:

- *Intrinsic cognitive load,* which is determined by the complexity of the learning tasks.
- *Extraneous cognitive load,* which is caused by suboptimal instructional design and associated processes that do not contribute to learning.
- *Germane cognitive load,* which is caused by appropriate instructional design and associated processes that directly contribute to learning (e.g., induction and elaboration) (van Merriënboer and Sluijsmans, 2009, p. 56.).

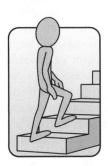
One of the many goals of instructional design is to plan for germane cognitive load and avoid overload, which renders learning a neurophysiological impossibility. Methods for minimizing intrinsic cognitive load include sequencing learning from simple-to-complex and by performance scaffolding. Going from simple to complex does not mean that the course designer must develop more and more cases that are each leveled in complexity but it might mean presenting a few pieces of information about a case, working through that much, problem solving, reflecting, and then adding in more information and essentially going through a series of "OK so now what should we do?" type of problem-solution building blocks. As learners move from more to less, dependent scaffolding is faded to the point where the learner is independent, self-directed, and self-evaluative without it consciously being stressful to get there.

Cautions to remember when lowering cognitive load include getting the load so low that the process becomes boring or forgetting to accommodate difference in learning needs among students. Making every student go through the same scenario in the same sequence will bore some students, be perfect for some, and too difficult for others. In didactic teaching, simulation laboratories using cognitive load to full teaching effect means being able to up the ante, or difficulty, for students who are catching on rapidly and pushing back on the intensity of a situation to allow slower students time to catch up. Building in learner-driven sequencing of tasks during both didactic and simulated learning, creates the opportunity for learners to develop their own systems and their self-directed learning that would be considered germane cognitive load. These problems should be taken into account in the instructional design to help create a balance between the ideal for individual students and what is possible for the whole of the class.

TEACHING/LEARNING STRATEGIES IN INSTRUCTIONAL DESIGN

Discussion-based Learning

Discussion-based learning is primarily a text-based phenomena in which learners are assigned some form of content, usually reading, and then directed to answer questions about what has been read or studied. True discussion is limited by several factors in the online environment. CMS are extremely limited in how discussion can be managed. One learner posts a reply to the assigned question and another student responds to the first student. Discussion-based learning helps learners to improve conceptual understanding, problem-solving ability, and communication skills, but leading a discussion under the best of circumstances is difficult (Bender, 2003). Active students jump into online discussion and share with abandon whereas passive students would not contribute a thing if left to their own devices. Open discussion rarely elicits response, but placing too many rules for discussion makes it a task to be done and checked-off rather than an opportunity for deepening understanding. All this must be taken into account by the instructional designer who is put in the position of trying to manage something that will be meaningful to learners while getting them to engage in content. Having stipulated what the content area for a course is, probably the most difficult challenge for instructional design is to find enough variations on the theme of discussion to keep learners interested. That means varying discussion assignments.

Bender (2003) suggests creating debates, using the Socratic method, answering questions with questions to elicit deeper thinking about an initial response, and having "guests" who are experts in a field of study to create interest. In addition, she suggests changing asynchronous discussion with a bit of synchronous discussion to enhance learning community development and foster a sense of belonging to a group. Another method that has been shown to work is assigning roles to students. For example, in a discussion of nursing theory each learner chooses to "be" a nursing theorist. The instructor then presented a patient case and asked each theorist how to address the case from the perspective of priority concerns, approach to management, and continuity of care. Learners became much more animated in their roles as theorists than they did discussing theorists' perspective and they reported spending much more time researching how the theorist actually translated nursing theory into nursing practice.

During the instructional design phase of a course, doing as much work as possible up front to manage all the details of discussion assignments will pay off a hundred-fold during the class. Having explicit directions for discussion-based learning includes provisions for mandatory response requirements, timing of response requirements, assessment criteria and weighing, tracking, and archiving of initial messages and then all the same things for student-initiated responses to fellow students (Ali & Salter, 2004). Ending discussions with an assignment related to thinking about thinking, what has been learned, and how learning can be used in different situations addresses metacognition. Asking learners to articulate what has been learned from fellow students motivates each learner to be more careful, knowing that they are responsible for assisting in educating their peers, and it sends the message that learning is suppose to occur through the process of discussion.

Problem-based Learning (PBL)

Problem-based learning (PBL) is a student-centered approach to learning in which the problem is the center stimulus to learning (Rideout, 2001). The conditions needed for problem-based learning to thrive include: "an instructional design centered around problems that are relevant to learning outcomes; conditions that facilitate small-group work; self-directed learning; and independent study, functional knowledge, and critical thinking" (Rideout, 2001, p. 23). All of these conditions are available in the online environment. In addition, working on solving problems is a great approach for keeping learners interested and motivated in their learning. The foundation that supports problem-based learning is creating rich contextual learning scenarios that are derived from real-life experiences and serve as the basis for complex multidimensional learning. Participating in these scenarios offers the learner the opportunity to integrate cognitive, psychomotor, and affective learning that simulates what is to be expected in real practice. Integrated learning allows learners to construct meaning and knowledge that can be transferred from the learning space to the practice environment (Merriënboer & Sluijsmans, 2009).

As students progress through a course, they will find themselves to be more and more autonomous in controlling their learning, choosing learning objectives, and planning demonstrations of competencies through fading-guidance strategies (van Merriënboer & Sluijsmans, 2009). Lest the faculty becomes too enthusiastic with the complexity of the problems and cases that serve as prototypes for the problem-based learning curriculum, the application of cognitive load theory, as already discussed, can be employed to avoid overstimulation and shutdown of executive and deep learning function. By decreasing cognitive load through scaffolding, moving from simple to complex in cases, and developing well thought out cases that are not presequenced for the learner, each learner is able to adapt learning goals to what they need instead of doing what everyone else has done. The learner can take on responsibility for assessing self-learning needs, plan for learning, implement learned strategies, and evaluate their effectiveness, which, in theory, will maximize learning (van Merriënboer & Sluijsmans, 2009). In terms of instructional design, the essence of what is necessary to facilitate PBL is well written cases that progress in complexity over time and direction for what is expected to validate the learning process and learning outcomes (Rideout et al., 2002).

EVALUATION

To meet learning unit objectives and avoid chaos in the classroom, it would well suit course developers and teachers to take the advice of Gronlund and Waugh (2009) and integrate curriculum, instruction, and assessment into the instructional design early, during the course development because these elements provide the support structure for maintaining and continuously improving the learning environment of learning units and the course.

Early in the development of a course, the developer draws links between the proposed course and the general curriculum. Having ensured a course fit, the developer considers the prior knowledge of perspective learners and builds upon that knowledge rather than repeating it. If the developer does not have a good idea of the learners' prior knowledge, she or he can do an assessment first thing in the class and then instruction can be modified as necessary. This, for example, would take the form of a pre-test, the final examination for the course, or a standardized examination related to the subject matter. As the course evolves, the instructor guides the learners through material in the form of instruction, coaching, demonstration, and so forth. During this time, she or he intersperses assessments to see if the learners are indeed learning what was intended. If the learners are proceeding according to the target plan, the status quo can be maintained, but if they are not, a remediation plan can be enacted early. This form of assessment is known as *formative assessment,* the purpose of which is to provide a mechanism for knowing if immediate course improvement is needed before the end of the course. According to Gronlund and Waugh (2009), formative assessments are used to meet the needs of learners by providing feedback to both learners and faculty to determine if learning is occurring along the anticipated trajectory of the class. Formative assessments take many forms including quiz questions, reflective exercises, and critical incident questionnaires (Brookfield, 1995). They can be used at any time during the delivery of course material. The role of formative assessment is to improve learning. Formative assessment differs in role from both benchmark assessment and summative assessment in purpose, timing, intensity, and use.

As formative assessments are completed the teacher can interpret appropriateness of instructional design for cognitive load, timing, effort needed to complete assignments, and for the level of learning that was intended by the written objective. She or he can determine the need to re-plan or further break down objectives so that learners are better able to understand what they are suppose to accomplish in their study time away from class. Classroom assessments will point out the need for remediation for the entire class, for a small group, or for isolated individuals. This gives the faculty information to work with regarding methods for remediation and it gives members of the school faculty information about learner needs in general. Doing classroom assessments has the added benefit of letting the learner know that they are important (Fig. 3.1).

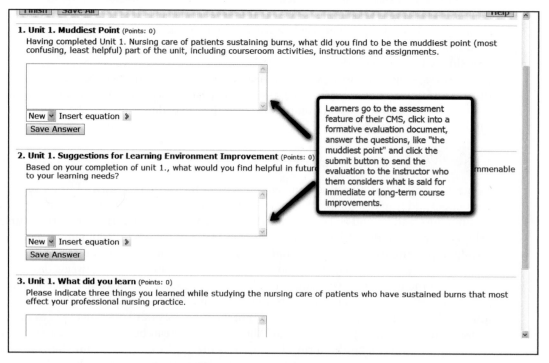

Figure 3.1   Screen shot—Formative evaluation tool.

They learn that a course is not written in stone and that what is happening is not happening to them but with them. They are reminded that they are a part of the course progress in helping to determine the flow, pace, and content coverage of the course to help them to become successful. As long as the assessment does not take over the course, this is a win-win situation.

Examples of Formative Assessments

Angelo and Cross (1993) provide an extensive review of close to 50 different assessments that can be used as formative assessments. These are categorized by what the instructor wishes to assess about a course or course learners. A few examples include techniques for assessing knowledge, recall, or understanding during a course, analyzing learners' critical thinking, assessing skills in problem solving, assessing learners' attitudes, values and self awareness, and assessing learners' reactions to instruction, a course, or the institution of a policy, procedure, or instructional method (Angelo & Cross, 1993, p. xi). A few favorite examples that are derived directly from Angelo and Cross's compilation follow.

The *muddiest point* is a simple-to-use, efficient, and effective method for finding out what learners understand and what they do not. As the name implies, at any time after a learning unit has started, the online instructor posts a discussion asking the learners to respond to the query, "What is the muddiest point in this presentation?" The learner then posts a response. The muddiest point is easily altered to get *the clearest point* and *the muddiest point* by asking just that. The hard part of the muddiest point is to gather the information, interpret it, and decide what to do to respond, which is not always easy in the online environment.

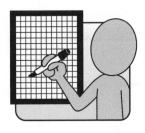

A *categorizing grid* is a type of sorting matrix and helps learners practice critical thinking and provides instructors information on student progress. When used with children, the teacher might ask learners to put all the circles into one bin, all the cubes in another, and so forth. In an online pharmacology class, the instructor could ask learners to move a series of words or phrases into a grid that has drug names, categories, therapeutic uses, and pharmacokinetics. The grid gives the instructor information about how the students are doing at keeping concepts straight or knowing "what goes with what." The matrix also has the advantage of letting students know quite clearly how they are doing with both memorizing and keeping concepts straight.

The *what's the principle assessment* helps instructors and learners assess how well they are able to recognize the effective use of problem-solving skills related to a particular area of content. Any content area that has a sequence of steps, structure, or principles that guide practice, such as aseptic technique, are appropriate for the what's the principle assessment. For example, a group of learners is doing an online unit in advanced assessment strategies. After going through the content, the instructor wants to know if the students can identify when and if some or all of the steps and strategies in the module are used at all and if they are used effectively. Several scenarios are presented and the student is asked to attribute principles to the scenario as appropriate. Another way to do this online is to use video clips of assessments and have the learners critique the video segment by attributing principles from the content module to the scenarios, demonstrating what is present and what is absent in applied situations.

The *double-entry journal* has the learner address assimilation of course materials from two sequential perspectives. First the learner answers a series of questions via the discussion board or in an online journal about unit content (Figs. 3.2 and 3.3). These may include items

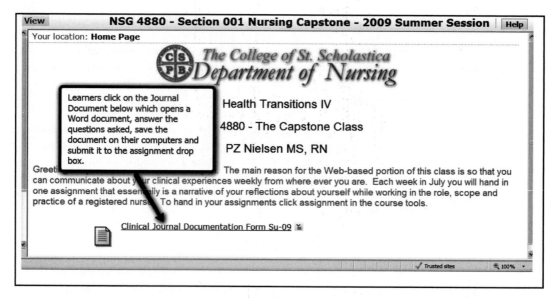

Figure 3.2   Screenshot—Form for online journaling.

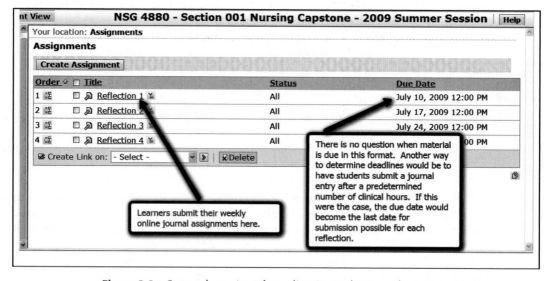

Figure 3.3   Screenshot—Area for online journal entry submission.

such as identifying the main principles in the content, attributing standards of care, theoretical or any type of principles to learning situations, or discussing the most controversial aspects of a passage from the reading. The second discussion response or journal entry then explicitly details metacognitive thinking by directing learners to reflect on what they have been thinking about the content, why they picked what they picked, why what they wrote about has meaning and is useful to practice, or how it would be possible to implement an idea into practice. The instructor then has the opportunity to follow cognitive, affective, and metacognitive development.

An additional classroom assessment that comes from Brookfield (1995) is the *critical incident questionnaire* (CIQ). There are many variations of this, but essentially, at the end of a learning unit the learner is asked to reflect on what has been learned, what was not clear, and what would have been helpful in making the module more meaningful. The instructor analyzes this feedback and makes a decision about making an immediate change, considering learner suggestions for the next time the course is taught, or making changes in future modules. The learner has the opportunity to reflect on the fact that learning has indeed occurred and they are allowed the opportunity to have a voice in the flow of the course.

Summative Evaluations

Graded learner evaluations come as either *benchmark assessments* and *summative assessments*. Benchmark assessments are used to predict learner performance. They might be used to predict scores on other tests, success in an institution, or the ability to complete a course of study. Summative assessments are designed and used to appraise learner performance and determine grades. They are usually used at a natural break in course material such as at the end of a learning unit or at the end of a course. Summative assessments assume many forms but can be used for cognitive, psychomotor, and affective learning and the form the assessment takes should follow the type of material, the way the material has been taught, and the level of learning that was expected to be achieved as articulated in the learning objectives.

In the online course room, the teacher can break up content and help learners get feedback before being graded by interspersing test questions that mimic those that will be on an actual test, or provide critical-thinking exercises that will lead the learner in the direction of information gathering and interpretation before writing a larger graded paper or developing a large assignment. This is done as the instructor leads learners through developmental steps by scaffolding learning so that by the time a graded evaluation comes around, the learner had a solid foundation upon which to draw conclusions. When it comes to actually doing summative assessments, one of the key factors to good instructional design is that the summative assessments match the level of learning that has been designated in the course and unit objectives and subobjectives. In other words, if an objective requires that the learner be able to apply a concept to practice then the assessment should reflect the objective by asking for an application response or test item. A table of specifications (ToS) (Table 3.4) provides a format for developing a table of specifications (Notar, Zuelke, Wilson, & Yunker, 2004). These can be used many ways. The one presented is only one page for the purpose of demonstration, but would be much longer for an entire course. When using the table of specifications before the course going live, the instructor and course designer work through every objective, level it,

TECHNOLOGY TIP 3.2

Building a rubric is not difficult, but it is time-consuming and getting started can be the hardest part. Rubistar (http://rubistar.4teachers.org/), an online program that provides step-by-step guidance for developing rubrics, puts a completed rubric into a premade useable form and allows the user to print and save the finished product. It is a great way to get started.

TABLE 3.4

Table of Specifications

Learning Outcomes Categories → Leveled Objectives ↓	Assessments for Remembering Learning Outcomes	Assessments for Understanding Learning Outcomes	Assessments for Application Learning Outcomes	Assessments for Analysis Learning Outcomes	Weighted Percentage For Outcome and Assessment
Course **Objection 1** **Subobjective 1.1** By the end of this unit you will be able to recall . . .	In this discussion you will need to recall several arguments made by . . .				2%
Subobjective 1.2 By the end of this unit you will be able to compare two theoretical frameworks		Compare the value of the transformative learning theory to the experiential learning theory for			4%
Course **Objective 2** **Subobjective 2.1** By the end of this unit the learner will be able to illustrate the concept of . . .		Using an example from your practice, illustrate how you use Watson's theory in your course work			4%
Subobjective 2.2 By the end of this unit the learner				Read articles A, B, & C and attribute	8%

Objective	Activity	Description	Weight
will be able to attribute ideas found in the reading to underlying theories of		the main ideas in each article to the underlying leadership theory that is represented	4%
Course Objection 3 **Subobjective 3.1** By the end of this unit the learner will understand how to use three models to complete family assessments	Make a table in Word and abstract the major points from each of the family assessment models you have studied		
Subobjective 3.2 By the end of this unit the learner will be able to apply Family Assessment Theory to traditional family situations		This week you will perform and record a complete family assessment using the systems model	6%
Total weight in percentage			

and make sure that every assessment, which in online learning takes the form of a quiz, a discussion board entry, an examination or an assignment, matches the level of the objective. Using the grid gives the instructor a visual image of how objectives are being assessed, that objectives and assessments match in terms of leveling of thinking, delivers a prompt for calculating grade points, and an assessment of the overall level of the course (Table 3.4).

Quite often, summative evaluations in nursing and in online instruction take the form of written work. This provides an opportunity to evaluate concept formation and provides an opportunity for reflective thinking. Table 3.5, Course Objectives and Clinical Journal

TABLE 3.5
Clinical Objectives and Online Journal Assignments for a Clinical Capstone Course

Learning Objective	Summative Evaluation of Learning Objective
1. The learner analyzes her or his ability to function as a care manager and care coordinator and reflects on possibilities for continuous improvement in this role.	Document the actions that were taken during the week that validate your ability to work as a care manager and care coordinator. Reflect on how your abilities as a care manager and care coordinator have improved beyond what they were last week. Provide one specific example of something you learned before your clinical experiences this week that you have used to improve your care manager and care coordinator role this week. Provide a specific example of something you have learned this week that will help you in the role of care manager and care coordinator in the future.
2. The learner analyzes her or his ability to function as a care provider and reflects on possibilities for continuous improvement in this role.	Document and reflect on your nursing actions as a care provider. Where are you confident and competent to work as an independent care provider and where have you found that you are in need of improvement? What actions have you taken this week to learn about and/or fill the gaps in your cognitive, behavioral, and affective knowledge that you have identified as personal learning needs?
3. The learner synthesizes classroom learning and clinical practice to appropriately delegate and prioritize patient care.	As a nurse you will be making decisions regarding delegation and prioritization several times a day. Discuss your nursing actions related to delegates and prioritization of patient care. Provide at least one example of what you chose to delegate, how you knew it was an appropriately delegated assignment, how you carried out the delegatory assignment, and how you evaluated that the assignment you had delegated was done successfully in a timely manner. Provide at least one example of what you chose to prioritize care, how you knew you appropriately prioritized care, and how you evaluated that your prioritization was done successfully for the patients involved.
4. The learner evaluates her or his knowledge of pathophysiology as a foundation for patient care and creates opportunities to improve practice by improving pathophysiological knowledge.	As an entry level nurse you will discover daily that you do not know something about the pathophysiology of a patient's condition that would make your care better if you knew it. What have you found this week, in terms of pathophysiology, that you have not known, or not known at a level that suits you, and what have you done to remedy the situation? (Takes the opportunity to improve knowledge of patient care—pathophysiology.)

TABLE 3.5—cont'd

Clinical Objectives and Online Journal Assignments for a Clinical Capstone Course

Learning Objective	Summative Evaluation of Learning Objective
5. The learner evaluates her or his knowledge of pharmacology as critical to patient care and creates opportunities to improve practice by improving pharmacology knowledge.	As an entry level nurse you will discover daily that you do not know something about the patient's medication that would make your care better if you knew it. What have you found this week, in terms of medications, that you have not known, or not known at a level that suits you, and what have you done to remedy the situation? (Takes the opportunity to improve knowledge of patient care—medications.)
6. The learner recognizes the importance of helping patients progress successfully to the next level of care, analyzes her or his role in this transitional process, and finds opportunities for continual improvement in this process.	Analyze your experiences with discharging patients this week. Reflect on the discharge process, transfer, or self-care management plan you have developed for a patient/client and provide an outline of your teaching plan for the patient/client. (There must be a different teaching plan each week.)
7. The learner recognizes the importance of patient advocacy in professional nursing, analyzes her or his role in this process, and finds opportunities for continual improvement in this process.	You will find many opportunities to act in the RN role of patient advocate. Reflect on how, when, and why you advocated for patients and their families within the context of the health-care delivery system or the community. (This, of course, must be part of your clinical from this week, not from your community as client projects.)
8. The professional nurse uses communication to the benefit of safe quality patient care and optimal collaboration with the care team.	You will spend a great deal of time as an RN communicating with patients, families, collaborative health-care team members, and members of the community. Analyze the effectiveness of your communicating, collaborating and/or negotiating with members of the health-care team. What are the successes and where are the challenges? What are the possibilities for improvement?
9. The professional nurse continually evaluates patient status and patient care to assess the achievement of predetermined outcomes and to redirect care if predetermined outcomes are not being met.	You will spend a great deal of time as an RN evaluating the effect of your and others' nursing and collaborative care. Analyze and reflect on your efforts at evaluating nursing care and patient care outcomes based on predetermined patient outcomes. In other words, how did your specific care and the care of the collaborative team help the patient to reach the predetermined goals of care for a particular day?
10. The professional nurse is actively involved in self-assessment as a nurse and member of the profession.	Self-evaluation is a life skill and you do it for all kinds of things. At this time, analyze and reflect on your professional growth this week and describe how you are experiencing this growth as part of becoming a member of the profession of nursing.

Documentation Elements, illustrates how an online journal can be used to elicit conceptual, psychomotor, and affective learning in a longitudinal fashion based on the objectives of the clinical aspect of course. Using a grading rubric for the evaluation helps enormously with faculty work load and with standardization of grading. It also provides the learner with an excellent idea of what is expected in each response. An illustration of a summative evaluation rubric for a course that is offered on the CMS Black Board can be seen in Figure 3.4.

CONCLUSION

By this time, anyone becoming involved in online nursing education will have surmised that preparing an online course gives an educator much to think about. Instructional design for each course will include an eye to instructional design models such as Gagne's nine events or the Dick and Carey model to system design to be sure that every aspect of what is needed on an online course has been achieved before the start of the course. The instructor will have the opportunity to reflect on pedagogy and choose when and how to use authority and constructivism in the best possible blend to create an environment. At the same time, instructional design should reflect a theme of inclusivity so that all learners share an equal opportunity to benefit from the online course. As planning for a course progresses, the focus of instructional design will necessarily turn to content delivery, at which time faculty and designers will worry not just about imparting information but at what level to best serve learners based on their previous experiences and education. Efforts will be made to incite students to reflect on not just content but on learning itself and, in the process, making meaning and transforming through education. To optimize conditions for learning, instructional design will include scaffolding to create a strong foundation for building, learning and cognitive load strategies to keep learners from being overwhelmed or underwhelmed. Instructional design necessarily addresses teaching and learning strategies. Problem-based learning is highly recommended for its fit with online learning, motivational factors, and benefit for creating nurses who are ready to assume responsibility for their professional roles upon graduation.

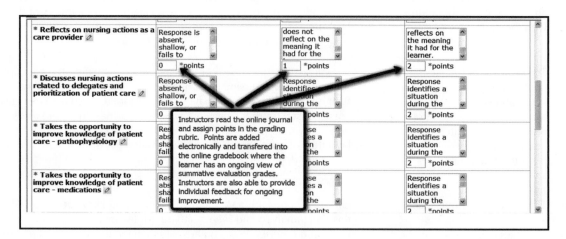

Figure 3.4   Screenshot—Summative evaluation rubric.

Evaluation, including preplanned formative classroom and summative course assessments are used harmoniously to improve the learning environment and to critique learner performance and achievement. Putting all the steps of instructional design together while referencing pedagogical frameworks for active learning in the clinical art, science, and practice of nursing will assist in developing an optimal online environment for learning success.

REFERENCES

Ali, S., & Salter, G. (2004). The use of templates to manage on-line discussion forums. *Electronic Journal on e-Learning, 2*(1), 11–18.

Anderson, L. W., & Krathwohl, D. R. (Eds.). (2001). *A taxonomy for learning, teaching and assessing: A revision of Bloom's taxonomy of educational objectives.* Upper Saddle River, NJ: Allyn & Bacon.

Angelo, T. A., & Cross, K. P. (1993). *Classroom assessment techniques: A handbook for college teachers* (2nd ed.). San Francisco, CA: Jossey-Bass.

Bender, T. (2003). *Discussion based online teaching to enhance student learning.* Sterling, VA: Stylus Publishing.

Brookfield, S. D. (1995). *Becoming a reflective teacher.* San Francisco, CA: Jossey-Bass.

Cagiltay, K. (2006). Scaffolding strategies in electronic performance support systems: Types and challenges. *Innovations in Education and Teaching International, 43*(1), 93–103. doi: 10.1080/14703290500467673

Coyne, P., Ganley, P., Hall, T., Meo, G., Murray, E., & Gordon, D. (2008). Applying universal design for learning in the classroom. In D. H. Rose & A. Meyers (Eds.), *A practical reader in universal design for learning.* Cambridge, MA: Harvard Education Press.

Dick, W. (1996). The Dick and Carey model: Will it survive the decade? *Educational Technology Research and Development, 44*(3), 55–63. doi: 10.1007/BF02300425

Dick, W., Carey, L., & Carey, J. O. (2006). *The systematic design of instruction* (6th ed.). San Francisco, CA: Berett-Koehler Publishers, Inc.

Freire, P. (1993). *Pedagogy of the oppressed* (30th ed.). New York: Continuum Press.

Gagne, R. M., Briggs, L. J., & Wager, W. W. (1992). *Principles of Instructional Design* (4th ed.). Fort Worth, TX: Harcourt Brace Jovanovich College Publishers.

Graessner, A. C., McNanara, D. S., & VanLehn, K. (2005). Scaffolding deep comprehension strategies through Point&Query, Auto Tutor, and iStart. *Educational Psychologist 40*(4), 225–234.

Gregiore, M. (2003). Is it a challenge of a threat? A dual-process model of teachers' cognition and appraisal processing during conceptual change. *Educational Psychology Review, 15*(2), 147–179.

Gronlund, N. E., & Waugh, C. K. (2009). *Assessment of learner achievement.* New York, NY: Allyn and Bacon.

Knowles, M. S., Holton, E. F., & Swanson, R. A. (Eds.). (2005). *The adult learner: The definitive classic in adult education and human resource development* (6th ed.). Woburn, MA: Butterworth-Heinemann.

Molenda, M., Pershing, J. A., & Reigeluth, C. M. (1996). Designing instructional systems. In R. L. Craig (Ed.), *The ASTD training and development handbook* (4th ed., pp. 266–293). New York, NY: McGraw-Hill.

Meyers, A., & Rose, D. H. (2005). The future is in the margins: The role of technology and disability in educational reform. In D. H. Rose, A. Meyers, & C. Hitchcock (Eds.), *The universally designed classroom: Accessible curriculum and digital technologies.* (pp. 13–16). Cambridge, MA: Harvard Education Press.

National Center for Universal Design. (2009). Introduction: UDL guidelines–Version 1.0. D.H. Rose & J. Wasson, compilers: Retrieved from http://www.udlcenter.org/aboutudl/udlguidelines/

National League for Nursing. (2005). Position statement: Transforming nursing education. New York: National League for Nursing. Retrieved from http://www.nln.org/aboutnln/positionstatements/transforming052005.pdf

Notar, C. E., Zuelke, D. C., Wilson, J. D., & Yunker, B. D. (2004). The table of specifications: Insuring accountability in teacher made tests. *Journal of Instructional Psychology*: Retrieved from http://findarticles.com/p/articles/mi_m0FCG/is_2_31/ai_n6130123/pg_4/?tag=content;col1

Reiser, R. (2001). A history of instructional design and technology: Part II: A history of instructional design. *ETR&D, 49*(2), 57–67.

Rideout, E. (2001). *Transforming nursing education through problem-based learning.* Sudbury, MA: Jones & Bartlett Publishers.

Rideout, E., England-Oxford, V., Brown, B., Fothergill-Borunnais, F., ...Coates, A.l (2002). A comparison of problem-based and conventional curricula in nursing education. *Advances in Health Science Education, 7,* 3–17.

Strampel, K., & Oliver, R. (2007). Using technology to foster reflection in higher education. Proceedings ascilite Singapore. Retrieved from http://www.ascilite.org.au/conferences/singapore07/procs/strampel.pdf

University of Illinois. (2010). Instructional strategies for online courses. Retrieved from http://www.uillinois.edu/resources/tutorials/pedagogy/instructionalstrategies.asp

van Merriënboer, J. J. G., & Sluijsmans, D. M. A. (2009). Toward a synthesis of cognitive load theory, four-component instructional design, and self-directed learning. *Education Psychology Review, 21,* 55–66. doi: 10.1007/s10648-008-9092-5

The Strategic Plan

Tim J. Bristol, PhD, RN, CNE

Ready, Fire, Aim! That is how I approached the use of online testing. I had heard about this great system and decided to use it with my students. We dove right in. Exam 1 was a nightmare. Between pop-up blockers and my lack of understanding of how to use the tool, we were all close to mutiny. After we got the information technology team in the loop, it started to go better. I also had to spend a little more time preparing myself to manage the tool during a live exam. If I had a plan in place and carefully analyzed what was needed, I would have realized the absence of key players (IT personnel) and my lack of training for the tool.

Effective implementation of e-learning in nursing education requires a methodical approach that helps the educator address the needs of the learners and the health-care system they aspire to serve. The approach taken to this implementation may unintentionally yield confusion and subsequent frustration. Using a strategic plan can help the educator move through the process of implementation in a way that yields the intended results.

Strategic plans come in many shapes and sizes. It is not the intention of this chapter to advocate for the one best plan. It is the intention of this chapter to recommend a structure that will help the educator (and other team members) realize success in the planning process. If your organization or department has a different strategic planning model, that plan may suffice. Simply apply the concepts of this proposed plan and transfer accordingly.

It also should be noted that the strategic plan is just as useful for the individual educator pursuing the use of a particular technological tool (e.g., the online discussion board) as it is for the nursing department that would like to offer an entire program online (e.g., an online associate degree RN program). The goal is to enhance the learning experience while decreasing negative impacts on the students and faculty.

STRATEGIC PLANNING PROCESS OVERVIEW

The plan is composed of five basic components.

1. Goal development
2. Plan development
3. Resource analysis
4. Plan implementation
5. Continuous evaluation

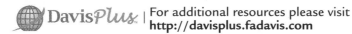
DavisPlus | For additional resources please visit
http://davisplus.fadavis.com

Strategic Plan Form-Details

Project Title _____

Goal Development/Congruence
Program _____
Course _____

Plan Development
Tool _____
Budget _____
Training Needed _____ (Release Time?)
Syllabus _____
Rollout _____

Give your students the **V**ery **B**est **A**lways!
Variety! _____
Build Community! _____
Active Learning! _____

Resource Analysis
Currently In-House_____
Hardware _____
Software_____

Plan Implementation
Who needs to hear from you as the implementation progresses?
Did you address the 4 Cs?

Continuous Evaluation
Formative?
Summative?

Strategic Plan Form-Open

Project Title _____

Goal Development/Congruence

Plan Development

Resource Analysis

Plan Implementation

Continuous Evaluation

Figure 4.1 Strategic Plan Form. An electronic copy of this form can be found at DavisPlus.

TECHNOLOGY TIP 4.1

Consider using the latest version of MindManager as it allows your planning team to work in real-time to organize, manage, and communicate ideas and information while developing strategic plans.

"MindManager is the ultimate tool for increasing productivity—for you or your entire team. Use it to visually connect ideas and information to help you save time, solve real business problems, improve business processes, and drive innovation. By visually organizing all your information, you'll have the big picture clearly before you, while still tracking the smallest details. Add images, hyperlinks, attachments, priority, and more to help you understand the structure, relationships, and importance of your information. Import and export Microsoft Office documents, including Word, PowerPoint, Visio®, and Project®. Link Excel files to topics. View and edit these files directly within MindManager." http://www.mindjet.com/products/mindmanager-8-win/overview

A Strategic Plan Form is shown in Figure 4.1 and also can be found on the companion Web site. The reader is encouraged to print that handout and have it nearby as you read. Consider the initial read of this chapter as a brainstorming session. As you read, write any ideas, thoughts, or concerns that come to mind. Then use a clean copy of the Strategic Plan Form as you work through the process with members of your planning team. Even though these steps are presented in a linear fashion, the wise team will review all areas of the plan often. It is a dynamic process that should be in a state of continuous improvement and revision.

GOAL DEVELOPMENT

As with any educational endeavor, the goals must drive the process. These goals can come from a needs assessment of a group of potential learners, a parent institution, an accreditation body, or an administrative need. Administrators and educators should be certain that they start here and make sure that goals are remembered at every step of the strategic planning process. The members of the team will do well to review the goals often as they progress through this journey.

NEEDS ASSESSMENT

As you consider a needs assessment, be sure to keep the end goal in mind. For instance, if you are embarking on the process of converting your traditional course into an online course, you may not need to conduct a fully developed institutional assessment. Keep in mind that needs assessments may have already been completed. Consulting with a colleague who has gone down this road before is often a good way to help ensure that your needs assessment is not prohibitively overwhelming while still being comprehensive enough for the strategic plan to succeed.

There are many stakeholders to consider in the needs assessment, including students, other faculty, and administrators. For example, assessment of student satisfaction data may reveal that learners find the face-to-face (f-2-f) broadcast lecture format boring. Faculty may indicate that learners are not engaged in the f-2-f classroom. Administrators may note that the discussion boards are not being used in most classes, even though the faculty have indicated that they need more learner-learner interactions in their online classes. The enrollment department has noted that many potential students are indicating that the f-2-f classroom schedule is prohibitive because of their children's schedule and a need to work

TECHNOLOGY TIP 4.2

There are many online survey tools that can be used to survey stakeholders. Some of them are free if the sample size is moderate and the survey tool has a reasonable number of questions. Online survey tools are a good way for the educational unit to quickly collect data related to the needs assessment. Contact your information technology experts (or buddies from other schools) to see if they can recommend reliable and inexpensive survey tools. Two possible tools are http://www.surveymonkey.com/ and http://zoomerang.com/

while going to school. The nurse managers at one of the clinical agencies continuously report that students and new graduates have a deficit in the area of critical thinking. The accreditation standards have been revised and now require students to demonstrate competency in informatics.

Data from the needs assessment should be evaluated with a critical lens. A collegewide committee was contemplating whether or not to recommend that all students be provided a laptop computer. A survey published in a technology journal revealed that the percentage of colleges doing this was small. The committee chose not to recommend this move. This simplified example demonstrates a good yet questionable assessment. It does not appear that the adoption of laptops campuswide is a common policy. However, if the school had adopted the policy, it could have gained prominence in this area compared with the competition. The other consideration, had this school required students to purchase laptops, students at this particular school may have been able to use financial aid to cover the cost of the computers. As these examples indicate, a needs assessment can come from a number of different stakeholders in multiple formats.

Program/Course Level Objectives

The school, program, and course level objectives (sometimes called outcomes or goals) are the starting point in the strategic plan. Learning objectives should be considered when developing a goal for the strategic plan.

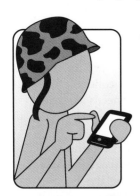

The focus of nursing education is not to use technology, but rather to develop the workforce of the future. A common error is to pursue technology irrespective of the learning objectives. To avoid this, the strategic planning process needs to begin with a careful review of chosen learning objectives.

An example of a program-level objective would be: "Graduates will function as providers of care in diverse health-care settings." After reviewing this objective, faculty noted that health-care settings require staff to use electronic medical records. In other settings, nurses are taking laptops to the clients' homes. Military RNs are required to enter client assessment data on handheld computers (e.g., tablets and PDAs) (Fig. 4.2). Other rationales for e-learning (based on the aforementioned program level objective) could arise out of the fact that students don't have adequate access to certain populations such as pediatrics. Hence, the school is pursuing adoption of virtual pediatric clinical simulation software for the computer.

An example of a course-level objective would be: "This course will prepare the student to effectively communicate to all members of the health-care team." The faculty for this course discovered that the nurse manager at the local hospital is sending out two e-mails a month to her staff to replace the monthly staff meeting. While on a trip to a developing country, the

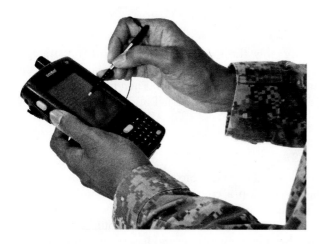

Figure 4.2 Handhelds in the military.

faculty noted that nurses in the hospital were text messaging each other as a means of calling for assistance and/or for client needs (e.g., to pharmacy). Based on these observations, faculty saw the need for teaching students how to professionally communicate via e-mail and text messaging. Having these skills would then allow students to effectively communicate with other members of the health-care team.

One consideration with college, program, and course level objectives is that these need to be developed independently of the learning tools (i.e., e-learning). The accreditation bodies and external stakeholders will need to see clear evidence that a learner in an online class is developing the same competency as a learner in a f-2-f classroom. If simulation is being used for a day of clinical, then those students need to be able to demonstrate mastery of the same skills as the students who complete their entire clinical in a health-care facility. To properly track this process for the external reviewers, the team should keep the final drafts of the strategic plan and any meeting minutes related to its adjustment and acceptance. Most accreditation bodies are open to questions related to this process and many have well-developed white papers that speak to this.

Administrative Goals

There may be other goals and objectives that are not directly tied to a program-level objective. This includes administrative issues such as enrollment patterns, access to faculty, and space limitations. For example, in a rural community college that serves three counties, access to faculty is always a concern. The same 6-hour class had to be taught on two different campuses by the same instructor on Mondays. Therefore, the class was converted into a hybrid course. It was offered for 3 hours in the morning in one county and for 3 hours in the afternoon in another county. As a result, the same faculty person was able to teach both courses.

Another example is that smaller private colleges often struggle with physical space if they are growing. As the registrar developed the course schedule for next spring, the classroom space became a significant issue. The administration asked each department to identify a course that could be converted to an online offering. The result was that students started requesting more online courses because of the convenience of this type of scheduling. These are just a few of the examples of what could arise administratively.

PLAN DEVELOPMENT

Developing the implementation plan is arguably the most important step of the strategic planning process. First, the make-up of the team should be considered. Next, a review of the literature will provide data to help ensure plans are evidence-based. Then the administrative support and timeline should be considered. Finally, both internal and external marketing strategies are addressed.

Team Development

As the team forms, multiple considerations should be made. First of all, a team of one is never a good idea. If the faculty member has to develop a course online without others in the department, consider a consultant from outside the department. These individuals can be the librarian (who may provide online resources to the students in this online course) or maybe a faculty member at another school who teaches this same course and has put it online already.

Another consideration should be the size of the team. Although you do not want to exclude certain individuals, you need to keep the team at a size that is manageable. In most situations, this author has found that strategic planning teams of 7 to 10 members seem to function the best. If administrators are not on the actual team, they need to be well advised of the process development. Subject matter experts help to ensure learners have access to current evidence-based content. Many times the subject matter expert is a faculty member. The subject matter expert should work with an instructional design (ID) specialist. If a team does not have access to this expertise, they can access a current text or Web site related to instructional design for e-learning. Although this is not an ideal replacement for this team member, it will help to improve the quality.

Assessment is important and the team should include (or at least consult) individuals familiar with institution- and department-level accreditation and assessment practices. Information technology and instructional technology staff are key because they understand the impact that new e-learning can have on the current infrastructure. Other support personnel

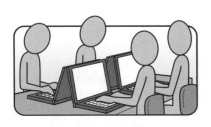

include library staff, registrar, financial aid, tutoring services, and student development. Consider asking vendors what supports they can provide. Often they give their customers access to certain expertise for no additional fees.

One final tip is to not avoid the "nay sayers." As noted in *Diffusion of Innovations* (Rogers, 2003), adoption of new technology is more likely to happen if the change agents are spending time with those who are not comfortable with the technology. So why not bring one of them along in the process?

Evidence-based E-Learning

Faculty should identify an evidence-base to support their plan development. This evidence-base can be found in various health-care resources (e.g., CINAHL) and educational resources (e.g., *Online Journal of Distance Learning Administration*). These assets often include books like the text you are reading right now. These authors have learned a lot by much study and even more through trial and error. These authors often list for you a number of resources and references that can assist faculty in making solid decisions. See the reference section at the end of the chapter for a number of important resources (Fisher, Newbold, & O'Neil, 2008; Jeffries, 2007; Pallof & Pratt, 2007).

Other resources can be the journals that faculty access often. At least once a month, *Journal of Nursing Education* or *Nursing Education Perspectives* will publish a journal article related to online learning and/or some other type of educational technology such as human patient simulators. These articles will not only help with developing a plan to implement e-learning, but also will demonstrate educational principles that can affect other parts of teaching such as the classroom or clinical environments. Many of these journal authors will present at various conferences. Watch mailers and Web sites for different conferences to identify ones that may address topics of interest.

Another source will be your accreditation bodies (see Chapter 17). Many accreditation bodies are implementing recommendations, regulations, and requirements related to the use of technology in nursing education. These printed resources are not only important because of the need to maintain good standing, but also because they have reviewed many professional resources to help craft their guidelines. In a sense, the authors of these various types of publications become your buddies in providing advice and bibliographies.

As for empirical research, that is an ominous source to help develop the evidence-base. It is ominous for two reasons. First, the research is often done with many overarching limitations. Often, research done on e-learning at a small private college will have few implications for the community college down the road that admits 80 nursing students twice a year. The other issue relates to the lack of empirical research. It is for this reason that all faculty developing and implementing e-learning of any type should start with research in mind. Collecting data through the entire process assists in improving the desired outcomes and adding to the knowledge base.

The next resource that can help to identify evidence-based plans and techniques is a buddy. They often have a different perspective and can provide many anecdotes that will help with planning. These buddies can be internal (i.e., the nursing department) or external. Don't hesitate to call on a colleague at another school or even from a non-nursing department. Most are interested in developing this relationship as the benefit is often reciprocal. Buddies can serve as a peer-review for syllabi and learning objects. They can give advice, and sometimes, more effectively, offer a sympathetic ear. More formal buddies can come in the form of consultants. These consultants can be identified through accreditation organizations, books, at conferences, and from colleagues.

Administrative Support

Administrative support is crucial for plan development. The first area of administrative support is enrollment. This includes admission to the college/university, admission to the nursing department, enrolling the student in the registration system (i.e., where one finds grades, class schedules, billing) and enrollment into the software used for e-learning (e.g., course management systems, online textbooks, clinical tracking software). The enrollment issues are very dependent on the type of technology being implemented. Here are a few examples:

1. Simulation implementation: Will students need to be enrolled in the software used to manage pre-, intra-, and postsimulation activities? Will laboratory faculty need access to the course management system (e.g., Angel, Blackboard) to enter grades for the simulation event?

2. Online course implementation: Will students have to log into a different Web site to get to the learning content and examinations? Will grades from the online course need to be manually transferred to the registrar's grading system?
3. Online program implementation: Can students pay their tuition, obtain a library card, and enroll for classes without coming to campus?

Support services are important in e-learning. These services help ensure that the learner has all they need to fully engage the learning environment. Areas of consideration include the library, information technology, and tutoring. Library support is important in providing access to content regardless of the delivery method of the learning. Videos are sometimes archived in the library. The vendor for these videos will need to be contacted to see if the videos can be streamed online. Another way to address this is to find a vendor that allows students to purchase a student copy of the videos. This single-user license allows students to download the videos and/or play them from a disc. Another library concern is external access to electronic print media. Library services will need to ensure that students from afar can access journals and e-books. When this is not possible, considerations will have to be given for mailing print media. Libraries also need to ensure that training provided for students (i.e., how to find journals and use databases) is accessible to students at a distance.

Information technology support staff (sometimes called instructional technology or IT Support) assist the learners and faculty in managing the different hardware and software involved in education. It is important to make sure they are accessible to students when students are using the technology to address issues.

The registrar and billing offices also may find interesting challenges in servicing students at a distance. They need to consider whether they will take payments via phone or will a Web form be developed. Another issue to consider is how will students register for classes? Will they still need a f-2-f meeting with an advisor before registration? Will original signatures work? Will e-mail count as official communication? How will these new policies affect the Family Educational Rights and Privacy Act (FERPA)? As the registrar and billing departments consider these issues, they should communicate frequently with their software vendors and their information technology department. Communication with vendors and technology personnel is important because many times, registration systems can interface with course management systems (e.g., eCollege, Desire 2 Learn).

Access to personnel is just as important as access to services. Will students have access to personnel who can train them on the new technology (i.e., PDA or simulator)? Sometimes these trainers can be other students (e.g., upperclassman needing training in education). If the student is not on campus, how will they receive support related to new e-books or new course management system? Does the information technology help desk understand the new technology enough to help students and faculty?

Tutors also play a role in the e-learning plan. Tutors can be IT personnel, faculty, other students, and even vendors. Tutors also need to be available to distance education (online) students just like they are available to f-2-f students. Tutors can help students with technology in addition to course content. Therefore, a system may need to be in place for phone calls, e-mail, and even online networking to connect students to tutoring services.

Most accreditation bodies also want to know plans for giving students access to advisors and administrators. Will advisors have virtual office hours? Will administrators have a toll-free number so that students can gain access when needed? Are there policies in place to govern virtual access and accessibility for faculty and students? Some colleges will put e-mail policies in place that direct faculty and students on how many times a week they need to check e-mail.

Faculty also are a key concern in the e-learning plan development. Administrators need to consider how the technology implementation will affect faculty shortages. When properly managed, the technology can enhance the learning environment and help moderate faculty workload. When improperly managed, technology can be a reason for some to leave the faculty role.

To avoid or minimize adverse effects on the faculty, administrators and planners might consider recruitment, compensation, and development. When recruiting faculty to any role, are they properly advised of the need to use technology? Faculty should be identified based on their interest and the departmental need. As Rogers (2003) aptly points out, adopters need to see and experience the value of an innovation before they can adopt it. This value can often be demonstrated through a conference or outside entity; therefore, if recruiting faculty to implement handhelds/PDAs, they may be persuaded to spend a few days at a school that is already using them well. If recruiting faculty for a fully online nursing program, emphasize that although the workload is still considerable, the hours can be flexible.

Compensation often accompanies recruitment. The compensation for e-learning development is as diverse as the types of e-learning. If grant sources of funding are being sought, generous amounts of compensation should be pursued for all parts of the strategic plan. If funds are quite limited, priorities should focus on faculty time, faculty development, and instructional design assistance. In many situations, motivated faculty will welcome the challenge of developing an online course or implementing another technology without pay (i.e., as service to the college). Although this seems noble at the outset, it often leads to a burned-out faculty member and an e-learning experience that is often labeled as unsuccessful by administrators, faculty, students, and other stakeholders. If an adequate instructional design process is in place, compensation for developing an online course can be the same as compensation for developing a f-2-f course (unless that compensation is zero). Incorporating simulation into the curriculum should be a completely different compensation structure and often includes a significant amount of release time and reallocation of staff.

Faculty development is a crucial component of administrative support for e-learning. Helping faculty understand the pedagogy for and management of technology in education is crucial for student success (Box 4.1). This training can take on many formal and informal venues. For instance, two faculty (sometimes referred to as "super-users") can go to the training on using the in-class audience response system (ARS) (e.g., clickers). Then they can provide a demonstration at the next faculty meeting by voting on agenda items with the ARS. Next, the super-users can implement functions in their classroom and serve as a coach to help other faculty use them (see Appendix C).

A more complicated implementation may include online examinations. Consider the following exemplar. The implementation could happen programwide. Training is provided at the "beginning of the semester" faculty in-service. The faculty are given a bit of "homework" after the in-service and they take a quiz or two online. Finally, the implementation happens when the first online examinations are given. Extra faculty and IT support staff are on hand to help with any questions that may arise.

Faculty development in the areas of andragogy (adult learning principles) and instructional design for e-learning is crucial (Sitzman, 2010). Training in how to use the course management system (CMS) is inadequate for success. This may include how to set up the

---

BOX 4.1
EFFECTIVE PEDAGOGY FOR ONLINE TEACHING

Bailey and Card (2009) conducted a phenomenological study of 15 instructors who were "recipients of the South Dakota Board of Regents' E-learning Award" (p. 153). As a result of the interviews, they identified "Eight effective pedagogical practices for effective online teaching . . ." (p. 154).

Fostering relationships—be personable

Engagement—help students contribute and respect the contributions of others

Timeliness—be there for the students

Communication—ability to connect with students

Organization—well-developed learning environment

Technology—be prepared

Flexibility—be patient

High expectations—clearly identify what is expected from the students

---

gradebook, upload PowerPoint, and create announcements. Although these skills are helpful, the importance of keeping learners engaged and how to successfully facilitate professional growth in a virtual environment are paramount. Faculty development in the areas of andragogy and instructional design will help faculty understand how to succeed in the online learning environment (Appendix C).

Faculty development is best accomplished when it is administrator supported, school funded, and policy driven. Administrators can support it by providing opportunities for training, encouraging workgroups and brown bag lunches around the topics of interest, and referring to if often in a variety of venues (Benner, Sutphen, Leonard, & Day, 2010). School funding for faculty development is a consideration that can come in the form of time or money or both. If faculty are not receiving compensation or assistance for training, they should strongly consider the risk of attempting to use e-learning without it. Finally, policies on training in e-learning are essential. They help to demonstrate the importance of training to faculty and accreditation bodies. Most accrediting organizations will want to see clear guidelines that help facilitate quality and success in e-learning.

Timeline for Implementation

Most people are familiar with the book *The Best Laid Plans of Mice and Nurses* (OK, we admit, this is a fictitious title of a book yet to be written). Most nurse educators have become experts in expecting the unexpected. It really is no different with implementing e-learning. As a timeline is considered, be mindful to provide adequate cushions on both ends of the plan. One timeline strategy that is particularly useful is the "pilot study" plan. This allows for the implementation to happen on a smaller scale and often is a bit more forgiving simply because it is a pilot study. If implementing simulation in the curriculum, maybe for semester one, the implementation could happen in two of the five clinical groups in the medical-surgical course (e.g., 10% of each clinical is conducted in the simulation center). In the next semester, implementation would occur in two of the clinical groups in medical-surgical and two of the clinical groups in maternal-child. The next school year, all clinical groups will use simulation.

If moving an entire program to the use of a course management system, take small portions at a time. Semester one, all courses will use the online gradebook feature. Semester two, all courses will use the online gradebook and put the syllabus online instead of printing it. Semester three, online examinations will be added. As you can see, the department is progressing as a team.

Another scenario includes the faculty member who is directed to put his or her class fully online (and the semester starts in 3 weeks). In this sort of a crunch, faculty would do well to remember that this semester may not be the best on record for this class. Although it is best to always have an online class fully written and ready to implement on day one, it may not be possible in this scenario. In this case, faculty should ensure course objectives are met (remembering that students can read and study independently to develop competency), key assessments are made (papers, projects, examinations), and key interactions are made (see the chapter on building community). Avoid pursuing highly technical learning objects (e.g., video and flash presentation) or interactions (e.g., instant messaging and chat). Priority must be given to the assessment plan (i.e., examinations and discussion grading rubrics). Then clearly outline these concepts in the syllabus. If at all possible, have a colleague or former trusted student review the syllabus for clarity. Next, ensure that adequate technical support and training is available to help students navigate the online environment. Do students understand where to go to access the syllabus, take part in discussions, and how to upload papers? More importantly, do they know when and who to call when they need help? As the calendar for this course is considered, be sure to give adequate time up front to develop any remaining learning objects. As for student assignment due dates, some grace should be given in the first half of the class as all parties involved acclimate to the new learning environment.

Instructional Design

The term "instructional design" rings the bell of intrigue (and sometimes fear) in the minds of many educators. The term used in this discussion will serve as a framework for a part of the plan development. This discussion is not meant to be an exhaustive exploration of instructional design for nursing education. The overall theme is "What will be the form of the learning interaction in which e-learning is used?" A simplified instructional design process includes analysis, input, process, and output.

One common theme in the instructional design should be consistency (Bailey & Card, 2009). The goal is to make the instructional design as unobtrusive as possible. By striving for consistency, the balance between "creativity" and "hindering learning" becomes a challenge. One example may be in due dates for discussion forum posts. If one professor requires all discussions be posted on Tuesday and another requires that all posts be made on Saturday, there is a risk of confusion and subsequent frustration. Another design issue could be related to submitting projects. If one design calls for papers to be delivered via e-mail in .RTF format and another design calls for assignments to be submitted in the dropbox in .DOC format, confusion will ensue (for students and faculty). Other considerations for consistency might include:

1. Instructors will respond to e-mails and discussion posts in _ _ hours/days.
2. Syllabi format and policies. (Do all syllabi include a statement on Netiquette?)
3. Technology requirements. (Windows 7.0/Vista/XP?)
4. Course management system layout. (Where is the dropbox located? Can faculty change the format from Weekly folders to Module folders?)

5. Students must check their e-mail at least once every _ _ hours/days.
6. PDA drug guides will be used in every laboratory scenario.
7. The presimulation quiz is due _ _ hours/days before the simulation test-out.

Many of the consistency issues may become departmental or collegewide policy. Consequently, the developers of the strategic plan need to consider the value of academic freedom. Many in academia may look at such guidelines (e.g., discussion posts are always due on Wednesday) as infringing on their freedoms. It is for this reason that a thorough explanation of the ID process and subsequent benefits be provided to all involved. Some key advantages of this ID process to faculty may include:

1. Faculty can focus on being the subject matter experts.
2. Quality of part-time or adjunct faculty may be less of an issue as they only have to bring their professional expertise to the classroom.
3. Students can focus more on learning and less on learning environment or faculty preferences.
4. Assessment can be easier to manage.

Analysis. The first part of the simplified instructional design process is analysis. As was noted in the beginning of this chapter, educators must always start with an analysis of the learning objectives. Understanding the learners and their environment also is an important part of analysis. Next, faculty (instructional designers) should be aware of variables that may arise regarding the technology available to the learners. In some simulation laboratories, the learners may have access to high-fidelity manikins that are very realistic in their response. In other laboratories, the manikins may be static and require the use of sticky notes (e.g., Post-it on the forehead of the manikin says "My head hurts"). Some learners may only have access to computers in the computer laboratory or library, whereas others may be required to purchase a computer for use at home.

Analysis should also focus on that academic structure. Syllabi and related policies that are currently used should be evaluated to ensure consistency. Current e-learning–related policies (i.e., no FERPA sensitive material can be e-mailed) need to be considered.

Input. Input includes all the different facets and modalities of data collection and concept discovery by learners. It also can include constructs and variables that affect the learning process such as the learning environment and peer interactions. The input should always be learner-centered. This means that students are engaged in the discovery process and not simply recipients of knowledge transmission. Discovery can happen through reading, exploring the Web, interacting with a PDA, discussing a concept, and watching a video. Input comes for some by taking part in a virtual simulation code in SecondLife. Input can be the prequiz phase of a learning object (e.g., "Watch this slide show and take the quiz in the examination section of Blackboard"). Input can be a f-2-f interview with a health-care professional in the community about teen alcohol consumption. It can be an instant message chat with a nurse in a missionary hospital in the African country of Togo. The variety of input modalities can be staggering.

Early in the planning phase (i.e., the first time simulation is used or the first time a course is taught online), the designers and educators should not attempt an excessive amount of variety with input modalities (i.e., there could be too much confusion for an initial rollout). For every level of complexity, there will be challenges to overcome. As previously noted, attempt to simplify the input phase by implementing consistency between courses or learning interactions. Here are a couple of examples.

1. Use the same vendor for PDA software in all classes (e.g., Skyscape, Pepid, Unbound).
2. Use the same layout for highlighting reading/resource/exploration assignments in each class.
3. Use the same electronic medical record software in each simulation experience.

Process. Process is the third part of instructional design and addresses the experiences that will help learners "make meaning" related to learning objectives and program goals. It should be noted that the different parts of instructional design can crossover. For instance, a discussion forum between learners and faculty can serve as input, processing, and output all at the same time. The discussion forum serves as input because learners may discover new concepts from their peers. It also is process as learners will dialogue and debate issues being learned. Finally, output is addressed because faculty can assess for competency and appropriate attitudes through a learner's participation in the discussion forum.

The process phase of instructional design can occur through individual and group activities. Individually, learners can process the input through writing, manipulating software, or developing a project to name a few. The strategic plan should try to identify a few key process activities that can be used in a variety of learning experiences. In the community health class, the learners may develop a Web site about a particular community health issue. In the following semester, these learners take nursing research. In nursing research, they will study the impact that the Web site has on viewers. Another process event could be developing a presentation, interviewing a professional (in-person or virtually), or creating a podcast.

Output. The final phase of the instructional design process is output. For the purposes of this discussion, the focus will be on assessing the learners for acquisition of competency and attitude. The output can come from part of the process phase or it can be separate. Consistency should be sought in the output phase. If a digital care plan format is used in one clinical, the same form should be used in other clinicals (except for content-specific variation—geriatric care plan versus family care plan). If a virtual reality experience is used in multiple courses (e.g., DxRor Virtual Clinical Excursions), the output should be similar in the different classes (i.e., print out the evaluation report or upload the answers to the post quiz to the dropbox).

Marketing

Plan development also should consider marketing. Marketing is the chosen term to describe how buy-in is solicited from internal and external partners. Marketing can affect funding sources, administrative support, and success at implementation (i.e., faculty/student support). Internal marketing will focus on controlled information dissemination. Understanding the attitudes, beliefs, and perceptions of stakeholders is essential. One example may be related to offering a course online in a traditionally f-2-f environment. Faculty in other departments may be concerned that they will be required to offer courses online. The library may be concerned that students can take the course who are not physically located on campus and will now require services at a distance. If a course shell (i.e., one course room in a course management system) is being open for each course on campus, some faculty may be concerned that their students will pressure them to use it as well.

Internally, there can be several ways to market the adoption of new technology or instructional design. First, understand perceptions that are out there. For example, if a nursing department decides to offer online courses, they should talk with the science department (where some prenursing courses are offered) about concerns that science faculty may have. The survey of science faculty reveals that they feel online learning cannot deliver the same level of quality as f-2-f learning. In response, marketing should cite credible sources about the research related to "no significant difference." Discussions with students about the adoption of PDAs may reveal that students see no value in using PDAs. In response, marketing to the students should focus on the use of PDAs on the battlefield by medics and in acute care for medication administration systems.

Externally, marketing may need to address similar concerns. Students have heard that online courses are easier. Because the courses were set up with a solid instructional design and more active learning, students should be aware that learning online could be very different. Alumni and donors may hear about online learning and think that it is not a valid mode for a rigorous education. Their concerns should be appropriately addressed. Clinical partners may think that the new simulator will completely replace clinical time. Although the new simulation center is highlighted, the marketing should focus on the fact that 15% of clinical time will be spent in the simulation center to enhance the training done at the clinical sites. Internal and external marketing can have an impact on the success of the strategic plan and plan implementation; therefore, they need to be addressed.

RESOURCE ANALYSIS

Key resources are necessary for the implementation of e-learning to be effective. The foci of resource analysis will be human resources, financials, hardware, software, and noncomputer-related materials. Understanding the acquisition, preparation, and maintenance of each resource will facilitate success.

Myths

Two key myths should be addressed immediately. First, e-learning does not save time. As for time, most e-learning takes an initial investment of time that is not regained until later in the process. For instance, if a school is adding online courses, setting up those courses will take additional time. Later, after the same faculty has taught the same online course a few times, they will become more efficient with managing the learning experience (just as we see in the f-2-f world). Overall, the time for implementation, management, and evaluation will be about the same. So why adopt e-learning?

The second myth to address is that e-learning will save the institution money. In the end, e-learning may demonstrate some financial benefit from increased or sustained enrollment and not having to build a new lecture hall to handle growth. However, initially the capital outlay can be daunting (depending on how technology adoption is monitored). Take for instance the school that adopts simulation to help with shrinking clinical sites. Initially, the cost of the technology and training can be extensive (grants are our friends). Next, the issue arises of how to manage simulations. After initial training is complete, scenarios have to be developed and adapted. Next, while the ratio in simulations is not as tight as clinical (1 instructor:10 students), it is still difficult to manage more than 20 students in one day of simulations.

With these myths addressed, consider first human resource analysis.

Human Resources

Human resources serve as glue for all parts of the strategic plan for e-learning. One key human resource to consider is the faculty. Depending on the institution, the faculty can serve multiple roles (project coordinator, instructional designer, subject matter expert). Although nursing faculty are prone to taking on multiple roles at one time, the potential impact of this move should be considered. First, the faculty need to be trained for the roles they are assuming. Secondly, their time availability must be considered. Often, an instructional designer or consultant can be brought into the mix for a reasonable cost (especially when the cost of having a faculty member burnout is considered) and this allows faculty to focus on other parts of the project that better suit them (e.g., subject matter expert). Another issue with time is to encourage faculty to consider all that they are attempting to add to their plates. For instance, one faculty member may decide to add a fifth paper (writing assignment) to the course. Although he or she may feel this paper adds a lot to the course, if he or she is busy developing a new simulation program, the faculty may not have time to grade that additional paper. Could that paper addition be put off until next year and could students demonstrate competency in that area in a way that is less taxing on the faculty member? The answer to both these questions is almost always, yes.

Other members of the team include the help desk staff. Do they understand what to do if students call and cannot upload an assignment? Do they know what to do if faculty call because the electronic medical record software is not working? These human resources are very important and there is usually need for extra support in the beginning of each term. Peer tutors for students also should be considered. They serve as great mentors and often know the technology from the student perspective. One possibility is having fourth-semester students (seniors) work in the simulation laboratory with first-semester students (juniors). For the seniors, this is a project in which they learn how to train others (they may even get leadership clinical hours for this). For the juniors, they have increased access to assistance in conquering this new and often intimidating technology. Peer tutors work great for a number of learning environments and technologies, and can be included in the online course management system, computer-based software, hand-held computers, and laboratory-related tools.

Speaking of the laboratory, the laboratory personnel are vital in today's nursing program. These individuals can serve multiple roles depending on their qualifications and the school's needs. For instance, in one state in a generic program the laboratory director was baccalaureate prepared. This person became the simulation expert and would set up training sessions for students to come in and have a day of clinical. Because of the laboratory director's level of training (BSN), this individual could also serve as clinical faculty in the hospital. In a different situation, the laboratory director was an associate degree prepared nurse (ADN). This person could not serve in clinical settings but could handle setting up laboratories for four different allied health majors to including respiratory technician and surgical technician. In one large university, the laboratory director was a doctorally prepared nurse with four masters prepared nurses as his staff.

Other human resources include admissions and library personnel, advisors, and the registrar. In one recent nursing program start up, the nursing program increased the size of the day program by 15% and the overall college by 10%. State, regional, and national accreditation bodies closely analyzed the infrastructure of this college to ensure that they could handle this program.

Finances

Financially, resource analysis should highlight access (real and potential) to funding sources. Often, the departmental budget has little if any ability to assist in implementation. One area that some departments find helpful with implementation is the faculty development budget. If each faculty member has a total annual allotment of $500, then the faculty of eight has a total of $4000. This would be just enough to have two faculty drive to the "big city" for training at the university on how to use the new simulator. Or if department has one fund of $2000, could they hire an e-learning specialist to do 10 hours of webinar training on how to create an online course? Given the importance of faculty development, creativity in meeting this need should be sought around every corner.

Economy of scale is the next principle to consider related to the budget. In some situations, doubling the number of users has little impact on the cost of the technology. When a college/university, division, or department evaluates adoption of a course management system (CMS) (e.g., Angel, Blackboard, Desire2Learn) they should consider all possible users. It is financially unwise for adoption of one CMS for the adult learning programs (i.e., evening/weekend program) and the generic undergraduate program. Likewise, if the medical school has a contract with one handheld computer software company (e.g., Skyscape, Pepid, Unbound), the nursing and pharmacy schools should strongly consider using that vendor as well (Fig. 4.3). Not

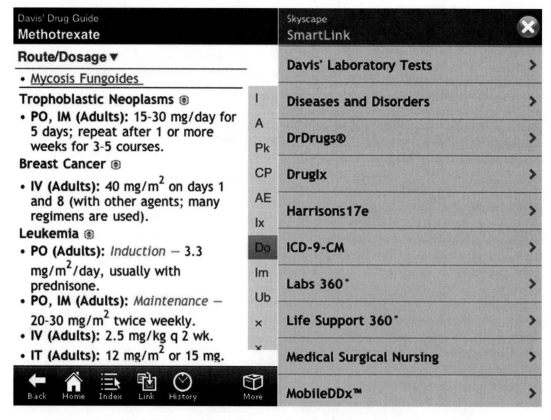

Figure 4.3 Davis' Drug Guide in Skyscape links to other Books on the same device.

only can the price be much more manageable, but also the collaboration between the disciplines could prove quite advantageous.

Sharing with students can have financial benefits on both sides of the desk. One example is in the area of videos. Many vendors in the nursing/medical video business are now offering single-use licenses. This means that instead of the nursing department spending $4500 to purchase a video series that lives in the nursing laboratory, the students can spend $50 and have the same videos bundled with their textbook. Now students do not have to sign up for a time to sit in the nursing laboratory and watch the videos. They can watch them anywhere and anytime. They also will have access to the videos after graduation.

Another financial consideration related to students is considering their financial burden. If adopting a new technology that requires them to make a purchase, is there something else in the curriculum that is not as necessary? For instance, why require the purchase of a drug guide to put on the computer or PDA and another paper copy? If a software program is being purchased for a class, could that class not require the study guide to accompany the textbook? These considerations can help the students.

Exploring vendor assistance and options often allows for savings as well. One example is the course management system (CMS). Many health-care book publishers will provide a CMS course room for the course in which one of their books has been adopted. If the nursing department were to subscribe to a single-use CMS course room, the cost could range from $250 to $4000 per course. The only caution with this example is that nursing programs should not use different CMS vendors for different courses. If one course is using Blackboard and two other courses are using Angel, mass confusion could result for the students, faculty, and staff.

Identifying external funding sources also can help with implementation. From the local hospital foundation, to longtime donors to the college, to major grants, there are often many external resources for funds. One favorite story relates to small town USA. The small nursing program sent out many applications for a grant to purchase a human patient simulator. Using a statewide common grant form, they were able to submit the same grant to dozens of foundations. A small town branch bank contacted the school for further discussions. Because the nursing department sent one clinical group of eight students to a nursing home in that community (town population of 4075), the bank's foundation gave the school $40,000 for the simulator. The local hospital agreed to pitch-in an additional $8000 for extras if they could use it as well. Chief avenues to explore when identifying funds include:

- National sources/resources (National League for Nursing, Robert Wood Johnson Foundation, U.S. Department of Agriculture).
- State and local public health departments.
- State nursing organizations (Nurses' Association, League for Nurses, Nursing Board/Board of Examiners).
- Local and statewide business foundations (many states have a "common" grant form/process).
- Clinical partners.
- List of foundations on the state's public radio station Web site.

As financial concerns are addressed, a budget for the implementation must be addressed. The budget should be clearly developed and reviewed by members of the planning team, administrators, and even vendors in some situations. By consulting other schools/departments that have gone through this process in the past, the team may be able to identify unforeseen budgetary issues before they arise.

Hardware

Hardware includes technology such as computers, servers, and handheld computers. Many schools have some or all of this in place. The key issue that can arise here is ensuring that software works with hardware and end-users have access to both. These issues can only be addressed if the strategic planning team has sought counsel from the information technology department, software manufacturers, and instructional designers. It also is essential for demonstrations to be done in-house so compatibility can be ensured.

One hardware-related problem became apparent when a medium-sized nursing program in a large community college system purchased a site license for a video series. The idea was to 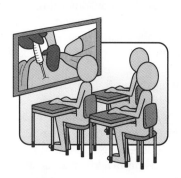 put the videos on the campuswide servers so that students and faculty could access the videos anytime/anywhere on campus. The vendor said this was a great idea. IT noted that their system met the vendor specifications. So the purchase was made and the videos were loaded. The instructor used the videos for the first time a week into the class and noted that the download was too slow. When IT was called, they said that was to be expected because they could only allow so much "bandwidth" at any given time throughout the network. The instructor said that is fine, I will just send all the students to the computer laboratory or library and let them watch the videos on their own. The IT department said this was fine but only two students could access the videos at a time because of these bandwidth constraints. Needless to say, with 60 students needing access, that would not work.

In a similar situation at a small private school, the department considered purchasing a video series that could be streamed from servers. In this situation, the faculty ordered a sample trial, had it loaded to the servers, then had teaching assistants (TAs) test multiple computers throughout the campus. They were all delighted to find that the videos would stream to five "older" computers at a time while simultaneously streaming to computers in the library. Teaching assistants then tried the videos from home and work and found they were functional there as well. The team then purchased the site license for these videos.

Other hardware concerns include compatibility issues. Will students' home computers run required software? Will the course management system (CMS) work with the new computers' operating systems. This was a challenge for one CMS with the new PC Windows operating system Vista. Some of the windows do not work on machines using Vista so "workarounds" had to be identified.

Hardware accessories such as built-in cameras, microphones, and wireless devices also should be considered. It is known that some wireless cards have better antennas than others do. That is why in wireless classrooms some of the laptops may not be able to connect. Some PDAs also have better antennas then others. As for audio/visual equipment, if a video is made by a faculty member, will her built-in Web cam work or should a better one be connected to the computer?

Handheld computers will usually need to synchronize with computers. This compatibility needs to be explored. Manikins and other simulators are controlled by computers as well. Having the right people at the table for strategic planning is critical.

Larger hardware considerations can include where the CMS is housed. For instance, some companies will host a CMS on their servers. This can be a bit costly, but the students and faculty off campus can access the CMS even if campus computer systems are down. The other benefit may be that there are additional technicians keeping a watchful eye on the CMS performance.

Software

Software includes programs that can run in a variety of machines and environments. This includes software for the internet, computers, simulators, audio/visual equipment, mobile/smartphones, and handheld computers (PDAs). As was noted earlier, the CMS needs to be compatible with the computer. Many PDAs and smartphones are now using the Internet. If PDAs are adopted, will they be able to access Internet-based software that is required? If a virtual reality world (i.e., SecondLife) is used for training, will the bandwidth of the college support 20 students online at one time? Will the graphics work with the computer available on campus? If students have Apple/Macintosh computers will the software work on their computers?

Other Resources

The other resources may include phone lines, phones, Internet connectivity (bandwidth), manikins, video recorders, audio recorders, and audience response systems (e.g., clickers, 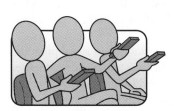 remotes). Phone lines are often used to facilitate the voice part of video conferencing. If there is an audio conference service used, the department may want to know if the audio can be recorded with the video for archiving. Will the phone lines and equipment work if there are 25 people on a call at one time? Internet connectivity is often a challenge. Many campuses will divide bandwidth between faculty/staff and students. This means that if multiple faculty are streaming, conducting webinars, instant messaging with colleagues/students and the like, they may run into problems with download/upload speed.

PLAN IMPLEMENTATION

The plan implementation is an exciting time. All the hard work is now being put to the test. The plan implementation involves the 4 Cs—communication, contingency plan, cooperation, and change.

Communication must be constant and clear (Bailey & Card, 2009; Sitzman, 2010). Think about who should be knowledgeable and how best to stay connected to those individuals throughout the implementation. For instance, if the first online course on campus is being rolled out in the nursing program, the faculty may want to stop by and talk to the students f-2-f in another course. Even though the course is fully online, if there is physical access to the students this is a great opportunity to communicate with them. Administrators and support staff should be in the loop as well. This communication will contain data related to issues that arise, success of certain aspects, and potential needs. It also may include data related to research or experience from others. One example is with the use of active learning. For online courses to work well, they need to follow an instructional design that facilitates active learning. It is noted in the research, however, that active learning can initially lead to lower student satisfaction (Lake, 2001). Administrators, therefore, should be in the loop about this phenomenon.

Frequent communication with vendors also should be maintained. Share with them the successes and the problems often. This may spark their memory of another customer who had similar issues and could help in preventing unwanted problems.

When considering communication frequency, caution should be given to balance. If a communication is coming out every other day, it could become "white noise," that is not taken seriously. Some consider it best to create a weekly update of some type. This allows for an expected communication point in time.

Communication tools can be diverse and sometimes add an element of fun to the process. For instance, in the CMS there is often an announcement tool that can be programmed with date/time on/off. So an announcement can be programmed to come on the beginning of the fourth week of class reminding students that tutors are available via e-mail and phone for preparation for the week six examination. This announcement also could include a picture of the faculty member's dog or something else fun. Other communications could come embedded in assignments. For instance, if this is the first time a manikin has been used for a test out, the faculty may want a certain cue or reminder to be placed in the patient's chart. "Remember that Mr. Claborn (the manikin) can only have blood drawn from the right arm because of the speakers in the left arm."

Contingency plans are vital during plan implementation. If giving tests online for the first time, do not hesitate to have a stash of paper examinations nearby. If you have the paper examinations nearby, then you will not need to use them (as noted in *Murphy's Law*). When using PDAs for medication "test outs" for the first time in the laboratory, have paper copies of the drug guide and diagnostics manual nearby.

Contingency plans also are sometimes required of students. Some distance education programs require students to identify a backup computer and location should they experience computer, Internet, or power failure (Box 4.2). The students inform the advisor and faculty that if something unplanned happens, they will go to the local public library, their parent's home, or at work.

Cooperation involves flexibility on the part of all involved. In the online classroom, there should be weekly or biweekly due dates. In the first part of the class, however, there should be grace periods given with these due dates. Toward the end of the class, the due dates should be strictly observed and tied to grades. Flexibility and cooperation should be sought with the information technology department. If a student has trouble with his or her PDA and calls the help desk, the student may not get a satisfactory response. Faculty and administrators should work together to identify systems that can support the students in these new ventures.

The final "C" of plan implementation is change. When an issue arises during implementation a decision will have to be made about an appropriate response. When the manikin breaks in the middle of test outs, the PDA crashes in clinical, or the Internet goes down during an

---

BOX 4.2
PODCASTS FOR CHAPEL

Data: Faith-based school required chapel attendance of students in a hybrid program. Students were not on campus enough to meet this requirement. They would need to come to campus during nonclass times to attend chapel. Chapel was considered an essential part of the college experience.

Action: Chapels were Podcast for increased access. "Internet" chapel attendance was accounted for through summaries of the chapel.

Response: The Podcasts were well received yet some students still came for f-2-f chapel.

examination, consultation with other members of the team is always indicated at some point. Although the initial response should be to minimize the impact on the students, this consultation with others will help to gauge the best course of action. As previously noted, team members can be from other departments and institutions.

Carefully consider how much change should take place in the middle of a class or semester related to an undesirable technology-related event because change often will add more confusion. It may be best to lighten the burden on the students (OK, everybody gets this examination as a take-home.) to allow for careful analysis and planning for the next time the technology is used. Another example may relate to grading technology-related events. In the middle of the semester, a faculty member concedes that the grading rubric is a bit problematic because of the online Wiki that is being used to facilitate the project. Instead of eliminating the whole project, reworking the grading rubric, or giving everybody an "A" for the assignment, work on a modification that will simplify the project for everyone. This will give the faculty member time to truly reflect on the issue, conduct some research, and plan for a better experience next semester. Remembering the 4 Cs, communication, contingency plan, cooperation, and change, will help plan implementation have a higher chance of success.

CONTINUOUS EVALUATION

Evaluation should be ongoing throughout the strategic planning process. Evaluation is so important to this process; the NLNAC (2008) even lists it in their standards. They require programs to train their faculty (full- and part-time) in "instructional methods and evaluation" related to distance education (p. 82).

Continuous evaluation does not wait for the end of the semester or before the self study is due, so the assessment can come in many different forms. The data can arrive sporadically (i.e., a phone call from a student, an incident in the laboratory); therefore, the strategic planning team may want to create a "Miscellaneous" file in which they can collect random comments and observations. More formal evaluation can be in the form of two- to three-question surveys handed out at different points throughout the process (Halstead & Billings, 2009). It can be done through focus groups led by a TA who reports data anonymously. Data can be collected through online survey tools (available as part of most CMS), anonymous discussion forum posts, and even paper/pencil surveys. If the student is submitting self-evaluations or reports related to the use of new technologies, faculty may want to add an event/tool evaluation section to the end of the form or report.

Evaluations should first assess attainment of academic and administrative goals. It is important to ensure that implementation of the new technology has had a null or enhanced effect on the attainment of learning objectives and goals. Of key importance is assessing for the possibility that the technology is having a negative impact on the learning experience and subsequently returning that information back into the strategic plan as soon as possible. Administrative goals also should be assessed. Flexibility for learners and faculty is often an administrative goal. Because of the newness of a technology, the added work of implementation and training may cloud the ability to assess whether or not the goal of flexibility has been met. Time may be needed for a complete assessment. Other administrative goals may include return on investment, or providing students and stakeholders with a more technologically advanced learning experience. As these examples highlight, some assessments can occur formatively, and some will need to be summative.

Accreditation concerns should be considered throughout the strategic plan. This involves ensuring that standards are being met and a program or collegewide assessment plan reflects any changes that may have an impact on learning or outcomes.

One example comes for the 2008 *Essentials of Baccalaureate Education for Professional Nursing Practice* (AACN, 2008). The *Essentials* stipulate that the generalist nurse needs to be able to use clinical decision-support tools. As a result, the nursing department decides to implement the use of PDAs (e.g., handhelds, iTouch) across the curriculum. The nursing department will want to use AACN verbiage from the *Essentials* when training students on the use of clinical decision-support tools. The department also will want to ensure that program and course-level learning objectives and assessment tools reflect these competencies. Finally, faculty meeting minutes and self-study documents will want to demonstrate this progression from identifying a need (based on the *Essentials*) to implementing a strategy and then evaluating the outcome (further discussion on accreditation considerations can be found in Chapter 17 Program Assessment).

Another area to consider is the satisfaction of faculty, staff, students, and other stakeholders. There are many key issues to consider. As for faculty, retention and continuous development is of concern. The surveys can focus on questions about workload, usability, and effects on the learning experience. Students need be queried in the same way. What are the impacts on students related to this new modality? Staff could have different questions in their assessments based on their areas. For this reason, they may need more qualitative assessments (i.e., surveys with open-ended questions). After assessments are complete, the strategic planning team should draft responses that highlight advancements being made (especially if they connect to data collected from the assessments).

Perceptions are very much linked to understanding the technology (Bristol, 2005). Keeping this in mind, satisfaction assessments should provide data that directly affects future planning for faculty/student development and staff processes.

One final mode of continuous evaluation is benchmarking with other departments and organizations. Comparing processes with other schools can be beneficial. It not only allows for identifying problems before they arise, it builds a network of individuals who truly understand the implementation process. The benchmarking might come in the form of using similar evaluation surveys and comparing data. It could be a comparison of student outcomes or even reports from clinical partners on new graduate performance. These partnerships can develop into a two-way experience that is quite engaging.

Other benchmarking can come from standardized testing services. These services offer data about a school's students compared with thousands of similar students across the nation. Although these services are not specific to e-learning, they are specific to monitoring for change in learner outcomes.

CONCLUSION

The key players in the strategic plan are a team that comes together with a clear set of goals. Team members should be properly developed, trained, and resourced in the areas related to e-learning implementation. This is often critical because a school or department may secure a fantastic new technology but neglect to adequately provide training. The results tend to be underuse and an adverse effect on student outcomes. The strategic planning team should consider bringing outside partners into the process. These can be formally hired consultants or colleagues from other departments or schools who have experienced the e-learning process. These consultants can prove to be invaluable and often appreciate the consultation, because they also tend to learn something.

As the plan progresses, all members of the team should write the 4 Cs (Communication, Contingency plan, Cooperation, and Change) on a small note card and carry it in their pockets, purse, or wallet. With communication, consistency and clarity should be sought. Attempt to use similar language when communicating with everyone involved. A discussion forum online should be called a discussion forum in the syllabus and on the course calendar. Often, the discussion forum online is called a discussion board in the syllabus and a threaded forum in the calendar. This not only leads to mass confusion, it also can affect success.

Do not forget to have a backup plan in place during the first few times a technology is used. Flexibility is also key to the implementation phase and includes everything from due dates to patience with others. Finally, discuss carefully plans to change the e-learning process in the middle of implementation. It may be best to wait until the end.

The continuous evaluation part of the strategic plan ensures that goals and outcomes are being met. Often, technology can be used to collect and assess this data. Evaluation should be considered in all stages of the strategic planning process and, in many situations, the data collected could quickly feedback to the plan development and implementation phases.

REFERENCES

American Association of Colleges of Nursing. (2008). *The essentials of baccalaureate education for professional nursing practice*. Washington, DC: Author.

Bailey, C. J., & Card, K. A. (2009). Effective pedagogical practices for online teaching: Perception of experienced instructors. *Internet and Higher Education, 12*(3), 152–155. doi:110.1016/j.iheduc.2009.1008.1002

Benner, P., Sutphen, M., Leonardson, V., & Day, L. (2010). *Educating nurses: A call for radical transformation*. San Francisco: Jossey-Bass.

Bristol, T. (2005). *Perceptions of E-learning in Iowa nursing faculty*. Capella University, Minneapolis.

Fisher, C. A., Newbold, S., & O'Neil, C. A. (2008). *Developing online learning environments in nursing education* (2nd ed.). New York, NY: Springer Publishing.

Halstead, J. A., & Billings, D. M. (2009). Teaching and learning in online learning communities. In D. M. Billings & J. A. Halstead (Eds.), *Teaching in nursing: A guide for faculty* (3rd ed., pp. 369–389). St. Louis, MO: Elsevier.

Jeffries, P. (2007). *Simulation in nursing education: From conceptualization to evaluation*. New York: National League for Nursing.

Lake, D. (2001). Student performance and perceptions of a lecture-based course compared with the same course utilizing group discussion. *Physical Therapy, 81*(3), 896–902.

National League for Nursing Accrediting Commission. (2008). *2008 Edition: NLNAC accreditation manual*. New York, NY: Author.

Palloff, R. M., & Pratt, K. (2007). *Building online learning communities: Effective strategies for the virtual classroom*. San Francisco, CA: Wiley, John & Sons.

Rogers, E. M. (2003). *Diffusion of innovations* (5th ed.). New York, NY: The Free Press.

Sitzman, K. (2010). Student-preferred caring behaviors for online nursing education. *Nursing Education Perspectives, 31*(3), 171–176.

UNIT 2

Online Learning

Chapter 5

Building Community

Tim J. Bristol, PhD, RN, CNE

OUR COMMUNITY

The idea of building community can really help learners connect and support one another. In a fully online masters of science in nursing (MSN) program, the students had an area called a cyber café. This is an area where they can share material that is not course-related. Susan (one of the graduate students) began sharing about the process of placing her father in a long-term care facility. You could feel the emotion and pain in the words she shared. It was amazing to see the outpouring of support from her classmates. They gave her links to support resources and some who were geographically close even offered to meet her and help her make some of the arrangements. This is the essence of community and an example of how building community can go far beyond the classroom.

Learning environments need to offer the learners much more than knowledge acquisition and psychomotor mastery. This is especially true in a complex field such as nursing in which the sheer volume of knowledge can be overwhelming to the point of fatigue. It is for this reason that nurse educators should seek to build community in all learning environments (especially e-learning) (see Appendix C). This chapter will help you explore what it means to build community in your nursing courses.

The three domains of learning are cognitive, psychomotor, and affective. The cognitive domain addresses the learner's ability to intellectually master bodies of knowledge. The psychomotor domain includes skill such as dexterity and manual manipulation. The affective domain addresses one's attitudes toward the content.

We all can think of a time when we were involved in a boring learning environment. This made the development of understanding and mastery of the content very tedious. The motivation to tackle the educational material was just not there and greatly affected our ability to truly grasp the content. No matter what theory or concept one uses to explain this phenomenon (adult learning, attrition, retention, change) all roads lead back to the idea that addressing the affective domain of learning can enhance motivation and encourage learners to master the objectives.

The best way to address this motivation is to help the learners find meaning through building community. The idea of community can be summed up as a group of individuals with common goals working together to meet those goals. This could be a group of neighbors attempting to get a pothole filled on their road; maybe a band of teens hanging out to see what others are talking about, or a team of students attempting to prepare for the next

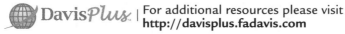

Davis*Plus* | For additional resources please visit
http://davisplus.fadavis.com

TECHNOLOGY TIP 5.1

Many learning interactions can be enhanced by inviting a guest. The mother whose son died from leukemia, the Director of Nursing from the long-term care facility, or the politician. Bring these guests to the online classroom by having them enrolled with special guest access. Most course management systems have a role called "Guest" that allows an individual to come in and participate only in select areas (such as the asynchronous discussion forum). This way, the guest can share lived experience with the learners without the constraints of getting the guest to campus at a time convenient for all. This is a great way to build community. See your facility's information technology director for more information.

examination. All of these groups are communities. Some are more formal; others are more spontaneous. Some aim for academic goals, others pursue self-worth, or fun.

To build community, the instructor will need to understand certain concepts. Preece (2000) offers a simple yet concise framework for building community. She talks about the people, the purpose, the policies, and the computer system that is used to facilitate a successful online community. The people are obviously the students who come to the learning environment with their goals and objectives. The people may also be the instructors and the guests who visit. Learners should realize that the instructors and guests have a vested interest in the learning environment because this helps to bring a sense of reality to learning. Striving for realism is one reason that many online schools will tell the online instructor, "you need to bring your professional experiences to the classroom." Instructors also may be encouraged to share information about their private lives (my mother had this disease . . .) When learners see that the instructor is sincerely interested in the topic, connections are made and motivation for the learner builds. As the instructor opens up, they too may have more motivation to contribute positively to the learning environment. Encouragement for guests to positively contribute also may be realized.

The next important part of the community framework is purpose. In nursing education, this purpose is development of new competencies or maintenance and enhancement of competencies already mastered. Any instructor, in any learning environment (face-to-face [f-2-f] or online), needs to remember the primary objectives for the learning encounter. All actions should help attain that end.

Preece (2000) also talks about policies for the community. This means that there are a set of rules that lead the group toward the desired outcomes. Learners often need the motivation of grades or compensation (tuition reimbursement) to attain a goal. As the instructor thinks of building this learning community (either f-2-f or online), he or she should seriously consider how this motivation can be incorporated. An example may include the instructor who develops an online asynchronous discussion. The instructor decides that adding a grade to the discussion makes the learning too artificial. After 2 weeks into the class; however, only three learners have contributed. The instructor spent a month developing this new learning strategy and had others review the content (i.e., discussion questions). So why did it fail? The policies were not realistic for the community. These learners are second semester junior nursing students and struggling mightily to keep up grades, work, and meet family responsibilities. The motivation to participate in this community was not great enough. For the next group of learners, the instructor makes the online discussions for the course count as 25% of the final course grade and every student participates in every discussion.

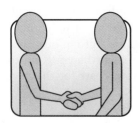

Other policies needed are dependent on the people and purpose of the community. For instance, in the practice environment, grades are not used, but the promotion committee assesses the learner's participation in the discussions. The nurse manager will evaluate who has been a leader in the community and who has just pursued the bare minimum. Policies in the area of Netiquette, schedules, and format also will help to enhance the community (Box 5.1). It is worth noting that the idea of people, purpose, and policies of communities can easily apply to the f-2-f or online learning environments. As instructors seek to develop this part of their practice for the online learning environment, they should consider these principles in their f-2-f practice as well.

The final component of the online community involves the technology needed to facilitate the interaction (Preece, 2000). Instructors should remember, that online community can enhance any learning environment. Whether it be clinical, laboratory, f-2-f classrooms, or completely online courses, the online community can prove to be a powerful tool to enhance learning (Sitzman, 2010).

As the technology is considered, it is best to remember that complexity is not needed. The idea of building community revolves around bringing people together. It does not need to be flashy to be effective. As a matter of fact, the bells and whistles may detract from the community or cause so many technical issues that learners may lose motivation (the opposite of our goal in this chapter). Basic chat, instant messaging, e-mail, and the online discussion board/forum are usually ideal.

LEARNER-TO-LEARNER

The importance of building community between learners cannot be overstated. Learners realize this (sometimes unconsciously) as they seek to find ways of maintaining their drive to meet the learning objectives. In a staff development session that is insanely boring, the learners may band together to complain (if only amongst themselves) that the learning is boring and dry. Nursing students may come together to divide and conquer the 100 terms that are going to be on the examination in 3 days. Clients with congestive heart failure may come

---

BOX 5.1

NETIQUETTE

- Rule 1: Remember the human
- Rule 2: Adhere to the same standards of behavior online that you follow in real life
- Rule 3: Know where you are in cyberspace
- Rule 4: Respect other people's time and bandwidth
- Rule 5: Make yourself look good online
- Rule 6: Share expert knowledge
- Rule 7: Help keep flame wars under control
- Rule 8: Respect other people's privacy
- Rule 9: Don't abuse your power
- Rule 10: Be forgiving of other people's mistakes

Visit the following Web address for further discussion on these areas. Instructors may even wish to put this link in their syllabi. http://www.albion.com/netiquette/corerules.html

together in an online discussion forum on the American Heart Association Web site to see how others are coping with the dreaded disease. All of these are examples of communities that may or may not have been intentionally "built" by an instructor.

Regardless of the theoretical base, learning while interacting with others is always paramount to a learning experience that is void of peer interaction. Critical thinking can be enhanced when learners appreciate the development of others in this area (Ignatavicius, 2005). Learning environments are enhanced when learners make meaning together (Horton, 2008; Jonassen & Land, 2000). Learners can better understand the navigation of the information age when they struggle together to accomplish academic (professional) objectives (Nelson, 1999; Palloff & Pratt, 2007; Reigeluth, 1999).

People

The learners in an online community can be students in a nursing program, professional nurses in need of staff development, or clients seeking to understand a disease process. The goals (purpose) of this community will help to define what people are appropriate for this learning environment.

One example to consider is the skills laboratory that accompanies a first semester nursing foundations course. The instructor does not have enough time in the laboratory to address all that he would like as part of the learning experience. For this reason, he has chosen to make an online discussion 10% of the skills grade. Students are required to go online (asynchronous discussion board) every Thursday and answer two critical thinking challenges (deep questions). Then by the following Tuesday, they must go back to the online discussion and critique two of their peers.

This online discussion, to accompany the first semester laboratory, serves an important purpose in facilitating the learning of the students. The learners see the content from a completely different angle. Rather than just memorizing the steps of a wet-to-moist dressing change, they have to critically analyze potential hazards and problems with this type of dressing (depending on the deep questions offered by the instructor). The learners may be required to discuss the fear a client with a wound, which has dehisced, may experience. Learners may have to come up with teaching material for this client or even recommend a Web site that will help the family manage this new task. What if the client was homeless, diabetic, missing a limb, or mentally incapacitated? Remember, this instructor in the skills laboratory barely has enough time to demonstrate the skill much less cover all of these areas; therefore, the online (asynchronous) discussion board will serve as a powerful tool to enhance the learning in the skills laboratory. Learner motivation will be enhanced as they see potential connections to the psychomotor skill and the client safety/outcomes. Instructor satisfaction may increase as they see more learners engaged and thinking about the far-reaching ramifications of the wet-to-moist dressing.

Purpose

As an instructor thinks about improving the learning environment through building community, the learning objectives need to be considered. Some communities need to focus on making meaning and striving for synthesis of knowledge level learning (new nurses being oriented to the intensive care unit [ICU]). Others need to practice directly with team work (nursing students in the leadership course). Still others may need to learn to cope with loss of function (young woman who is now paralyzed from the waist down).

In the example of the new ICU nurses, the staff development coordinator has decided that they will practice with Virtual Clinical Excursions (VCE) and share their results in an online asynchronous discussion (AD) board. The AD is important because the learners are on multiple shifts and getting them all together at one time would be impossible. The staff development specialist decides that the VCE is due on Mondays and peer replies are due Fridays.

Building community among the new ICU nurses is crucial. The hospital will put significant resources (personnel, time, financial) into the orientation of these professionals. If they are not motivated or don't have adequate moral/emotional support, the new recruits may be less likely to progress. This AD assignment allows them to connect with others going through the same thing (a rigorous orientation program). Learners can share not only their learning with the VCE, but also their feelings about being yelled at when staffing is low. Feelings of frustration and fear can be shared and support/encouragement received from those who know exactly what is happening (Sitzman, 2010). Even though the learners and educator rarely meet f-2-f, they are creating bonds that can get them through the learning process.

In the leadership course, the nursing students need to develop team-building skills and practice group dynamics (even though this is a fully online course and two of the students live in other countries). Due to the learners being spread out, they are prone to feeling isolated and alone. Using the AD is a great way for them to come together, share, learn, and disagree as they grow into their new professional roles. Students also may attempt to use a synchronous chat (be online at the same time talking in a text-based window). Although it was difficult to get time zones to work between Hawaii and London, the eight students were able to accomplish a meeting and they reported great satisfaction with meeting in real-time. "It helped to build our sense of teamwork and reminded all of us that we are not alone here in cyberspace."

The following scenario illustrates the importance of "purpose." Josie was in a serious car accident last summer. As a result, she was paralyzed from the waist down. She has been home from Neuro rehab for 2 weeks and has not gone out. She talks with the nurse at the rehab clinic and that is about it for social interaction. The nurse explains to Josie that there is this online group who uses AD and synchronous chat. After a few days of "lurking" (watching the discussion and not participating), Josie decides to introduce herself. Five months later, Josie is taking training to be an online moderator for one of the discussion forums. She went on to college and now has a degree in social work.

Josie found community in the online discussions. Initially, she was embarrassed to go out in public, which greatly inhibited her social interactions. For this reason, she was at significant risk for all the complications of isolation. The community of individuals who had suffered a similar fate, was able to help Josie cope, and even encouraged her on to greater accomplishments.

Policies

The policies of the online community are very important. The main reason for this is that social interactions are not only encouraged, but altered from what we may normally be accustomed. The young adult may have been using instant messenger and cell phone text messaging for the past 7 years of adolescence and young adulthood; however, IMHO (in my humble opinion), d^_^b (listening to music), and LOL (laughing out loud) don't work well in a professional discussion on the implications of teaching clients who have congestive heart failure. For the older adult who is returning to school or considering continuing education, communication in a text-based environment may be something they have never tried and is very confusing.

One very important policy in all online communities is Netiquette (Palloff & Pratt, 2007; Shea, 2005). Observing Netiquette reminds the participants of what text-based communication can do to intentions and thoughts being shared with others (see Box 5.1). Jokes are often not taken as intended. Slang is confusing. Cultural context causes well intended thoughts to become distorted. By using a policy of Netiquette, the members of the online community are all aware of the possible shortcomings of digital communication.

Another area of policy is peer interaction. The learners are to offer a critique of one another's posts. This is a vital policy to the building of an online community. By requiring thoughtful interaction, the learners develop competency in professionally encouraging and challenging others. Given the growing intricacy of the nursing profession, peer evaluation is a critical competency of the nurse of the 21st century.

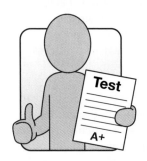

Instructors should remember a few simple, yet significant, concepts in peer interaction. First, if there is not a grade attached, the participation will dwindle immediately, or not begin at all. Anecdotally, participation rates in ungraded discussions for undergraduate nursing students is about 10%. Requiring the peer interaction and showing the students it is important (i.e., attach a grade) brings quality and quantity to the AD. For staff developers and faculty development, many organizations will use a raffle (participation means learners could win one of four prizes) or a promotion-related incentive to encourage learners. The other issue with peer reply is that most learners (even at the graduate level) do not know what appropriate professional feedback involves. Because many courses do not focus on this topic (e.g.., interpersonal communication, management, human resources techniques), it is best to give your learners some simple and effective guidelines.

In one example, the instructor requires a minimum number of words in the peer reply and discusses the concept of a 2+2 (2 positive comments and 2 challenges or concerns) (Allen & Allen, 1996). The use of these basic principles has been proven to give the learners enough guidelines to create effective feedback in most learning situations. The other important element is due dates. E-learning is meant to be flexible; however, the learners need due dates. In one nursing department in all courses, the main post is due on Thursdays and the peer replies are due on Tuesdays. This keeps all students on track and gives them someone with whom they can interact for their peer reply. It should be noted however, that this usually only works in the AD. It would be hard to implement and monitor this type of feedback mechanism in a synchronous chat.

One final issue regarding policy is that all courses in a program of study or staff development department should attempt to develop community in a similar fashion. If there is great flexibility and variation among instructors, the learners may become frustrated at learning the different preferences and setups. This will detract from building community. In Box 5.2 is a list of community building ADs from Indiana Wesleyan University that encourages learners and instructors to interact on a professional and personal level. In each course in the graduate nursing program, there is an AD called Facilitator's Forum, Autobiographies, Prayer Requests, and a Café. Learners and faculty know what to do in each of these areas and use them often because they are in every course in that exact same order. These are great tools to build community.

Computer Systems

Multiple computer systems or technologies can be used to facilitate a learner-to-learner online community. Community is better developed if the complexity of the technology is kept relatively low. One of the more basic tools is *e-mail*. E-mail lists and groups can be used to share

---

BOX 5.2

FACILITATOR'S FORUM AND TOOLS FOR BUILDING COMMUNITY

- Facilitator's Forum: Is similar to office hours. Learners go into this area and post a question. The instructor or another learner will answer the question. This is very useful, because that question and the answer can be seen by the entire course. This also is a great place for the instructor to clarify assignments and make announcements.
- Class Autobiographies: In each class, the learners see the instructor's biography and are expected to post their own biography with an update from the previous class (e.g., I just got a new job in home health). Some instructors also will ask a question of the group related to the content of the course (e.g., What will your retirement look like?).
- Prayer Requests: Indiana Wesleyan is a faith-based organization and all instructors follow the Christian faith. As a result, instructors post an opening prayer. Learners and instructors will go into this area and ask for prayer or share praises with one another (e.g., Our house just sold and my husband found a new job).
- Café or Student Union: Learners and instructors can share funny stories and images with each other. They will often post Web links and talk about issues that are not necessarily connected with the course content. Learners also will encourage one another (e.g., We can't let Statistics get us down; we are half way through this program).

---

information and allow teams to work on projects. The e-mail can be easily sorted and using "reply" and "reply all" allows the participants to control who in the discussion receives the e-mails. At first glance, this seems like an efficient way of building community. That is not the case.

Most participants will discover that the volume of e-mail they receive from those not involved in the community is too distracting to the development and flow of the community. Spam and junk mail can easily infiltrate most e-mail systems and causes clutter that is distracting. From an instructor's perspective, the e-mail system is usually not in a format that allows the instructor to monitor all communications. This does not allow the instructor to adequately monitor the building of community.

The synchronous chat is a tool that usually resides in conjunction with a group of online (Web-based) tools. The chat may be found in a course management system (CMS) or as part of a Web site with other goals (major league sports teams allowing fans to chat with one of the players). Chats are synchronous because all of the participants must be logged on at the same time. In a chat window, one will see the sentences of the discussion pop up as each person types. This is great for real-time discussion and may even have advanced features such as file sharing, real-time video, or a white board that allows participants to draw or type together. Because this technology is usually in a password-protected environment, unwanted intrusions are usually few.

Where the chat may be problematic is if there are more than 10 participants. The screen fills up quickly as most screens can only handle 20 lines of text. The readers may get confused as they are trying to answer questions from multiple individuals at the same time. The other issue is related to bandwidth. Those whose Internet connection is fast will have messages popping up at a quicker rate than those with a slower Internet connection. Nonetheless, this tool does have its use. Many instructors like to have this tool activated for virtual office hours (e.g., Hi Class, I will be on chat from 8 pm to 10 pm CST). Some groups of learners like to use it for group-related work (e.g., the budget proposal that is due Monday morning).

Instant messaging (IM) is another tool that does have some utility in building community. This tool tends to stand alone and runs on a computer connected to the Internet. Individuals create a group of people that are electronically identified as "safe/acceptable" partners for the purpose of a project or course. While the person's computer is on and connected, they will receive a signal that others are "present." They may send each other messages that can include text, images, audio, and even video.

As with chat, IM technology works well for office hours and small-group work. The technology tends to live outside of a tighter password-protected environment (some more than others); therefore, there is a greater chance for unwanted participants and transmission of malicious code (viruses). Instructors also will find it difficult to manage and monitor activity so they have no clue how the community is developing.

The AD is an area where the instructor/facilitator posts a series of questions or assignments. Each area has a place for participants/learners to reply to the main question. The participants also can see the other learners' replies. The participants can then give each other feedback. Most AD tools allow the person creating the post to attach a file (e.g., image, audio clip, PowerPoint, document, spreadsheet). Because the AD is asynchronous, the learners and instructors are not bound to time (however, weekly due dates are important). For instance, the instructor may post the questions on Monday. Tuesday night, three learners reply, Wednesday afternoon four others answer. Then five of the learners go in Friday and offer peer replies. The rest of the learners stop back on Saturday.

The AD seems to be one of the best tools for building community (Yukselturk & Top, 2005–2006) (EBP Box 5.1). First of all, the control for most discussion boards lies in the hands of the instructor. The instructor can open certain ADs to the whole class and allow access to only two or three students for others. The AD will usually take place in a CMS that is password protected and, therefore, only learners with permission can enter the discussion (no spam or lurking). The AD can be organized by topic, author (posts are listed by students), date, or thread (progression of the conversation with responses, see Fig. 5.1). In certain CMS, the instructor also can access the AD through an electronic grade book that will allow for quick, effective grading.

The blog format is similar to the AD. The main variation is that the blog tends to be a stand-alone Web-based tool. Blogs are often more vulnerable to "hackers" and are usually found in an environment that does not require a password for access unless associated with a course management system.

Twitter is a type of "microblogging" in that the blog posts must be 140 characters or less. This tool allows one individual to provide information to all who are following. Some

TECHNOLOGY TIP 5.2

There are many chat and instant messaging tools that are free. These include Yahoo and MSN. You should be careful to turn on all settings that restrict participants. Never allow "guests" to sign in and never accept invitations from an e-mail address that you do not know. Many of these tools have features that require you to invite participants. This prevents unwanted intrusions.

EVIDENCE-BASED PRACTICE BOX 5.1

Asynchronous and Synchronous Discussions

Issue: What Is the Nature of Interactions in Asynchronous and Synchronous Communication?

The study analyzed asynchronous and synchronous discussions in an online information technologies certificate program using Bales's Interaction Process Analysis model, which focuses on social-emotional (SE) and task-oriented (TO) areas.

Study Findings

The content analyses of asynchronous and synchronous communication transcripts showed that posted messages were related to both task- and social-oriented areas, but mainly to task-oriented ones. The instructors' and participants' TO messages are mainly related to attempted answers to the questions. Instructors and the participants posted more positive reaction messages than negative reaction messages in the SE area. Also, semi-structured interviews with participants and instructors were conducted to investigate findings, which revealed complementary results to the content analysis. In addition, the discussion list was used primarily by participants for asking questions or getting answers and instructors' guided chat sessions to discuss critical issues in course topics by asking questions.

Nursing Implications

- Both asynchronous and synchronous discussion should be used complementarily in online learning environments.
- Both task- and social-oriented messages should be posted; however, emphasis is expected to be on task-oriented ones.
- In online environments, synchronous communications (e.g., chat) can be directed or facilitated by instructors and asynchronous ones (e.g., discussion list of questions) by students.
- Time and number of synchronous communications should be arranged based on students' needs and expectations. (Yukselturk & Top, 2005–2006)

---

may wish to follow Tweets from a certain organization or person depending on their interests. Instructors may use Twitter in class as a way to get instant feedback from a group of students. Each student who posts a tweet includes a "hashtag" that is specific to that class (e.g., #nur340). The instructor then displays these tweets on the screen and discusses questions and comments. Twitter can be considered both synchronous and asynchronous.

LEARNER-TO-INSTRUCTOR

Instructors are people too. This concept is vital to building community. Instructors needs to remember that they are human and their emotions/mental state and affect can be influenced by the goings-on of the learning environment. Keeping this in mind is important for two reasons. First of all, if instructors feels like part of the community, their motivation to contribute and strive for excellence may be enhanced. Secondly, if the learners see instructors as a real people (i.e., with weaknesses, competing interests, strengths), they too may be more likely to contribute to the building of community.

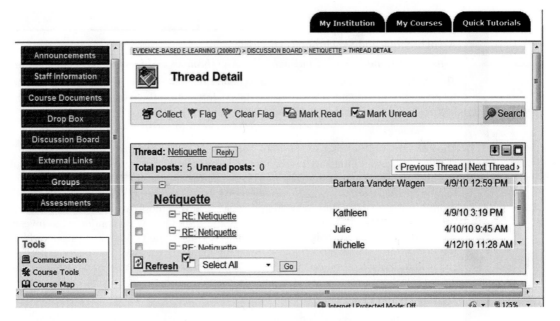

Figure 5.1   Asynchronous threaded discussions.

People

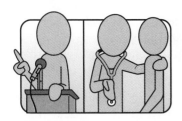

Professionals of the information age must be lifelong learners. This is vital to the professional nurse. One way of facilitating this is the role shift for the educator. The instructor online must transition from "sage on the stage" to "guide on the side" for effective community building to take place (Palloff & Pratt, 2007). This can be very difficult for nursing instructors and staff development professionals as they struggle with an incredible sense of responsibility to ensure that the appropriate knowledge is attained by the learners.

For the active learning to take place, for the lifelong learning to be practiced, and for the learners to build community, the instructor needs to get out of the way and facilitate the process for the learners taking control (Royse & Newton, 2007). By instructors being more of a guide on the side, they will not only facilitate all that was mentioned, but also could promote enhanced outcomes (Lake, 2001).

Purpose

Instructors often talk about teaching as being enjoyable because they like learning. This is a fortunate attitude for the online instructor, because if they can capture that mindset, building community becomes that much easier. In many online learning environments, the administrators are discovering that if they have a lead faculty and lead instructional designer develop all sections of the same course, the quality is much better across the board.

Administrators can then say to the instructor/facilitator "You bring your talents and professional experience to the discussion." This allows the instructor to share what the textbooks cannot—his or her experience. This allows the instructor to step beside the learners and become one of them in learning and discovering new concepts and ideas.

Two words of caution for the instructor seeking to become more of a facilitator and less of an orator. First, do remember that there does need to be some boundaries and space to effectively provide solid and useful assessment (See "Grading the Discussion" in Chapter 10). Being a guide on the side does not mean giving the entire class an "A" just for showing up. Second, the instructor will need to be careful not to shut down the discussion. When an instructor gives a thought or comment on a topic of discussion, that can greatly hinder the creativity from the learners. When the instructor speaks, it is obviously the right answer so there is no longer a reason for learners to struggle with the content and make meaning.

Policies

Just as the learners need guidelines to keep the community going, so do the instructors. As this discussion begins, some will become concerned about the principles of academic freedom. Whether they are concerned with their own academic freedom or the academic freedom that others may demand, this is bound to be a concern. Academic freedom should be sought for the lead instructor in charge of controlling the subject matter for a course or continuing education offering. When discussing the concept and importance of building community; however, it is vital that certain concepts be remembered.

When there is great flexibility in course structure, the students will often become confused and frustrated. If pharmacology and med-surg require that all online discussions be completed in APA format, and maternal-child and leadership don't even consider grammar, students are going to have a difficult time. When the nurse manager from the hospital serves as an adjunct for two different lead faculty, and they both have a completely different take on instructional design, that adjunct is likely to either choose one over the other to work for or quit altogether and find another hobby.

Based on observations of hundreds of students, instructors, and courses, the best at building community adopt the following model. The department has adopted an instructional design that is a compromise of the best of the best in their program. They have decided that it will be the one format that is used in all courses (e.g., In every nursing course, all main posts are due on Thursday at midnight and peer replies are due on Tuesday at midnight). The department then decides on a subject-matter expert who is in charge of each course. No changes can be made to the content of the course without approval of that expert and/or the entire faculty. This not only decreases variability and frustration, it also maintains quality and shows the accreditation bodies that outcomes are the primary objective.

There are many different variations of policy structures for instructors using online technology (see one example on DavisPlus). There needs to be delineation between a class that has f-2-f time and a class that is completely online. There also needs to be simplicity in that the same policy works for adjuncts as will work for full-time instructors. This will decrease confusion and help the focus to stay on building community and developing high-quality professionals who are ready for the health-care industry.

Computer Systems

The technology discussed under learner-to-learner is quite similar to what is needed in learner-to-instructor interactions. There are a few tools; however, that instructors will be able to use to help build community. One is the announcements section of a course management system (CMS). In most CMS, the instructor can program announcements (e.g., The examination will be in room B345 at 2 pm on Friday) to turn on and off on certain dates. When students log into the CMS and click on their course, they will usually see the announcements first thing. This also can be used as a community-building tool (Fig. 5.2).

The instructor can post a picture of something funny/interesting/mysterious and describe/challenge with the announcement text. The instructor may post a picture of a tool from a physician's kit in the 1800s and see if the group can guess what it is. The instructor may ask the students for baby pictures and post one and see if the group can guess who it is. If a CMS is not being used, the instructor could e-mail the image or post it on a Web site. Instructors should be careful to adhere to all copyright and fair-use laws when using photos or links from other organizations/individuals. These are just fun ways of using the technology to help build community.

INSTRUCTOR-TO-INSTRUCTOR

What is an instructor? In nursing this has many different answers. Is it the social worker that the students "happened" to talk to at clinical? Is it the PhD-prepared director of the Health Sciences Division of the school? Is it the LPN that stocks the laboratory? Is it their grandmother who birthed all eight of her children at home with the help of a friend? We know that all of these individuals can contribute to the learning of the student (whether it is positive or negative is situation dependent). For the purposes of this section, we will focus on full-time, part-time, adjunct, and preceptor faculty who contribute to the learning of the student.

People

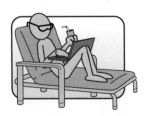

In 2006, we learned some startling facts about the nursing professorate. Although the vacancy rate in nursing education programs grows, many schools are looking to part-time and adjunct faculty to fill the void (National League for Nursing, 2006). Overall, nursing programs across the nation have seen an increased use of part-time faculty by 72.5%. With increased retirements of faculty and the need for increased enrollments to meet market demand, this trend will not change anytime soon.

The increased use of part-time faculty brings about some important issues for nursing education. First of all, nursing education needs to be mindful of the people involved. The faculty who are retiring often welcome ways of staying involved in academia while still having the time to relax and enjoy the retirement they have earned. Another group is the professional nurse who is working in a high-paying and high-stress clinical environment. This person often has little extra time for academia, yet holds vital experience that could revolutionize the learning of the student.

The other major person to consider in building instructor-to-instructor community is the current full-time faculty member. This may be the new faculty member who had no training as an educator. This may be the faculty member that teaches alone at a remote site. The full-time faculty member may be responsible for the quality of the clinicals taught by the preceptors.

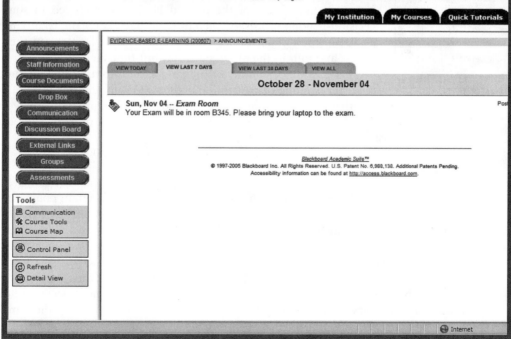

Figure 5.2 Online announcements in CMS. Notice how the announcement can be programmed to turn on and off at certain times/dates. This allows for preplanning on the part of the instructor that can facilitate learner success.

Purpose

The purpose of building community between instructors is important for two main reasons. Instructors need a solid support system to successfully navigate the academic domain. The program needs to ensure that quality education is being provided in all situations.

Teaching nursing is a tough undertaking, no matter who you are. The rewards are great and so is the price paid by those who provide it. These individuals need a strong support system that can get them through the tough times and celebrate with them in the high times. Building online community for these individuals can prove invaluable.

Nursing instructors can collaborate in the AD where no students are allowed. They can share ideas, concerns, and jokes. A lead faculty member could have preceptors online in a synchronous chat at a couple of different points throughout the semester. This not only allows the instructor to know what is happening in the preceptorships but will also allow preceptors to interact and support one another.

Quality is another reason to build community among instructors. Instructors are often separated by time and geography. A program cannot afford to send a lead faculty to every clinical preceptorship. Some students are fulfilling course requirements in other states/countries. Some instructors are teaching the on-campus students from a distant location. Regardless of the scenario, the nursing program needs to ensure that quality outcomes are maintained. The process of building community online can facilitate this.

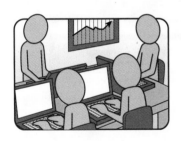

One example might be online mentoring. The CMS is loaded and being used for pathophysiology. The course is for students who are on-site but the faculty member teaching it lives in a different state. This online adjunct will feel more like a part of the team if he can be included in some of the decision-making processes; therefore, the agenda for the faculty meeting is posted in the online AD for faculty. The adjunct faculty can then post at leisure and join in the discussion with full-time faculty.

This previous example allows the adjunct from a different state to not only feel like one of the team but allows him to identify areas of his practice that may not quite meet the standards of the program. He would then be able to enhance his academic practice while learning from the pros who are doing the work on a consistent basis.

Policies

As with students, the faculty's time is very limited and valuable and certain policies may need to be in place that encourage them to actively participate in the community. This can be done in a number of ways to include incentives and mandates. The incentives may include a game or prize. The faculty with the most hours spent in the online discussion wins a prize. All AD Team Meeting discussion participants are enrolled in a drawing. All faculty must participate in the continuing AD on at least two different days within 2 weeks after the f-2-f faculty meeting.

Although it would be nice if faculty could just participate in the process without these policies in place, they do have to prioritize their time and these may help them make decisions that could help to build community for the whole group.

Another similarity between students and faculty involves the decrease in social inhibitions in the online environment. Faculty (especially those not used to e-learning) may need a brief primer/reminder of the importance of Netiquette (Palloff & Pratt, 2007). Anyone who has been a part of a faculty meeting can tell you that there can be moments of significant tension. It is for this reason that all members of the online community be reminded of the best way to communicate in a digital environment.

Finally, policies around the interactions can also be important. Are there limitations to the size of the files that can be shared? If the online community is sharing documents, is it important that they all use Microsoft Word? Do participants need to have an up-to-date virus scan done on their computer?

Computer Systems

The computer systems and technology needed to connect instructors is similar to that of learners. Instructors will all need access to the CMS. This may be challenging when you think about the RN in the ICU who is serving as a preceptor. She could make some great contributions to the online community/faculty meeting but the school has a strict policy that only faculty and students can access the CMS. The best way to address this is to have administrators sit down and talk about the process that identifies a faculty member. This could include a new type of faculty such as a professional faculty or teaching assistant role.

Another area to consider involves roles in the CMS. In most systems, there are one or two instructors in an online course room (where online tools are located; such as gradebook, AD, exams, documents, dropbox, chat). It is important to note that if 10 faculty are enrolled in an online course room, only one or two should be identified as the instructors for the course. This prevents all the participants of the online community from having complete access to all aspects of the control panel or author tools. This can allow the participants to feel like true participants (as opposed to the instructor/facilitator role that they possess in all the other online environments). Keeping their roles limited also can prevent accidental or intentional alteration of the online community (e.g., erasing a post from another participant who does not share one's own philosophy).

GUESTS

Guests can include anyone from a patient to a missionary to a politician. These individuals will enhance the community and education. The school chaplain may stop into the online discussion to offer a thought for the week and learners can ask questions. Patients may login, which can allow students and instructors to really understand the pros/cons of certain treatments related to the diseases that affects the patient. The night nurse who serves as the emergency department, ICU, labor/delivery, and supervisor at a small rural hospital can be a guest speaker for a week in the leadership course.

All of these examples can help to really enhance the sense of community among the learners and faculty. Don't forget about the guest. For clients to be able to share experiences may help them to find meaning and experience a great sense of well-being. Clients may be too weak to leave the home or not able to risk sharing germs in a crowd. But the Internet may allow them to tap into the students' online community. The nurses and administrators of smaller facilities often feel slighted by academia as fewer students and groups frequent their facilities. By bringing these amazing professionals into the online community, they too can experience many of the same benefits that learners and instructors report.

CONCLUSION

Building community is an important part of any learning environment. This chapter has demonstrated the ability of the online community to enhance any learning environment (clinical, laboratory, lecture, Web). The community can motivate the learner to aim higher and persevere even in the most rigorous of courses. The online community can bring satisfaction to the faculty and encourage their commitment to student outcomes. Online community can bring guests from far and wide who contribute as much as they receive from the interaction.

Policies must be in place to manage and encourage the building of online communities. Policies will direct participants in participation expectations, interactions with others (Netiquette), and activities that can promote learning and growth of all involved. The policies will also help to clarify a uniform process across the academic environment. A uniform policy of community building will help faculty and learners in multiple courses to make smoother transitions between the classes.

REFERENCES

Allen, D. B., & Allen, D. W. (1996). *2+2 equals better performance: Alternative performance appraisal with feedback and encouragement.* Beijing, China: Author.

Horton, W. (2008). Knowledge management: From the graveyard to good ideas. In S. Carliner & P. Shank (Eds.), *The e-learning handbook: Past promises, present challenges* (pp. 77–107). San Francisco, CA: Pfeiffer.

Ignatavicius, D. (2005). An introduction to developing critical thinking in nursing students. In L. Caputi, & L. Engelmann (Eds.), *Teaching nursing: The art and science* (Vol. 2, pp. 622–633). Glen Ellyn, IL: College of Dupage Press.

Jonassen, D. H., & Land, S. M. (2000). *Theoretical foundations of learning environments.* Mahwah, NJ: Lawrence Erlbaum Associates.

Lake, D. (2001). Student performance and perceptions of a lecture-based course compared with the same course utilizing group discussion. *Physical Therapy, 81*(3), 896–902.

National League for Nursing. (2006). *Nurse educators 2006: A report of the faculty census survey of RN and graduate programs.* New York, NY: Author.

Nelson, L. M. (1999). Collaborative problem-solving. In C. M. Reigeluth (Ed.), *Instructional design theories and models* (Vol. 2, pp. 241–268). Mahwah, NJ: Lawrence Erlbaum Associates.

Palloff, R. M., & Pratt, K. (2007). *Building online learning communities: Effective strategies for the virtual classroom.* San Francisco, CA: Wiley, John & Sons.

Preece, J. (2000). *Online communities: Designing usability, supporting sociability.* New York, NY: John Wiley.

Reigeluth, C. M. (1999). *Instructional-design theories and models.* Mahwah, NJ: Lawrence Erlbaum Associates.

Royse, M. A., & Newton, S. E. (2007). How gaming is used as an innovative strategy for nursing education. *Nursing Education Perspectives, 28*(3), 263–267.

Shea, V. (2005). *The core rules of netiquette.* Retrieved from http://www.albion.com/netiquette/corerules.html

Sitzman, K. (2010). Student-preferred caring behaviors for online nursing education. *Nursing Education Perspectives, 31*(3), 171–176.

Yukselturk, E., & Top, E. (2005-2006). Reconsidering online course discussions: A case study. *Journal of Educational Technology Systems, 34*(3), 341–367.

Chapter 6

Web-Supported Learning Environments

Ellen Cummings, MSN, RN, CNRN, CNE • Margi Schultz, PhD, RN, CNE

Two students make separate appointments to see the Director of a large nursing program. Both students have complaints about the same issue—each from a slightly different perspective. The first student arrives, in tears, stating that no one had ever, during the entire admission process, made any mention of assignments or testing being done on the computer. Having truly no experience with computers and not even sure how to use the mouse, the student is sure that this is a hurdle that cannot be overcome, a true barrier to learning, a disaster of epic proportions, why was this not carefully detailed in all published materials about the program so that the student could have chosen a different program—one that never uses computers?

The second student arrives at the Director's office—angry, sputtering, demanding to know how on earth a student could be expected to attend class 3 days a week when reading, reviews, and discussion could just as easily be done online? Are the instructors so out-of-touch, the school so out-of date that no one realizes that students have to take care of family, work full-time, and cannot be expected in this day and age to put in "seat time" as the only learning environment? Having only a few assignments online is unacceptable!

The answer to both students is the same. Technology and computers are definitely a part of the new learning environments and many schools are struggling to find the right balance between too much and too little technology. The curriculum is designed to promote student learning and the value-add of Web-enhancements is a natural extension of the learning process.

Web-supported, computer-enhanced, "webademia" instruction, techno-learning, virtual classrooms, computer-assisted learning, computer-supported collaborative learning—all are buzzwords for a teaching modality and authentic learning environment that has exploded over the past few years. Web-supported learning is different from a "pure" distance learning class or a hybrid course. In an online or Web-based course, all of the course content is offered online. Web-supported learning also differs from a hybrid or blended course, where a percentage of the course content is online and a portion taught in the face-to-face (f-2-f).

A general definition of a Web-supported learning environment is one in which the course content is taught in a traditional f-2-f method and uses technology to facilitate learning, such as posting specifically developed content and activities in a course management system

Davis*Plus* | For additional resources please visit
http://davisplus.fadavis.com

(CMS). The Web-supported content is designed to illustrate concepts, increase attainment of course objectives, supplement instruction, and provide an avenue for the student to submit assignments via a dropbox in the CMS. A Web-supported course may be the first experience that a student has using computers in a class and can be the beginning of a great new adventure in learning.

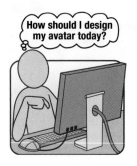

The use of Web-supported learning can range from relatively minor usage such as a learning platform that is primarily used to post grades, announcements, and share a few links for students to explore, to a well-developed learning site that includes rich discussion on content topics, streaming video, interactive modules and games, avatars, and enough electronic gadgetry to keep today's technologically savvy student entranced for hours while still engaging the technological newbie in such a manner as to not intimidate or overshadow the learning that must take place.

Along with the new technology and the many online opportunities that faculty have to enrich and explore new learning avenues with students, it is important to maintain the structure of the class, offer concrete information for accessing and using the online components, and use a variety of teaching and learning strategies including active, cooperative, reflective, constructive, and authentic strategies for both the f-2-f and Web-supported course components that yield meaningful, measureable outcomes.

A student needs to have access to a computer that can quickly retrieve the information that is provided and he or she also must have thorough, clear, concise instructions on how to manipulate and use the online components. The student will require access to technical help when needed—preferably not the instructor, but a dedicated department, live chat, or online help desk who can respond in real time when the help is needed. The information may be rich, the activities well-planned, and the graphics amazing, but this is only true if the student can find and successfully navigate through the resources. Keep in mind that if a student gets lost in the maze of a technical manual or is unsuccessful after several attempts at accessing information, the value of the Web-enhancement will be lost and the student will be frustrated and discouraged from trying again.

If the course outline in the syllabus is not concise and does not give clear direction for use, requirements, and evaluation criteria of the online components, the student may feel that he or she is floundering among all of the information not knowing how to prioritize the elements that are intended to enhance the learning environment. Spending time during the f-2-f portion of the class explaining the Web-supported resources to students and making sure that they know what is expected of them is definitely time well-spent. The first assignment using the online components should be something fun, introductory, and nongraded. This decreases fear about the experience and gives the student a sense of competence with the online environment. Web-supported environments should be an enhancement for the student, and preparations carefully crafted by the faculty member can make a big difference to the students.

This chapter reviews authentic learning and how Web-supported learning environments can have an impact on all of the learning domains. It also discusses benefits, best practices, and perilous pitfalls to this dynamic teaching and learning modality, and explores the practical applications of Web-supported learning environments for nursing education in the laboratory, clinical, and classroom settings. Assessment techniques of student learning in the Web-supported environment also are detailed.

AUTHENTIC LEARNING AND LEARNING DOMAINS

As faculty create innovative assignments for the Web-supported environment, they should be mindful of not falling into the trap of assigning "busy work" for students. The study time or activities devoted to online components are intended to add quality to the Web-supported class and should offer authentic learning and tasks, add value to the student's learning, and not simply include random items that do not contribute to the attainment of course outcomes. As described by Lombardi in a 2007 Educause Learning Initiatives white paper, authentic learning is learning by doing, a type of learning long considered by educators as the best way to learn and retain course content. With the help of current technology, the Internet, personal communication devices, and the rapidly expanding amount of software designed to replicate patient care scenarios and increase critical thinking ability, students have a wide range of authentic learning tools at their fingertips.

Students acquire a skill set through authentic learning that is normally acquired through on-the-job experiences. These skills include the ability to make thoughtful clinical judgments, the flexibility to adapt and generalize situational learning, the patience to think through and follow more complex arguments, and the ability to recognize patterns and syn-

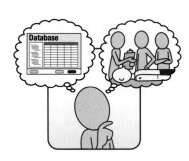

thesize prior learning. Nursing students are not simply expected to read, remember, and regurgitate facts. Students are being asked to create, analyze, and to evaluate their learning.

Authentic tasks are structured to extend beyond the traditional textbook and be relevant in the real-world applications in which students will find themselves. Students discussing an intense simulation scenario that they have just completed no longer ask the question "Is this really something I have to know?" The learning is real time, genuine, the reinforcement occurs in the debriefing, and, best of all, the "patient" can duplicate scenarios or create scenarios time and time again that are difficult to find in the land-based clinical setting.

Learning Domains

Well constructed Web-supported learning environments can involve the three basic learning domains, cognitive, affective, and psychomotor. The cognitive domain, which is integrated in all learning domains, involves the capacity to think and problem solve, sometimes known as the knowledge domain. The six levels identified within this domain are: remember, understand, apply, analyze, create, and evaluate (Krathwohl, 2002).

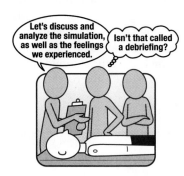

The cognitive domain is well served in Web-supported environments as concepts are illustrated in a variety of ways such as games, visual graphics, matching components, and case studies. Sadly, much of what is taught and the level the material is assessed at in many nursing schools is that of applying, understanding, and remembering. Although it is true that it is easier to identify and test to these levels, the learning involved at the levels of analyze, create, and evaluate is truly where the students need to be.

Cognitive learning tools are spreadsheets, databases, discussion forums, embedded learning objects, simulations, or other electronic platforms where students use technology to learn *with* rather than learning *through*.

These examples of cognitive tools are the backbone of Web-supported learning environments. Students are actually able to construct their own learning with cognitive tools, encouraging critical thinking, and partnering with technology to increase learning and problem-solving abilities.

Cognitive tools help the students to scaffold (construct knowledge based on the student's own experiences with assistance and guidance from the instructor) knowledge leading to reflection, generalization of learning, and ultimately, the student's ownership of that knowledge (Brush & Saye, 2002). Kim and Reeves (2007) defined cognitive tools as "technologies that learners interact and think with in knowledge construction, designed to bring their expertise to the performance as part of the joint learning system" (p. 224).

The affective domain is the domain associated with feelings, caring, therapeutic communication, listening, advocacy, and attitude. Learning in the affective domain is dependent on the student's willingness to participate and desire to see things in a different manner. An excellent way to incorporate the affective domain in a Web-supported environment would be to embed short streaming video clips, use social networking sites judiciously, and to provide open-ended discussion board questions where the students can interact, learn from peers, and obtain insights and feedback from the faculty.

The psychomotor domain is the action or the "doing" domain. Hands-on learning in laboratories, simulation, and clinical experiences demonstrate the learning accomplished in this domain; however, Web-supported environments also support this domain. Interactive games, videos, drag-and-drop activities, and online clinical scenarios involving avatars (an electronic image that is created and manipulated by a computer user) in which the student guides the avatar through case studies and skills can all involve psychomotor skills (Table 6.1).

BENEFITS, BEST PRACTICES, PERILOUS PITFALLS TO WEB-SUPPORTED LEARNING

Effectively using Web-supported learning requires an understanding of benefits, best practices, and perilous pitfalls.

Benefits

From a student perspective, Web-support offers a flexible learning environment. The student can choose the time, place, and setting for engaging in learning opportunities. Web-support can increase student satisfaction with a course. Salyers (2005) compared student satisfaction with a traditional and a Web-supported graduate-level nursing course. Increased student satisfaction was found with the Web-enhanced course. In particular, students commented on the course flexibility and independent learning.

Lim, Kim, Chen, and Ryder (2008) compared online, traditional and Web-enhanced courses and discovered that the Web-enhanced students reported higher satisfaction levels for overall learning than their peers in the other groups. In addition, students in the online and Web-enhanced classes had higher achievement scores than students in the traditional courses. Bartini's (2008) comparison of traditional and Web-enhanced students revealed higher examination scores and satisfaction with the learning experience in the Web-enhanced group. Another study supports supplementing lecture and laboratory with Web-enhanced interactions including gaming, quizzes, and case studies to improve student examination scores (Allen, Walls, & Reilly, 2008).

TABLE 6.1			
Assignments That Address the Learning Domains			
	Cognitive (Thinking)	**Affective (Feeling)**	**Psychomotor (Doing)**
Characteristics	• Collaboration to support construction of knowledge • Authentic, problem-based activities to simulate real world application • Scaffolding of information to create complex strategies • Integrated learning and assessment • Outcome based learning	• Willingness to entertain a new perspective • Desire to listen, learn • Ability to debate concepts • Consistently acts from a value set • Acts based on motivation and emotion • Attitudes for caring	• Skill acquisition • Willingness to act— to do • Problem solve through action—from simple to complex • Active mental attention to event • Coordination • Scaffolding of skill set • Perfection of techniques
Possible Assignments	• Games • Puzzles • Streaming video • Critical thinking questions • Online discussion boards/forums • Chat—both synchronous and asynchronous • Drag and drop activities • Matching answers • Creation of online concept maps • Teleconference • Podcasting • Microworlds • Second Life	• Surveys and questionnaires • Case studies • Online discussion boards and forums • Role playing • Second Life • Streaming video • Concept papers • Online debates • Dilemma discussions	• Microworlds • Second Life • Animation • Creation of student video • Podcasts • Interactive modules • Virtual clinical experiences • Drag and drop activities

Lashley (2005) evaluated the Web-enhanced delivery of a health assessment course. Students had weekly Web-based assignments and reviewed Web sites covering assessment skills. In addition, the faculty produced streaming video of a complete health assessment for the students to view at any time. Evaluations were favorable, particularly for the assessment video, which was found to be very helpful as students could watch the video as many times as needed to reinforce the skill.

Another benefit to Web-supported environments is that carefully selected Web-enhancements liberate faculty from the dreaded "sage on the stage" and "tyranny of content" by freeing class time that would ordinarily be spent in a race to cover announcements, testing, and content and instead engage in richer class discussion, activities, and meaningful interaction. Bowen (2006) coins the term "teaching naked" to describe the idea that technology can be used outside of the classroom to help better prepare students before the classroom experience.

Preclass online activities, quizzes, games, and podcasts can be used to help the student actively prepare for the classroom experience—an experience that will be richer and more engaging because the faculty will not have to spend valuable time on humdrum activity, announcements, and all the preparatory content that normally occurs before the student is ready and able to actively engage in classroom discussions and active learning. Faculty and students will have more time to problem-solve, critically think, discuss, and clarify complex concepts.

Best Practices

Learning outcomes, student learning styles, and technological issues guide the selection of learning activities. Faculty must choose learning activities that will best meet the outcomes and engage the learner in a rich and meaningful way. Consider key concepts, learning domains, learning styles, and available resources (Billings & Halstead, 2009).

Technology must also be considered when preparing a Web-supported course. Both faculty and students will need to know what hardware, software, and technological support are available and how to access this support. There needs to be a course entry point for student access and a platform for the instructor to organize content and activities. Faculty who have relatively little computer experience can use software such as Dreamweaver or SharePoint to create a course homepage.

Learning or course management systems are packaged programs used to support the organization, delivery, and management of Web-supported or online courses (Billings & Halstead, 2009). Course management systems such as Blackboard (WebCT, ANGEL), PageOut, and eCollege® provide a template and easy-to-use tools so faculty can readily construct and manage a course. Students access the course and materials by logging on with their own username and password. Course management systems provide a wide variety of helpful options including communication, assessment, and tracking tools.

Communication tools generally include an announcements section, e-mail, threaded discussion board, and chat areas. Students can create assignments either within or outside of the management system and submit to a digital drop box. There is an option for students to do group assignments. Student tracking, online testing, and a gradebook also are available and enhance the Web-supported environment. Assignments can be sequenced, selectively released based on date/time, and there also is an option to set a completion date. Students can set up their own portfolio or personal home page for self-assessment. The consistent template and layout of the learning management system helps the student to feel at ease navigating the course components that the instructor designates (Billings & Halstead, 2009).

Whatever platform is chosen, faculty and students will need thorough orientation to the system and adequate technological support. In general, 24-hour support is desirable because students will want to take advantage of the ability to access information on their own time—even if that is at 2 a.m.! Most course management systems provide technological support for their systems but additional support may be provided by the institution. Instructional design support for faculty is helpful. Ongoing education on the technology and development of course materials will be needed.

Perilous Pitfalls

Pitfalls that can occur in Web-supported environments include resistance to changing pedagogy, faculty reluctance to create online learning objects or use of other enhancements, and issues surrounding enhancements, and technology. Moving from a traditional classroom to Web-enhanced course will be a learning process for faculty. Pedagogical approaches to facilitate student learning will need to be modified. Faculty may be unsure about how to create and use online activities.

Faculty assistance in the form of mentors and instructional design support will be necessary. Some faculty have created technology groups to work together to learn, share, and discuss new technology and share best practices. The Wisconsin Technology Enhanced Collaborative Nursing Education (WI-TECNE) is an example of a collaborative group of nursing faculty from five colleges who united for just such a purpose. Each of the individual colleges has taken on different aspects of technology including simulation, virtual reality, problem-based learning, e-learning, telehealth, and informatics (Schmidt & Stewart, 2009).

Many faculty are afraid to incorporate Web-enhancement because they are concerned that it will be too difficult to create the kind of quality educational materials they feel are necessary to achieve student learning outcomes. Materials do not have to be studded with technological wizardry to provide a pedagogically sound, engaging learning experience. In fact, there is a very real danger of information overload when too many resources are provided (see Evidence Based Practice Box 6.1). A very simple case study can engage the student in authentic learning. Fortunately, there are many wonderful, fully developed educational materials already available on the Web that can be easily incorporated into a course. The key is learning where and how to find these little goldmines and determining how best to match them to student learning outcomes for your program, and adapt them to different student learning styles.

When Web-based materials are used, it is important to review them carefully and critically for content accuracy and bias. Material supported by commercial enterprise is likely to be biased. Even material from a professional organization or government agency may contain bias. The bottom line is that careful appraisal is necessary to determine the appropriateness given the educational topic and objective (Wink, 2009).

EVIDENCE-BASED PRACTICE BOX 6.1

Danger, Danger—Resource Overload!

Be cautious of giving your students too many resources, Web sites, games, and other enhancements in the Web-supported environment. If a student gets lost in too much information, he or she will not know where to focus and this can lead to fragmentation of their study time, making it virtually impossible to prioritize learning objects or content. Instead, review the content that you want the student to focus on and map it all back to a course competency, outcome, or learning goal. Although a Web-part or learning object might be fun, interesting, or really flashy to a student, it can be an overwhelming cyber-jungle of information that students will get lost in and preventing them from achieving the end result that the faculty intended. Give your students a road map of how the Web-supported material is intended to be used, tell them what they need to do and when it is due, tell them how and if they will be evaluated on the material, and always provide a clear vision of what is expected. It also is a great idea to give the students a list of the module or unit objectives and student learning outcomes as their blueprint and then align your Web-supported activities with those for clarity (Simonson, Smaldino, Albright, & Zvacek, 2006; KnowledgeLoom 2006).

It is important for faculty to be knowledgeable about copyright rules to avoid problems with copyright infringement in the Web-supported environment. Copyright laws protect the author or original work, either published or unpublished. Under the law, only the author has the right to give permission to others to copy, reproduce, distribute, or display original work.

The Technology, Education, and Copyright Harmonization (TEACH) Act enacted in 2002 clarified language in the U.S. Copyright Act allowing nonprofit institutions to use copyrighted materials under certain circumstances: educational application, fair use, or with copyright holder permission (Rhoads & White, 2008). Work used must be part of an educational offering, incorporated into the course either by or under supervision of an instructor, and must be directly related to the learning outcomes for the course. Only students registered in the course should have access to the materials; students may not copy and disseminate the work to others outside the course. Because copyright guidelines and fair use issues are not well defined, the bottom line is that if there is any question about copyright violation, faculty should seek permission from the copyright holder. Table 6.2 lists selected online resources for copyright questions.

Some material available on the Web is under creative commons licensure, which allows the original author to keep the copyright but permits others to copy and distribute original work under specified conditions. The author or license holder determines whether commercial use is allowed, whether any modifications to the original material can be made, and how the work will be attributed (Creative Commons, 2009). Copyright is not a predicament when the Uniform Resource Locator (URL) is provided to the students to access or when a direct link to a Web site is embedded within online course work.

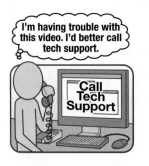

Other pitfalls that can occur relate to the technology. There can be technical problems with the hardware or software, issues with Internet connections, and student computer literacy. Technology often comes with a high cost and it takes time to develop appropriate Web-based learning activities. It is important to have good technical support. Students should be well oriented to the technology; be sure and

TABLE 6.2	
Copyright Resources	
http://www.copyright.gov/circs/circ01.pdf	Copyright information
http://www.copyright.gov/legislation/ pl107-273.html#13301	The TEACH Act (Technology, Education, and Copyright Harmonization Act)
http://www.copyright.com	Information about copyright, licensing, and permissions
http://www.techlearning.com/section/ copyright	Articles regarding copyright and fair use for education
http://www.universityofcalifornia.edu/ copyright/permission.html	One of many university Web sites with information about copyright, fair use, and obtaining permission
http://creativecommons.org	Information about Creative Commons licensure

plan adequate time at the beginning of the course for this. Review Web sites periodically to be sure the URL is correct and that the content is still there and appropriate (Wink, 2009).

WEB-SUPPORTED LEARNING ENVIRONMENTS: LABORATORY, CLINICAL, CLASSROOM

The decision to use Web-supported learning in the laboratory, clinical, or classroom could start with something very simple such as placing the class syllabus and information online or could involve a fully Web-supported course with multiple, rich, Web-based learning activities threaded throughout. Whatever is chosen should be student-focused, guided by student learning outcomes, and supported by appropriate technology and faculty expertise.

Laboratory

The laboratory was historically the place where nursing students had the opportunity to acquire knowledge and practice the psychomotor skills needed to perform in the clinical area. The lab experience has expanded into so much more incorporating human simulation, case studies, procedural simulation, virtual reality, gaming, role-playing, observation, and critique thus fostering not only psychomotor but also affective and cognitive skills (Billings & Halstead, 2009). A Web-enhanced laboratory experience fits nicely into this rich, expanded concept.

There are many options for a Web-enhanced laboratory experience. On a minimal level, skills lists and/or performance guides could be available online. Some easy-to-use additions to that include providing links to one or more of the many well-made, easy-to-navigate, pedagogically sound Web sites. There are a number of excellent Web sites where the student can view physical assessment demonstrations, listen to heart/lung sounds, learn and practice ECG skills, or view nursing skills. A common laboratory activity is medication administration. The student could be directed to a Web site to review selected medications or practice medication calculations. Table 6.3 illustrates a sample pre-laboratory reading and activities assignment.

TABLE 6.3		
Sample Laboratory Assignment		
Date	Topic	Prelaboratory Reading and Activities
Wednesday 10/21/11	Cardiac Assessment	Prelaboratory Reading: MedSurg text: read pages. 750–751; review Table 32-5 *Common Assessment Abnormalities* on pages 749–750 Blackboard: Cardiac Module: Heart Sounds Practice listening to selected sounds on *"The Auscultation Assistant"* Complete prelab quiz: Heart Sounds Print or download to your PDA: Cardiac Assessment Skills Checklist

On a more advanced level, faculty may want to construct a comprehensive module for the laboratory experience. Such a module could be very structured including pre- and post-testing, selected reading, skills demonstration and review, case study, learning objects, streaming video, and other rich resources. Discussion boards could be used to pose clinical questions or problems related to the learning objective.

Simulation is increasingly used in the laboratory and can vary from assessment practice and interactions with a low-fidelity mannequin to an entire clinical scenario with a high-fidelity mannequin. Other types of simulation include computer-based case study, procedural simulators, or even virtual reality. Whatever simulation type is chosen, a Web-enhanced assignment can enrich the experience. Presimulation preparation can include selected reading, skills review, online review of the simulation patient's medical record, and care plan/care map preparation. Other presimulation exercises could include discussion questions and pre-/post-assessment questions. Post-simulation should include a debriefing session. Part of the debriefing could include having the student complete an online post-test, contribute to a threaded discussion board, submit a completed care plan/care map, and/or journal about the simulation experience.

There are many advantages to the Web-enhanced experience for laboratory. From the student perspective it provides flexibility and learner control. The student can work at his own pace and practice or go over the material multiple times if needed in a nonthreatening environment. Pre- and post-laboratory preparation free laboratory time from some of the more mundane chores and facilitate active learning by allowing more time for students to practice nursing process, decision-making skills, and engage in critical thinking.

Clinical

Clinical experience is a vital part of nursing education. This is where the rubber meets the road and the student is truly required to combine knowledge and skills in a complex environment. Clinical locations and environments vary and during the course of the nursing program a student may go to a variety of clinical locations and interact with several clinical instructors and/or preceptors. A Web-enhanced environment can greatly improve student/faculty communication and support success in the clinical environment.

Communication is a fundamental part of any educational experience but can be a problem in clinical where clinical instructors often are not full-time faculty and may only teach a group of students for a relatively short period of time and in varying locations. Clinical instructor contact information, clinical schedule, expectations, and agency-specific information can be posted on the course Web environment. Students can post information about themselves for the clinical instructor and vice versa. E-mail, chat rooms, and threaded discussion also can provide a forum for students and instructors to meet.

Clinical agency information also can be made available on the course home page. Often, agencies have specific mandatory requirements over and above that of the school. Links to agency paperwork can be made available; the student can download, complete, and submit paperwork before the start of the clinical rotation. Some agencies have a Web-based mandatory requirement site for students. The link and instructions for accessing such a site can be placed online. Parking information, agency maps, and agency orientation materials also can be posted online for the student to review before the first clinical day. This information would be not only beneficial to the student but also to the clinical instructor.

Preclinical assignments can be placed online to assist the student with preparation for a particular clinical experience. An example would be to have the student practice listening to heart/lung sounds online or to watch physical assessment on streaming video on another Web site. Preclinical assignments may involve preparation for specific patient populations. For example, before an obstetrics clinical experience a preclinical assignment may include online assignments and activities covering such topics as stages and phases of labor, post partum normals, and newborn assessment. Students preparing for and engaged in a community clinical experience will find the Web-supported environment an ideal place for research and to document findings on the selected experience.

A discussion board is another useful adjunct to clinical. Threaded discussion boards can be used either in lieu of or as an adjunct to pre- or post-clinical conferences. In many clinical situations, such as community or preceptorship, students are not all at the same agency and there is no convenient way to get them together to share and reflect on their experience. Faculty could facilitate a synchronous or asynchronous threaded discussion board that would allow the students to reflect on clinical learning, problems, or other key concepts. Journaling and reflection, which have been shown to enhance higher-level thinking skills (Billings & Halstead, 2009), also could be facilitated through e-mail or the course management system.

The Web-enhanced environment is conducive to document management. Care plans or care maps can be electronically submitted, reviewed by the clinical faculty and returned to the student with feedback. An online skills list could be updated by the student and reviewed by faculty. Student sharing and collaboration can be facilitated on the Web. Students can use a Wiki to work together on clinical assignments such as care plans and care mapping. They can also team up on patient teaching projects, community assignments, or even share self-created medication cards.

Course, faculty, and agency evaluation is an important part of the clinical experience. Links for all can be placed online allowing the student easy accessibility. Many of the course management systems have evaluation and survey capabilities that allow confidentiality for the student and ease of accessibility of data for the faculty and nursing program. This also provides an opportunity to summarize and share information with all involved faculty and the clinical facility.

Classroom

As in laboratory or clinical, the Web-enhanced class promotes flexibility and an interactive learning environment by allowing faculty to shift from the usual content-delivery mode to

---

BOX 6.1

HIPAA CAUTION

Caution! Patient Privacy in Cyberspace

Online journaling and collaboration is wonderful but the Health Insurance Portability and Accountability Act (HIPAA) of 1996 privacy guidelines for protected health information (PHI) must be maintained. Be sure to reinforce guidelines for HIPAA related to online activities. There have been some legal issues and lawsuits filed against nurses related to potential violation of PHI in online blogging and social networking (McBride & Cohen, 2009).

active and collaborative learning. At a minimum, the course syllabus, announcements, and contact information can be placed online. Handouts and PowerPoint presentations also are commonly made available online. Audio can easily be added to PowerPoints with free tools such as Audacity. From those basic changes, the possibilities are endless and exciting as faculty begin to discover, explore, and use different methodologies to engage the students in active learning and accomplish the student learning objectives.

Preclass assignments can be designed to prepare the student for the classroom. The assignment could be as simple as a focused reading assignment and a post quiz. The quiz gives immediate feedback so the student can review content not fully understood before to class. A preclass assignment could be in the form of a self-contained module complete with objectives, focused learning activities, and some type of evaluation. "Muddiest Point" and "Minute Paper" (Angelo & Cross, 1993) are examples of traditional classroom assessment techniques that can also become part of the Web-enhanced environment by incorporating on a threaded discussion board (Billings & Halstead, 2009).

Faculty may feel overwhelmed at the thought of creating pedagogically sound Web-based learning materials. The good news is that there is a plethora of wonderful items already available on the Web. Learning objects are "small, reusable components of instructional media" (NEAT, 2006). Learning objects can be games, simulations, images, sound, pictures, streaming video, or modules that can be modified and repackaged to be used in different courses and contexts. They are generally self-contained, retrievable, and designed with a specified learning objective or outcome (Whitsed, 2004).

Learning objects can be created by faculty or found on the Web in a number of places but the most convenient is a learning object repository. An example is the Nursing Education and Technology (NEAT) repository, available at http://webcls.utmb.edu/neat. In partnership with the University of Texas Medical Branch, NEAT provides access to a number of learning objects including nursing-related objects focusing on nursing theory, education, and patient safety (NEAT, 2006). There is no fee to use the Web site but registration is required. The available learning objects range from simple, using graphics and/or pictures, to very interactive and complex. Recommended software and technical information are all listed on the Web site.

Multimedia Educational Resource for Learning and Online Teaching (MERLOT) is another example of a learning object repository. MERLOT, available at http://www.merlot.org, is a huge collection of peer-reviewed learning materials and activities in a wide variety of disciplines. There are many nursing-related topics including *The Auscultation Assistant* with heart and lung sounds, a 12-lead EKG tutorial, and an interactive tutorial on assessing blood pressure. The content is licensed under Creative Commons license conditions. Registration is free and there is the option to submit your own learning objects or become a peer reviewer.

Professional organizations are a superb source of educational material. The American Heart Association and the American Diabetes Association both have excellent educational resources including guidelines, statements, clinical updates, patient educational materials, lectures, and slide sets. The Society of Critical Care Medicine offers educational material for the critical care environment. The variety of offerings includes slides, podcasts, vodcasts, and clinical guidelines. One example is the Pulmonary Artery Catheter Education Project (PACEP). This educational offering is free; the user will need to register, however. Interactive lessons are designed to advance from novice to expert and include pre- and post-tests, case studies, and audio lecture. PACEP would be effective in a beginning critical care course or preclinical/clinical preparation for an intensive care rotation. PACEP is endorsed by the American Association of Critical Care Nurses and is available at www.learnicu.org.

Another abundant source of educational materials is government agencies. The Centers for Disease Control and Prevention (www.cdc.gov) is loaded with information on disease conditions and other topics such as emergency preparedness and bioterrorism. Educational resources include webinars, slide sets, pod casts, PDA applications, reports, articles, patient teaching guidelines, and fact sheets. The Institute for Health Care Improvement offers online learning modules with topics including patient safety, teamwork and communication, quality improvement, and health-care leadership (http://ihi.org/lms/onlinelearning.aspx).

Publishing companies generally provide rich support for their textbooks. Instructor resources often are online and include downloadable PowerPoints, pictures, graphs, animations, streaming video, case studies, and other interactive activities that easily can be linked to a learning module or Web site.

Faculty may want to explore creating his or her own learning activity or learning object. There are many wonderful tools to assist with this; some of them are free and some are quite expensive. SoftChalk is an example of a Web lesson packaging tool that is easy to use and allows faculty to create learning objects and easily add content, create games, and add images and Web links. Evaluations can be created in multiple choice, multiple option, true/false, matching, and ordering format. Feedback can be embedded into each evaluation. Faculty can choose from a number of different templates, layouts, and styles (http://www.softchalk.com). The modules are packaged and easily uploaded to a Web site or course management system. A free 30-day trial is available and can be downloaded from the Web site.

TABLE 6.4

Practical Tools: Examples of Learning Sites

Inner body—Human anatomy • Point and click • Explanations, video clips	http://www.innerbody.com/htm/body.html
The virtual body (in English and Spanish) • Brain, skeleton, heart, digestive tract • Information, animations, games	http://www.ehc.com/VBody.asp
BBC Science and Nature • Body—senses, skeleton, muscles, nervous system • Psychology • Fun games	http://www.bbc.co.uk/science/humanbody/index.shtml
Physical examination • Video clips showing selected adult physical examination	http://opeta.medinfo.ufl.edu/
Cincinnati Children's Hospital Cardiac anomalies/defects • Information: s/s, diagnosis, TX • Flash movies • Illustrations	http://www.cincinnatichildrens.org/health/heart-encyclopedia/anomalies/asd.htm

Continued

TABLE 6.4—cont'd

Practical Tools: Examples of Learning Sites

Cardiac cycle • Animation with explanation of EKG, heart sounds, cardiac pressures	http://library.med.utah.edu/kw/pharm/hyper_heart1.html
Heart sounds and cardiac arrhythmias • Tutorials, animations, quizzes • Fun online tools	http://www.blaufuss.org/
The auscultation assistant • Practice listening to selected heart/lung sounds	http://www.wilkes.med.ucla.edu/inex.htm
Acid-base tutorial	http://www.acid-base.com/
Eye simulation • See how problems with cranial nerves and eye muscles affect eye movement	http://rad.usuhs.mil/rad/eye_simulator/eyesimulator.html
Critical care medicine tutorials • Variety of critical care case studies	http://www.ccmtutorials.com/
University of Missouri-Columbia virtual health care team • Wide variety of case studies	http://www.vhct.org/studies.htm
Nobel Foundation—education based on past Nobel Prize awards • Games include blood typing, diabetes, EKG, tuberculosis	http://nobelprize.org/educational_games/medicine/
Health Education Assets Library • Variety of reusable learning objects	http://www.healcentral.org
Nursing Education and Technology NEAT • Nursing education learning objects	http://tlcprojects.org/NEATarchive/learningobjects.htm
Wright State University College of Nursing • Shareable Learning Objects	http://www.wright.edu/nursing/shareableobjects
MERLOT • Wide variety of learning materials	http://www.merlot.org/merlot/index.htm
Wisconsin Technical College • Learning objects	http://www.wisc-online.com/ListObjects.aspx
University of Nottingham • Learning objects	http://www.nottingham.ac.uk/nmp/sonet/rlos/

Podcasting is becoming more popular as an enhancement to educational technology (see Table 15.2 in Chapter 15 for keys to creating a podcast). Unlike using a tape recorder to record a lecture, a digital recording is downloaded to either a desktop computer, iPod, or other MP3 device. Forbes and Hickey (2008) suggest that a lecture be divided into smaller files to help with ease of loading and to make it easier for the student to find a particular topic. Podcasting lectures or chunks of learning material make learning portable and accessible.

YouTube is a technology that is also becoming more accepted in the education arena. The audience for video sharing sites such as YouTube and Google Video has grown phenomenally. A Pew Internet report stated that 62% of all adult Internet users have watched a video on one of the sites (Madden, 2009). Although this popular technology is typically thought of more as a social phenomenon, it can and is being used for educational purposes. A professor at Berkeley University found herself getting fan e-mail for her lectures on anatomy and neuroscience (Young, 2008). Faculty could record a lecture or demonstration, download it to YouTube and put the link on the course access site. Students can use YouTube to collaborate on a learning project. There are also a number of interesting, well-done nursing-related videos already on YouTube that could be linked into a course Web site.

Virtual reality has interesting potential for the clinical, laboratory, or classroom experience. Within a virtual environment, a student has the opportunity to apply knowledge through participation in simulated real-life learning in a safe environment. Virtual reality can be as simple as an instructor-created role play to a three-dimensional (3-D) world such as Second Life. Second Life has not only peaked the interest and imagination of millions of individuals but companies, industries, and institutes of higher learning are all interested and excited about the potential for learning, communication, and collaboration.

A participant in Second Life is symbolized by an avatar that can move through the 3-D environment and interact with other people and objects. The University of Wisconsin Oshkosh (UWO) implemented a presence in Second Life as enhancement for clinical in an online accelerated nursing program. Students were provided an orientation to the virtual reality environment that was initially used for group discussion, case study analysis, and faculty virtual office hours. UWO faculty and student presence in Second Life has increased and interactive scenarios are being developed for disaster planning and public health (Schmidt & Stewart, 2009).

This type of technology, although it has amazing possibilities, can seem complex and overwhelming to the student. Lessons learned by UWO staff include the importance and timing of orientation and preparation for students. Orientation should include specifics about technical specifications, navigating the system, class expectations, and technical assistance (Schmidt & Stewart, 2009). These lessons can be applied anytime very technical approaches are launched. It is important to plan for both the expected and the unexpected and be prepared to make changes and adapt to feedback as necessary. Be patient! Much of the aforementioned technology comes with a learning curve and jumping off the ship too quickly can cause faculty and students to miss out on a wonderful, exciting learning experience.

ASSESSMENT IN WEB-SUPPORTED ENVIRONMENTS

Assessment is a dynamic process that can be both formative and summative and is designed to evaluate student learning. In a Web-supported environment, the instructor may elect to perform many assessments in the traditional, f-2-f manner with multiple-choice, fill-in-the-blank, or other common types of examinations as well as practicum and clinical evaluations. These are effective and if thoughtfully constructed, will adequately assess the student learning outcomes of the course.

As with any assessment, it is vital to make sure that the material that is being assessed is meaningful, the assessment itself is thoughtfully created, and the purpose of the assessment is clearly defined. It is important to specify the criteria that will be used for judging student performance on an assessment. Instructors should be as specific as possible and provide a sample or rubric whenever possible to give students a better idea of exemplary work. An assessment should be used to refine the assessment process, revise curriculum and instruction, and provide feedback to students.

There also is a great opportunity for instructors to assess the student's ability in the Web-supported portions of the course. Whether or not these assessments are part of the final grade or simply included as activities or extra points, that is up to the instructor, but the richness of this type of diverse assessment should not be dismissed!

Assessment in Web-supported environments may include evaluation of the student's ability to interact with peers during either online group activities as part of the ongoing assessment process or in an online discussion board, peer evaluation, and self-evaluation. Evaluation of the student also may involve the review of an online e-portfolio that tracks the student progress through several courses and houses artifacts or learning objects that the student has completed as part of her or his coursework.

Faculty also may elect to have "open book" (or open computer) quizzes, papers, or other types of online assessments for students. In Web-supported learning environments, the instructor usually creates, defines, and facilitates the evaluation, but the student may have a more participative role in defining the process and play an active role in group assessment, peer assessments, self-evaluation, and the creation of an online e-portfolio.

An electronic or digital portfolio, commonly called an e-portfolio, is used to maintain a record of student work over a period of time (process or developmental portfolio) and also may be used to allow the student to review his or her own work and observe the learning that has occurred (personal reflective portfolio). It also may be used as a showcase portfolio to highlight exemplary work or projects that are selected by the student to showcase his or her work to potential employers or colleges/universities. E-portfolios also are used for peer and self-review as well as group projects and can provide an excellent means of alternative assessment. E-portfolios benefit students by showing learning progression, focusing the student on learning outcomes, and organizing assignments and projects so they may be easily retrieved and reviewed (Abrami & Barrett, 2005).

TECHNOLOGY TIP 6.1

Will it be on the test? NO! It is the test! Assessment in a Web-supported class can involve many formats. The instructor may want to offer pre- and post-tests, multiple-choice, fill-in the blanks, matching, or drag and drop types of quizzes. These can be a great way to use the alternate format style questions. Many learning platforms offer ways to make these more challenging. You can do a limited-time, password protected examination in which all students have a window of time to sign on, put in a unique password, and then complete the assessment. Although not totally secure, this environment can add a different dimension to the testing toolbox!

Assessment of Student Interaction With Peers

The assessment of interaction among peers can be difficult. Some instructors elect to mandate the number of postings/replies, number of days that the student participates in a discussion forum, or the number of words necessary to formulate a substantive reply. Assessment may range from the assignment of points for participation to simply making it a course requirement to access the Web-enhancements that are provided.

There is research to support the analysis of computer-supported collaborative learning (CSCL) and the concept that knowledge can be developed and retained as well as critical thinking fostered based on social interaction with peers and instructors (Garrison & Anderson, 2003; Pozzi, Manca, Persico, & Sarti, 2007). In collaborative learning in the Web-supported environment, the instructor may elect to use a discussion board for frequently asked questions, to provide a space for students to post concepts and ideas, or the instructor may elect to use the discussion forum to provide another avenue for assessment of course concepts. A record of student interaction, collaboration, and participation can be part of a grading rubric. It also is an opportunity for instructors to observe the student's time management abilities, respect for another's opinions, observe problem-solving skills, and the ability of the student to achieve consensus among group members.

Peer-evaluation

Peer evaluation is an interactive process and a type of formative assessment that can be valuable in the Web-supported environment. The assessment performed by peers involves the student in the evaluation process and provides the student with a different perspective encouraging reflection, thoughtful inquiry, and critical thinking. When using peer review, it is vital to involve the students in creating the assessment criteria, obtain student input in developing the form or rubric used for review, and providing examples of evaluations to model the assessments for students.

It is important to keep in mind that peer evaluation does not replace the evaluation by the instructor, nor should it be heavily weighted in the overall course grade. Ideally, it can be a formative assessment that is well developed and clearly defined by the instructor, encouraging independence in the student. It should be noted that there is research both for and against the use of peer evaluation. Issues with reliability and validity have been cited and concerns have been voiced about the fairness in one student evaluating another student's work (Bouzidi & Jaillet, 2009). In a 2003 article, Charles Juwah reported that participation in peer evaluation contributed to increased self-assessment by students, leading to a higher quality standard of practice and a higher level of performance.

Self-evaluation

Self-evaluation in any type of class environment is a great method for students to reflect on what they have learned, what they realized they need more practice with, and the attainment of learning goals that they have generated for themselves. There are a wide variety of self-assessments available for use in the Web-supported environment. These assessments include pre- and post-tests, simulations, formative grading rubrics, and multiple-choice practice examinations, as well as activities and exercises that are designed to give immediate feedback and rationales to the student.

TABLE 6.5

Checklist for Designing Self-Assessment Tools

- Select meaningful topics for the assessment, don't select minor concepts or unimportant content.
- Be clear with your instructions!
- Design the self-assessment so that the student is ready to assess a "chunk" of information and not be distracted by too frequent or too large of an assessment.
- Give meaningful feedback because this is what will either correct the information or reinforce the learning.
- Give feedback at the appropriate time—in simulations it might be more suitable to wait until the end of the activity and then provide a comprehensive review; in a multiple-choice quiz, it is usually more appropriate to provide immediate feedback right after the question is answered.
- Self-assessment should have an element of fun and be a good reflection of student learning.

Self-evaluation is an excellent way for the student to spot-check his or her own learning, focus on what has been learned, engage in application of new content, and it provides another avenue for instructors to gauge the extent to which students are meeting the learning outcomes of the course. Self-assessment and peer evaluation, can be part of both the formative and summative assessment in a Web-supported environment, adding another dimension to the traditional testing strategies used by the instructor.

No matter what type of assessments the instructor and student engage in, the evaluation of student learning and the relationship of the assessment to the attainment of the student learning outcomes is of primary importance. Assessment can be both formative and summative and the assessments related to the Web-supported content can truly add value for the student and help to foster independent, critical thinking.

CONCLUSION

The goal of this chapter has been to give a broad overview and provide some practical strategies for instructors who wish to add Web components to their course. Web-supported environments have the best of both worlds. The students have the benefit of f-2-f learning with the instructor present and they also have the value-add of all of the Web-enhancements that are now available. Authentic learning is "real world" application and provides nursing students the exposure and experiences that they need to be successful in land-based clinical and practice settings. Technology has created a wonderful platform for authentic learning and scaffolding of knowledge. Students now can experience access to tools and resources that were simply not available just a few years ago.

Web-supported learning can have an impact on all of the learning domains and there are a variety of items available to address the way that students learn and retain knowledge. Cognitive learning tools assist with knowledge construction and expand the opportunities for all students to practice new skills and learn new concepts.

Adapting a new pedagogy like Web-enhanced learning can be both exciting and terrifying at the same time. Instructors need to begin with something small, and be sure to match planned activities to learning outcomes. Web-supported environments encourage creativity and can provide solid content and information in addition to making learning fun! Web-enhancement increases communication, collaboration, authentic learning, and critical thinking in laboratory, clinical, and the classroom and, equally important, it helps the student work more independently to achieve student learning outcomes.

Assessment in the Web-supported environment should not be discounted. Even though instructors will still provide traditional assessment in the f-2-f classroom, the online evaluations can provide variety and offer opportunities for peer input and in-depth self-evaluation. There are a variety of assessments now available in the online classroom and instructors can proffer a different perspective on assessment by including the student in both the formative and summative process of evaluation.

For the instructor, the first step in offering students a new learning adventure in a Web-supported environment can be the most difficult, but it is time to take the plunge! Select one learning object or Web-enhancement to add to a current course. Tell the students what to do with it, how to do it, and how it will be evaluated. Solicit feedback, make revisions, and add another component to the next course. Before long, you will have created an innovative, dynamic course that will provide a rich, invigorating learning environment for your students.

REFERENCES

Abrami, P. C., & Barrett, H. (2005). Directions for research and development on electronic portfolios. *Canadian Journal of Learning and Technology, 31*(3).

Allen, E. B., Walls, R. T., & Reilly, F. D. (2008). Effects of interactive instructional techniques in a web-based peripheral nervous system component for human anatomy. *Medical Teacher, 30,* 40–47. doi: 10.1080/01421590701753518

Angelo, T., & Cross, P. (1993). *Classroom assessment techniques.* San Francisco: Jossey-Bass.

Bartini, M. (2008). An empirical comparison of traditional and web-enhanced classrooms. *Journal of Instructional Psychology, 35*(1), 3–11.

Billings, D. M., & Halstead, J. A. (2009). *Teaching in nursing: A guide for faculty* (3rd ed.). St. Louis: Saunders.

Bouzidi, L., & Jaillet, A. (2009). Can online peer assessment be trusted? *Educational Technology & Society, 12*(4), 257–268.

Bowen, J. A. (2006). Teaching naked: Why removing technology from your classroom will improve student learning. *The National Teaching and Learning Forum, 16*(1).

Brush, T. A., & Saye, J. W. (2002). A summary of research exploring hard and soft scaffolding for teachers and students using a multimedia supported learning environment. *The Journal of Interactive Online Learning, 1*(2).

Creative Commons. (2009, October 11). Frequently asked questions. Retrieved from http://wiki.creativecommons.org/Frequently_Asked_Questions

Forbes, M. O., & Hickey, M. T. (2008). Podcasting: Implementation and evaluation in an undergraduate nursing program. *Nurse Educator, 33*(5), 224–227.

Garrison, R., & Anderson, T. (2003). *E-learning in the 21st century. A framework for research and practice.* London and New York: Routledge Falmer.

Good models of teaching with technology. (2009). Retrieved from The Knowledge Loom: http://knowledgeloom.org

Juwah, C. (2003). Using peer assessment to develop skills and capabilities. *Journal of the United States Distance Learning Association, 17*(1), retrieved from http://www.usdla.org/html/journal/JAN03_Issue/article04.html

Kim, B., & Reeves, T. C. (2007). Reframing research on learning with technology: In search of the meaning of cognitive tools. *Instructional Science, 35*(3), 207–256.

Krathwohl, D. R. (2002). A revision of Bloom's taxonomy: An overview. *Theory Into Practice, 41*(4), 212–218.

Lashley, M. (2005). Teaching health assessment in the virtual classroom. *Journal of Nursing Education, 44*(8), 348–350.

Lim, J., Kim, M., Chen, S. S., & Ryder, C. E. (2008). An empirical investigation of student achievement and satisfaction in different learning environments. *Journal of Instructional Psychology, 35*(2), 113–119.

Lombardi, M. M. (2007, May). Authentic learning for the 21st century: An overview. *Educause Learning Initiatives*, white paper.

Madden, M. (July 2009). The audience for online video-sharing sites shoots up. *Pew Internet & American Life Project.* Retrieved from http://pewinternet.org

McBride, D., & Cohen, E. (2009). Misuse of social networking may have ethical implications for nurses. *ONS Connect, 24*(7), 17.

Nursing Education and Technology (NEAT). (2006). Learning object repository. Retrieved from http://webcls.utmb.edu/neat/

Pozzi, F., Manca, S., Persico, D., & Sarti, L. (2007). A general framework for tracking and analyzing learning processes in computer-supported collaborative learning environments. *Innovations in Education and Teaching International, 44*(2), 169–179.

Rhoads, J., & White, C. (2008). Copyright law and distance nursing education. *Nurse Educator, 33*(1), 39–44.

Salyers, V. L. (2005). Web-enhanced and face-to-face classroom instructional methods: Effects on course outcomes and student satisfaction. *International Journal of Nursing Education Scholarship, 2*(1).

Schmidt, B., & Stewart, S. (2009). Implementing the virtual reality learning environment: Second life. *Nurse Educator, 34*(4), 152–155.

Simonson, M., Smaldino, S., Albright, M., & Zvacek, S. (2006). Teaching and learning at a distance: Foundations of distance education (3rd ed.). Upper Saddle River, NJ: Merrill Prentice Hall.

Whitsed, N. (2004). Learning and teaching: An introduction to re-using learning materials in learning and teaching. *Health Information and Libraries Journal, 21*, 201–205.

Wink, E. (2009). Sources of fully developed course materials on the web. *Nurse Educator, 34*(4), 143–145.

Young, J. R. (2008, January 25). YouTube professors: Scholars as online video stars. *The Chronicle of Higher Education.* Retrieved from http://chronicle.com

Chapter 7

Hybrid Environments

Margaret Blodgett, PhD, EdS, OTR

"Since I started using online activities as a part of my course, students now come to class prepared to do more active learning. They review the lecture information online and participate in an online discussion prior to the class where we apply the concepts. So during our face-to-face classes I now spend most of the time on active learning and lab activities. I've been able to work with students at a more in-depth level on the course content than ever before. Now they are spending more time applying clinical concepts than just listening to me talk about them."

. . .Allied Health Faculty Member

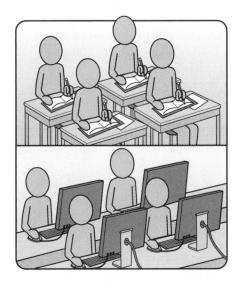

Hybrid (also called "blended" or "multi-modal") learning environments are those that incorporate both face-to-face (f-2-f) and online learning methods within one course (Reynard, 2007). The intent is to provide active, collaborative learning experiences in a manner that keeps students engaged in the learning process between f-2-f meetings and in contact with instructors. In some cases, the online activities provide a means of reducing the amount of f-2-f time needed to accomplish in-depth learning. The learning experiences are, thus, more accessible to students who might otherwise not be able to participate in such courses because of time or geographic obstacles.

As with all educational strategies, a theoretical framework provides guidance in enhancing the learning experience. Chickering and Gamson's (1987, para. 1) "Seven Principles of Good Practice" have long been referenced as the ideal way to design higher education courses, no matter what the discipline. These good practice principles encourage student-instructor contact, cooperation among students, active learning, and time on task, among others. More recently, Chickering and Ehrmann (1996) extended the use of these principles to describe ways to effectively implement technology into educational experiences. Today these principles and their application to technology implementation at all levels of education are widely accepted (Ehrmann, 2008). A hybrid approach to teaching can provide several opportunities to implement these principles while assuring effective use of technology to meet learner's needs.

DavisPlus | For additional resources please visit
http://davisplus.fadavis.com

Chickering and Gamsons's (1987) 7 Principles of Good Practice in Undergraduate Education are:

1. Good practice encourages contact between students and faculty.
2. Good practice develops reciprocity and cooperation among students.
3. Good practice encourages active learning.
4. Good practice gives prompt feedback.
5. Good practice emphasizes time on task.
6. Good practice communicates high expectations.
7. Good practice respects diverse talents and ways of learning.

An important technology to help facilitate these principles is the Learning Management System (LMS). The LMS includes Internet-based software such as Blackboard, Angel, and eCollege. The LMS can be acquired through a site license for an entire college, free from a book publisher for one course, or as a free (open-source) system such as Moodle (http://moodle.org/about/).

The typical LMS will provide a number of tools that emulate a classroom environment. These include the folloing:

Secure login: Only students and faculty assigned to a particular course will have access to the course Web site and materials. Although technical support may be provided to assist the faculty, generally only the person teaching the course can make changes to the course Web site. Note that the typical setup of LMS courses is through the college or university, with access provided only to faculty and students enrolled in the particular course. However, special arrangements can be made to provide access to other individuals involved with the clinical experience. This would be arranged through the Instructional Technology systems manager at the school.

Folders: Folders are used to organize the course materials. Typical folder arrangement will be by weeks or units of the course or by types of materials (assignments, lectures, tests, resources).

File upload: Word processor documents (.doc, .docx, .wpd), portable document format (.pdf) files, or HTML (Web page format) pages are the typical format for posting files within an LMS. Although other file formats are allowed, it is generally suggested the files be posted in a universal format to avoid software incompatibility issues for students.

E-mail: The LMS provides an e-mail system that is contained within each course. Student e-mail to the instructor is easy to follow-up and track. This avoids tracking personal e-mail addresses and avoids loss of student communications amidst other professional e-mail in one's personal account. Each school or department should have policies on the use of e-mail. Policies should specify the following:
- Approved e-mail system (LMS, university, personal)
- Need for antivirus and spyware software
- Acceptable maximum size of attachments
- Expected response time for student and faculty

Discussion forum: This tool provides a means to set up threaded discussions, personal journals, weblog (Blog), and WiKi formats for communication among course members. Discussion forums provide an interactive component to the online activities.

Assessment tool: These include quizzes and tests that can be developed using multiple-choice, true/false, matching, fill in the blanks, and essay questions. Testing can be set up as self-study quizzes or timed tests that are taken on a specific date and time. Anonymous surveys also are a typical option for assessment setup.

Assignment dropboxes: These tools allow for electronic submission of files. Typically, these dropboxes are used for graded assignments such as papers, worksheets, and pictures. Dropboxes provide a means for students to attach files, make comments, and submit the assignment. The instructor can then download assignments and return them to the students in the same dropbox with feedback and grades.

Electronic gradebook: All LMS provide electronic gradebooks. As long as the instructor regularly enters assignment grades, the students can easily keep track of their progress. Typically, grades entered through the quiz tool, discussion forum, and assignment dropboxes will automatically submit to the gradebook, reducing the time instructors need to communicate grading information to students. When tracking nongraded items (e.g., CPR expiration, TB skin test expiration), the gradebook also can be used. Assign these nongraded items a value of zero. When the student has met this requirement, enter a zero in the gradebook. To ensure privacy, students can only see their personal grades in the electronic gradebook.

Access to other resources: Multiple types of resources can be posted within an LMS course. These may include video presentations by faculty or guest lecturers, video demonstrations of treatment techniques, chat boards for quick, real-time Q&A sessions with a few students, and Web links to a multitude of resources.

The following discussion describes ways that instructors can use LMS tools to support f-2-f learning with online activities that provide effective ways to enhance communication, assessment, and organization/management. Instructors can add any or all of these features to a f-2-f course as a means to increase students' time on task, encourage contacts between students and faculty, and provide feedback. Although it may be appealing to add all of these techniques to courses, a suggestion is to implement a few at a time. Developing the use of these tools will require an investment in time but the resulting engagement of students in the learning process will be well worth the effort.

HYBRID APPROACH TO SUPPORT CLINICAL EXPERIENCE

The use of a hybrid environment as a support to faculty and students during clinical nursing experiences enhances quality and efficiency (Ireland, Martindale, Johnson, Adams, Eboh, & Mowatt, 2009). Most students, agencies, and clients now have computers with access to the Internet; therefore, it is possible to keep all the persons involved in students' clinical experience in close communication through the use of electronic tools such as e-mail, an LMS class Web site, and even video.

Communication

Good practice encourages contact between students and faculty. Faculty should clarify expectations on response time for communication and grading (e.g., all e-mails will be addressed within 24 hours Monday–Friday). The LMS provides a secure location for

EVIDENCE-BASED PRACTICE BOX 7.1

Blended Learning in Nursing Education

Issue: What Are Students' Evaluation of Gained Knowledge and Level of Satisfaction Following Completion of a Blended Learning Course Addressing Research and Evidence-based Practice Principles?

The study used a mixed-methods design to complete a longitudinal cohort study of nursing students who participated in a course on research and evidence-based practice that was presented in a blended (online and f-2-f) format. The study was done in three phases—a questionnaire, a focus group, and telephone interviews.

Study Findings

This study measured both knowledge gained and satisfaction with a blended learning approach to the topic of research and evidence-based practice for a second-year undergraduate nursing course. Participants submitted quantitative and qualitative data that gave evidence of positive attitudes toward both f-2-f and online activities and satisfaction with learning on most of the course content. Knowledge gained was reasonably high in comparison with previous presentation of this content in only lecture format.

Nursing Implications

- Blended learning courses are seen as a positive way to learn by students.
- Blended learning can address the range of learning styles of nursing students.
- Acquisition of knowledge, particularly of difficult or abstract concepts, may increase when taught through a blended approach.
- Experience in a blended learning course may encourage life-long learning skills (Ireland, Martindale, Johnson, Adams, Eboh, & Mowatt, 2009).

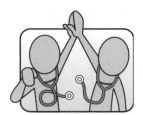

exchange of information. The e-mail system provides a means for personal interactions throughout the week and may be the easiest way for an instructor to share information outside of class and clinical time. A chat tool may be used to hold "virtual office hours" allowing students to ask quick questions without having to stay on-campus and find the instructor in his or her office. An advantage to this type of office hours for the faculty is that they can be available from any location (home, office, clinical agency).

If the desire is to have communication with clinical preceptors (if they are not the course instructor) and other agency personnel, consider inviting them to participate in short online sessions. Most LMS administrators have a process that allows for guest accounts. Guest logins can allow access only to specific parts of the online course while protecting private information such as student grades and communication with the instructor. Typically a preceptor or agency representative will be invited to participate in or facilitate a discussion forum or host an online lecture or meeting. Be sure to provide the guest lecturer with training on the system tools and give them a chance to run through their activity before the actual session that they will provide. Arrange this with your Instructional Technology support staff as early as possible to avoid problems and to allow for training time.

Preclinical Preparation and Assessment

Good practice encourages high expectations. Preparation for clinical can be done through the use of tools such as discussions, webinars, and even electronic books. The discussions can happen in an online forum where students share their findings while preparing for clinical. Some faculty may even ask students to post their care plan or medication cards to the drop-box before clinical. Webinars may be used as a way to have a live online discussion (with or without video) to address any concerns before clinical. Electronic textbooks can be used by students and faculty to bookmark, highlight, and even share important information that may need to be quickly accessed during clinical (Fig. 7.1).

Good practice encourages active learning, and gives prompt feedback. The use of the assessment tool in the LMS provides faculty and students with a convenient way to evaluate student preparation for clinical experience through the use of preclinical assessments. These assessments can be developed by the faculty or taken from textbook test banks and practice examinations for national boards. LMS assessment tools provide options for a variety of question

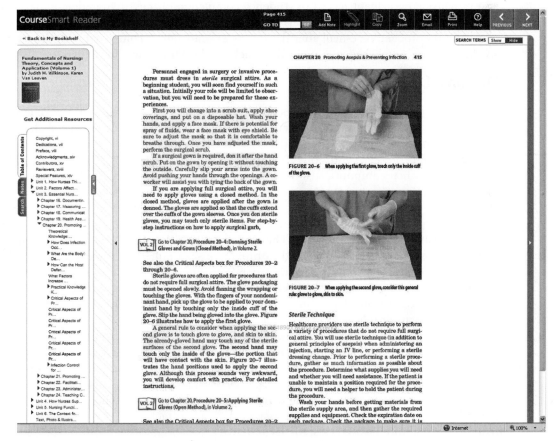

Figure 7.1 Electronic textbooks can be used by students and faculty to bookmark, highlight, and even share important information that may need to be quickly accessed during clinical.

types (multiple choice, true/false, matching, fill-in-the-blanks, essay) and can be automatically graded by the system, manually graded by the faculty, or a combination of those options.

Testing can be set up in multiple formats. Self-study quizzes can be completed by students in time frames that are convenient to their schedules and can be repeated multiple times. This allows students to check their understanding frequently as they prepare for clinical experiences. Timed testing gives students the experience of taking certification examinations and reduces the opportunity for students to look up answers as they take the test. Depending on what outcomes are desired, testing can be proctored in an on-campus computer laboratory or completed asynchronously (i.e., in the student's preferred time) online.

In addition, most LMS provide an option to do surveys, or anonymous testing. This format can be useful for getting feedback from students about how prepared they feel or to let them make comments and ask questions that they might not feel comfortable asking in class.

Interactive media also can be an important part of clinical preparation. Video or audio lecture information can be posted on such topics as universal precautions, blood-borne pathogens, or patient handling techniques. Some presentations may need to be viewed annually and followed by an online quiz or survey. This format not only saves f-2-f course time but also provides a permanent record of students' completion of these required activities. Automated "agents" in some LMS programs (such as ANGEL) can even send a certificate of completion to the student via e-mail after the review examination is completed with the required score. This is accomplished automatically, which can be a time-saver for the instructor.

Document Management

Good practice emphasizes time on task and communicates high expectations. The use of a hybrid approach to support document management provides students with a clear message that work is expected throughout the time they are enrolled in the course, not just during f-2-f meetings. In addition, providing access to course activities in an organized, professional format communicates the high level of work that is expected in clinical practice. During clinical experiences, students may or may not have regular contact with faculty; therefore, a clear process for keeping track of documents is essential. These may be assignments that must be submitted to the instructor or documents that the instructor needs to distribute to the students. The use of an LMS is an ideal way to conveniently deliver documents to students as well as provide a secure method for students to submit their work. Documents posted on the course Web site are available to the students 24/7, as long as they can access the Internet. Students also can submit required coursework to the instructor right from their clinical site, as they complete a requirement, through the use of assignment dropboxes.

There are several advantages to using a class Web site for document management during clinical experiences. Students are in multiple locations throughout the week and may or may not be in f-2-f contact with faculty at specific times. Electronic submission of assignments and online discussion about clinical experiences provides all participants with the same information and instructor access without requiring extra trips to the school campus. In addition, electronic submission avoids lost assignments, easy tracking of submission times, and reduces the amount of materials students and instructors need to carry with them from location to location. Finally, a well organized course Web site will provide students with a vision of the type of document management that is required in professional practice.

Online Post Conference (Synchronous/Asynchronous)

Good practice gives prompt feedback. The use of online tools to provide post conference feedback provides students and faculty with a format for accomplishing this important learning activity in a timely format that allows for an interactive process. Upon completion of a clinical experience, the student needs clear feedback on his or her performance before moving to the next level of training or graduating. Several players need to have input on this feedback process, including the student, preceptor, course instructor (if different from the preceptor), and other professionals involved in the students' training.

The ideal tool for this process is a webcasting program. Each individual can be in their location and only need access to the Internet and a Web-camera/microphone to accomplish an interactive synchronous (real time) interview. Systems such as Adobe Connect Pro (www.adobe.com) or Citrix GoToMeeting (https://www2.gotomeeting.com/en_US/pre/productOverview.tmpl) provide a rich environment for discussion of how the student participated in the clinical activities. An open discussion can be completed with all of the invited guests while also recording the session for future reference by faculty or student. So, the student not only can get prompt feedback during the time of the meeting, but that feedback also is available, asynchronously, for them to review at any time.

Postclinical Assessment/Study—Papers, Projects

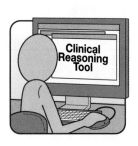

Continuing with the practice of giving prompt feedback, instructors can use a hybrid approach to accomplish postclinical assessment. This set-up allows the students to have easy access to assessment activities at the time they finish their clinical activities. The use of the LMS assessment tool can provide the students with both practice quizzes and more formalized testing for evaluating clinical competence. These electronic tools allow the inclusion of pictures, video, and sound, which can be used to develop comprehensive testing activities. In addition, faculty can add questions to these assessments that emulate questions on national certification examinations. If student evaluations and feedback need to be submitted to on-campus faculty, assignment dropboxes provide a means for timely submission.

HYBRID APPROACH TO SUPPORT LABORATORY ACTIVITIES

Hybrid learning for laboratory activities can be arranged in several ways. Programs may choose to have students complete a number of activities outside of the laboratory either before or after the f-2-f learning experience. Some schools have students come to the laboratory once every 2 weeks for extended hands-on practice and assessment. Outside of the laboratory, students study videos, computer-based simulations, and text materials. Another approach is to have students attend f-2-f laboratory sessions at the beginning and end of the semester or term. The rest of the term is spent completing learning activities online. Multiple strategies can be used to manage the hybrid laboratory course. These include prelaboratory preparation, communication, computer-based simulation, debriefing, and postlaboratory write-ups

Prelab Preparation

Good practice encourages active learning. Preparing for a laboratory session requires that students know the content and process required for successful and timely completion of laboratory activities. This may involve providing access to evidence-based practice literature, laboratory instruction notes, and lecture presentations. These may be in the form of links to library electronic databases, files posted in PDF format, or recorded video and/or audio presentations. Even when students are in regular f-2-f contact with faculty, having procedural information recorded and posted can avoid miscommunication or confusion. Precious laboratory time can be preserved for working on the required tasks if students have detailed instructions before the laboratory session.

Communication

Good practice encourages contact between students and faculty. To effectively integrate the lab experience, communication about the activity is needed. Discussion of activities prior to and after laboratory can lead to a deeper level of understanding of the laboratory activity concepts. The instructor also can evaluate student understanding of the laboratory learning objectives through the students' responses during such discussion. However, in the f-2-f environment, even if time allows for such discussion, there is limited opportunity for every student to participate and for the instructor to record or grade such participation.

The LMS discussion tool is an effective means to accomplish this in-depth communication in a timely and comprehensive manner. All students can participate equally in the discussion process. Generally, a required online discussion involves each student posting an initial response to a discussion question and then students respond to each other's postings for a specified period of time (e.g., during the days between each laboratory session). The intent is to have the students ask each other questions and compare/contrast their experiences in laboratory with that of their peers.

The instructor's role in this discussion is that of facilitator. Although the temptation may be to respond to each student's post with feedback on the "correctness" of their information, that feedback should be saved for private feedback during the grading process. Instead, the instructor should focus on keeping the discussion on topic and making inquiries to move the students' understanding to a deep level. Discussion questions can be developed using terms that reflect the desired level of comprehension. Bloom's Taxonomy of cognitive levels is an effective structure for developing questions that promote

TECHNOLOGY TIP 7.1

Webcasting programs such as Adobe Connect provide an easy way to record comprehensive lecture/instruction sessions. This program has the capability to record video of a technique being performed, with audio instructions. At the same time, a PowerPoint file or other document can be shown to highlight steps of the process. This can be accomplished using a web-cam and laptop in a classroom laboratory or instructor's office. The instructor can develop a recording just for posting online for student review, or if desired, the instructor could host this session as a live meeting where students can observe from a distance by accessing a Web site. They can submit questions/comments via the chat tool or microphone. This live session can be captured as a video recording for later viewing by students who did not attend the live session.

discussion at the level of understanding required (Churches, 2008). These levels were originally defined as knowledge, comprehension, application, analysis, synthesis, and evaluation. A more recent revision uses more descriptive terms of remembering, understanding, applying, analyzing, evaluating, and creating. Using verbs that address the desired level of learning is suggested for writing effective discussion questions.

HYBRID ACTIVITIES TO SUPPORT CLASS ACTIVITIES

When a f-2-f course replaces a portion of the seat-time with online activities, many opportunities arise. Students may have the opportunity for more active learning outside of the classroom. The faculty and students may have fewer limitations on their schedule (e.g., class is only once a week as opposed to two or three times a week). Programs could have fewer classroom space issues.

Organization

Good practice communicates high expectations. A well-known concept in education is that students will rise to or surpass identified expectations if they are clearly communicated. A hybrid environment allows the course instructor to maintain a high level of organization of class materials and experiences that will support students' success. Posting the course syllabus, schedule of activities and assignment due dates, grading rubrics, and other learning resources on a course Web site provides students with the information needed to meet such expectations.

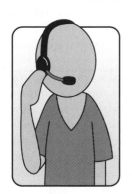

Within the LMS system the instructor can post assignment descriptions and grading rubrics. The information is then available to students no matter where they are, as long as they have Internet access. This avoids the problems of students losing assignment information or misunderstanding verbal directions given in class. Some instructors may even explain these tools and assignments in a brief video (www.youtube.com) or podcast (www.yodio.com). These recording tools allow the instructor to simply upload the video/audio directly from a camera-microphone attached to his or her computer (see Table 15.2 Keys to Creating a Podcast).

In addition, course e-mail or discussion forums can be used to post questions about the assignment. When a student asks a question via a discussion forum the instructor can answer in some depth, but only has to address that question once. The next student with the same question can read the previous posts. Clearly defined rubrics for all assignments are a key component to keeping class activities organized. When students can review a clear description of what is expected, less time is taken from class activities to explain and answer questions. Students also will be less frustrated because they know what is expected and where to find the information they need, when they need it.

TECHNOLOGY TIP 7.2

There are multiple resources for applying Bloom's Taxonomy including suggested verbs for each level of the taxonomy. One that provides a good overview and descriptive verbs in tutorial format is Colorado Community College System Colleges Faculty Wiki (http://faculty.ccconline.org/index.php?title=Blooms_Taxonomy_Tutorial_FLASH). Muilenburg and Berge (2006) provide an excellent overview of online discussion question development (http://www.emoderators.com/moderators/muilenburg.html)

TECHNOLOGY TIP 7.3

How Does a Discussion Forum Work?
All learning management systems provide a system of posting messages (called threaded discussions) that allow one person to post a public message that others can reply to. The result is a flow (or thread) of messages and replies to one topic. Each person can log into the course site, read what has been previously posted, and respond to any posts of interest. Such discussions are completed asynchronously, meaning each person works on their own schedule. No one has to be present at the same time for the discussion to continue.

One way to identify high expectations is to post examples of previous students' work (be sure to obtain permission). Sharing examples of exemplary work gives students a clear picture of how to achieve top grades and may even communicate a challenge to raise the bar for a new level of excellence. Using the course Web site as a showcase of student work can encourage excellence. Examples can be shared via the discussion tool or by posting in a public area of the course Web site. Students can review these publications and ask questions or give feedback and complete peer-review activities on each other's work. This provides a high level of sharing in each other's work as well as keeping all student work organized in one place for ease of retrieval and grading.

E-mail provides a means for organizing course information. Instructors can make use of the LMS e-mail system to communicate with students outside of class and thereby maintain an archive of all course communications. Although instructors can choose to do this type of communication through personal or professional e-mail accounts, the advantage of using the e-mail system within the LMS is that all information related to one course stays encapsulated within the course.

Good practice emphasizes time on task and respects diverse talents and ways of learning. Through the use of threaded, asynchronous discussion forums, students can discuss course information between f-2-f class meetings at times that are convenient to their schedules. They remain engaged in the course content and with each other through interactive discussions that can go into more depth than in f-2-f classes. This opportunity particularly benefits the student who prefers longer processing time before speaking up in class. Having time to read the course materials at one's own pace, search for other related resources, and then think about comments or questions to share with peers gives a voice to students who might otherwise not participate.

Communication

Good practice encourages contact between students and faculty, develops reciprocity and cooperation among students, and gives prompt feedback. These practices identify the need for a high level of clear communication between students and faculty, students and course content, and student to student. Courses developed using hybrid environments significantly increase all three type of communication. Students have a means to contact faculty through the course e-mail and chat or discussion tools. Students can engage in the course content at any time during or outside of the f-2-f class time because it is posted in an organized manner on the course Web site. With the use of asynchronous threaded discussions, they also can be in communication with classmates on course topics between class meetings.

Engagement

Good practice uses active learning techniques and respects diverse talents and ways of learning. The use of hybrid environments allows for more time in class to be spent with hands-on, active learning tasks because the students can be introduced to the content of a given learning unit through materials posted online before class. Handouts, presentations, and interactive online discussions with fellow learners and instructors before attending the f-2-f meetings can be used to accomplish initial understanding of course topics. Students then come to the f-2-f session with the same level of preparation, ready to apply their understanding by engaging in laboratory activities, simulated case planning, interaction with sample patients, or other active learning activities.

ADMINISTRATIVE TOOLS

Instructors are usually drawn to the use of hybrid environments to support f-2-f classes because they appreciate the benefits the tools provide for their students. What they might not discover, until they have adopted these tools, are the administrative benefits. Although most instructors have good organizational skills and develop their own record keeping and file management processes, the tools in a typical LMS provide a high level of organization that most instructors cannot accomplish on their own.

Organization

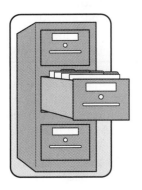

The use of an electronic gradebook alone might convince some instructors to use the features of an LMS. These gradebooks not only record grades but also figure assignment weighting, student grade comparisons, and make mathematical adjustments (adding extra credit, subtracting minimum/maximum scores, determining averages). Depending on the LMS, many, if not all, of these activities are provided and require minor set up in comparison to managing a spreadsheet file.

Another feature of the LMS that aid in course organization is the electronic calendar. The calendar provides two types of entries, public and private. Typically the instructor has the option to do both types of entries and students can do only private entries. The instructor will enter all assignment due dates and other reminders on the calendar; this can be done by simply checking a box when adding assignment dropboxes or tests to the course. Then students can add to those entries with their own appointments and structuring of how they will accomplish assignments. If changes in the schedule are needed, the instructor can easily update the calendar and notify students by the use of the announcement tool. When students next enter the LMS class Web site, the announcement will appear in a pop-up box, alerting them to the change in the schedule.

As previously described, assignment dropboxes, discussion forums, and electronic assessments all provide efficient means of grading and giving feedback to students. These tools also provide the instructor timesaving ways to keep student submissions organized. Assignment dropboxes feature the ability to download all students' submissions in one process and will automatically create a separate folder for each student in that process. Discussion forums provide the ability to review all posts submitted by one student, in a separate window, for ease of grading the quality and timeliness of that student's work. The assessment tool provides statistical information for each test question, providing the instructor with immediate feedback on what concepts the class, as a whole, understood or not. These statistics also help the instructor to recognize which questions need to be deleted or revised for future tests.

These features are but a few of the organizational capabilities available through the use of LMS tools. Instructors and program administrators will want to review the capabilities of the LMS with the instruction technologists at their school for more options and training in the set up of courses. Attending user conferences for the particular LMS that the school subscribes to is another way to get ideas and training in the use of these features.

Communication

Although the very nature of a course Web site and LMS tools is to communicate more effectively with students, faculty may feel overwhelmed by students having nonstop communication access. One option that may be of particular interest to nursing faculty to reduce the demand on instructors' time while maintaining a high level of communication, is to use the automatic capabilities of LMS tools. This is the capability to customize the course setup with the use of "agents" or "action" features. These features allow the instructor or course designer to set up a series of actions that will happen automatically based on activities that the student completes. Even though the instructor may feel that the set up of the hybrid environment has greatly increased his or her ability to communicate with students, the individual student may still want a more individualized communication process. Nursing educators are in demanding roles of teacher, preceptor, and clinical practice. They do not have much time to be available for drop in office hours or individual e-mails to confirm to students that assignments have been received or to tell them when those assignments will be graded. Individual communication should be encouraged, however, it is recommended that those contacts be done when a student needs specific feedback or assistance. The use of automated "agents" can assist by providing the student with confirming messages, saving the instructor's time for more personalized communications.

Agents, or automatic actions, are features in some LMS that provide a means to set up actions, such as sending an e-mail message when another action is completed. A student submits an assignment through the assignment dropbox and an e-mail that the instructor has previously written, is generated to confirm to the student that the assignment has been received and will be graded by a particular date. The message also can include information on how to retrieve that feedback. Submission of an assignment, such as a completed review of chapter questions, can generate the opening of a quiz on that chapter and send an e-mail to the students telling them to take the quiz. There are a wide variety of uses for these tools and although they require some "up-front" time to design, the time is well spent if it relieves the instructor of doing repeated versions of these activities while teaching the course. The impact on the student is that they feel in closer communication with the instructor and may find it easier to stay organized and on-task.

Even if agents are not included in the school's LMS, some planning before the start of the class can provide the instructor with similar automated features. Develop a file with answers to questions that get asked repeatedly throughout the course. That information can be easily copied into an e-mail message whenever it is needed. Use the announcement tool to tell students when assignments will be returned. Announcements can be written ahead of time and set to release on a specific date. Any activity that helps the students to see that the instructor is active and available, while decreasing the instructor time spent in routine activities, will improve both the students' and instructor's experience.

Engagement

Engaging today's student requires a multimodal approach. The typical nursing student is not typical! Not only are classes filled to capacity and beyond, but students represent multiple age groups, ethnic/cultural backgrounds, and are preparing to work in complex environments. These are not easy influences to address when there also is considerable content to provide in each course. Younger students are used to information delivered in short "sound bytes" whereas older students may prefer more written and paper-based course materials. Although each group needs to learn to manage information in multiple formats, an individual instructor has only a limited time to prepare course activities that address these diverse talents and ways of learning. A hybrid environment can provide the tools that will provide this multimodal approach and engage students of all backgrounds and learning styles.

Effective student engagement requires that the course be designed with an understanding of the needs of prospective students. In the past, the development of a f-2-f course had typically been up to the individual instructor. A course syllabus including objectives based on required standards may have been the only structure provided to the individual instructor. All presentation of content, learning, and assessment activities were at the discretion of each instructor. It is possible for an individual instructor to take on the development of a hybrid course; however, many schools are now engaging instructional designers to assist in developing the sophisticated design that is needed to engage today's students and address the new environments of clinical practice. If an instructor only has f-2-f learning and instruction experience, an instructional designer can provide the insight needed to develop effective and creative tools for a hybrid environment. Instructional technologists can help with training on the use of the tools of an LMS and be better able to translate the use of these tools to address learning objectives. If an instructional designer with online experience is not available at the school, the nursing department may want to hire a consultant to help in the development of a hybrid approach to program courses. The investment will be worthwhile when student course evaluations reflect better engagement and higher levels of satisfaction.

ASSESSMENT AND ACCREDITATION

The use of assessment and evaluation criteria in nursing accreditation standards (NLNAC and CCNE) is an important component of nursing education. Additional standards for e-learning and how the LMS can assist nursing programs to collect, analyze, and report data are discussed next.

Standards for E-learning

The question of whether learning accomplished in an online format is equivalent to that done in a f-2-f setting has been long established (Russell, 1999). Known as the "no significant difference phenomenon" this body of research addresses the effectiveness of courses held in a distance learning format. It can, therefore, be assumed that a hybrid approach to learning provides the best of both worlds to students needing to learn the demanding content of a nursing curriculum. Following established standards for curriculum development, a course built using a hybrid environment will include a design that is well laid out and addresses multiple learning styles.

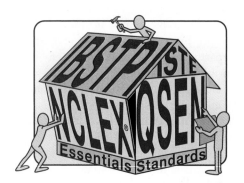

Typical standards that a nursing course would follow include those established by the nursing profession and nursing education accreditation bodies. Standards for online learning should be reviewed when developing the online aspects of a hybrid course. These may include the International Society for Technology in Education (ISTE) National Educational Technology Standards (NETS) (http://www.iste.org/AM/Template.cfm?Section=NETS) and International Board of Standards for Training, Performance and Instruction (IBSTPI) (http://www.ibstpi.org/competencies.htm). Use of these standards will provide course designers and instructors clear methods for development of learning activities that meet required guidelines and ensure student learning.

Student and Course Assessment Plan

Having a structured plan for assessment of student learning is critical to the success of any course. A hybrid approach to course design provides several tools to accomplish a variety of assessment activities, in addition to providing effective methods of data collection. A number of assessment tools are built into any LMS, such as quiz/test tools, threaded discussion forums, and assignment dropboxes. Additional tools can be incorporated as needed such as webcasting. Understanding the wealth of activities that can be accomplished with these tools can provide an instructor with more options for providing authentic assessment. According to Mueller (2008) authentic assessment is "a form of assessment in which students are asked to perform real-world tasks that demonstrate meaningful application of essential knowledge and skills." Examples of authentic assessment in a nursing course might include: student discussion of clinical cases through a threaded discussion forum with classmates and instructor; demonstration of proficiency with clinical tasks such as taking blood pressure readings, through the use of webcasting tools; or preparation of a plan of care for a home-health care client can be submitted to the instructor by assignment dropbox. Many instructors in nursing and allied health fields prefer to incorporate authentic assessment in their course design.

Assessment activities cannot only be delivered via electronic tools but they can also be evaluated with the use of rubrics that provide students with clear expectations for level of proficiency. Depending on the type of assessment given, the rubrics may be incorporated into the assessment tool to provide immediate feedback to the students. If the instructor incorporates a grading rubric and feedback into a quiz or examination, the tool can then generate grades and feedback to the student automatically as soon as the student finishes the task. The instructor is then freed to focus on grading authentic assessment activities. The use of electronic assessment also frees f-2-f class time for more in-depth exploration of course topics or other authentic assessment activities, such as laboratory examinations.

A good assessment plan also includes summative and formative course evaluation. Although most colleges and universities have a formalized plan for collecting summative student evaluation of courses, many instructors prefer to have some additional types of feedback from students. Brookfield and Preskill's (2005) Critical Incident Questionnaire (CIQ) is one example of formative evaluation because it provides regular feedback from students as to their understanding of course concepts as well as feedback on the course process. This assessment consists of five short questions, such as "At what moment in class this week were you most engaged as a learner" (p. 48) and "At what moment in class this week were you most distanced as a learner?" (p. 48) and is conducted anonymously at the end of each class session or week. It can take as little as 5 minutes to complete. This can be done on paper but the survey tool of the LMS can provide the opportunity for easier data collection and analysis. In addition, this information is then easily stored for use in future planning. If students have computers available during class, they can submit these questions immediately, or reflect upon the week's class when they are in the school's computer laboratory or at home.

Data Collection, Data Analysis, and Data Reporting

The LMS is an effective data collection tool. Even if an instructor decides that they only want to use a hybrid approach for collection of assignments, testing, and posting grades, he or she will have enhanced course communication and the ability to track student progress more effectively than in a typical f-2-f course. Many instructors do not have the time or the experience with data collection software to keep effective electronic data on each student. An LMS will provide not only data collection but also sophisticated analysis of the students' activity without excessive time and work by the instructor.

LMS systems track every activity that students do, whether it is the number of times that they access a particular item or each grade that they received on a test or an assignment is entered in the dropbox. The gradebook tool will typically tell students not only a grade on a specific activity but also their current course grade as well as their standing in comparison to the rest of the class. The use of the electronic survey tool (similar to the quiz/testing tool, but does not track who is making the submission) can be an easy way to collect student feedback.

CONCLUSION

The use of a hybrid environment within a nursing curriculum provides students and instructors with multiple advantages. Improved course organization, effective record keeping, increased communication, multimodal learning experiences, and multilayered assessment activities are some of these advantages. Faculty and students will likely feel a higher level of satisfaction with such courses as a result of the increased levels of interactivity with each other, the course instructor, and the course content, whether they are engaged in f-2-f or online activities. In addition, students using these technology-rich learning tools are more likely to be ready to handle the demanding environments and tools required in future nursing clinical practice.

REFERENCES

Brookfield, S. D., & Preskill, S. (2005). *Discussion as a way of teaching. Tools and techniques for democratic classrooms* (2nd ed.). San Francisco: Jossey-Bass.

Chickering, A., & Ehrmann, S. C. (1996). Implementing the seven principles: Technology as lever. *AAHE Bulletin, 48*, 3–6. Reprinted on the The TLT Group. Retrieved from http://www.tltgroup.org/programs/seven.html

Chickering, A., & Gamson, Z. (1987). Seven principles of good practice in undergraduate education. *AAHE Bulletin, 39*, 3–7. Retrieved from http://www.aahea.org/bulletins/articles/sevenprinciples1987.htm

Churches, A. (2008). Bloom's digital taxonomy. Retrieved from http://media.ccconline.cccs.edu/ccco/FacWiki/Blooms_Taxonomy_Tutorials/Churches_2008_DigitalBloomsTaxonomyGuide.pdf

Ehrmann, S. C. (2008). New ideas and additional reading. The TLT Group. Retrieved from http://www.tltgroup.org/programs/seven.html

Ireland, J., Martindale, S., Johnson, N., Adams, D., Eboh, W., & Mowatt, E. (2009). Blended learning in education: Effects on knowledge and attitude. *British Journal of Nursing, 18*(2), 124–130.

Mueller, J. (2008). Authentic assessment toolbox. North Central College. Retrieved from http://jonathan.mueller.faculty.noctrl.edu/toolbox/index.htm

Muilenburg, L., & Berge, Z. (2006). A framework for designing questions for online learning. Retrieved from http://www.emoderators.com/moderators/muilenburg.html

Reynard, R. (2007, May 23). Hybrid learning: Maximizing student engagement. *Campus Technology.* Retrieved from http://campustechnology.com/articles/2007/05/hybrid-learning-maximizing-student-engagement.aspx

Russell, T. L. (1999*). The no significant difference phenomenon as reported in 355 research reports, summaries and papers.* Raleigh, NC: North Carolina State University Press.

Chapter 8

Web-Based Environments

Erich Widemark, PhD, FNP-BC

I e-mailed a student the other day to request that he submit a paragraph describing a recent event that occurred during his clinical rotation. He replied, "Not sure what format you would like, but I could e-mail it in an MS Word document, submit it on the Online Learning System, or perhaps share it from Google documents. If you don't need that much information, I would be more than happy to text it to you. I would send via a tweet, but don't think I can limit myself to only 140 characters for your request. If you don't mind, because there are some visuals I would just as soon put together a media file using my Web camera. Do you prefer MPG, AVI, or RM format?" It was about this moment that I feared I might be getting too old for this job.

Recently, a friend completed coursework for his graduate degree. The facilitator for the course was living in Australia. A student left a message about her clinical day on Facebook, while still at the site. Web-based environments have gone through a significant evolution. The connectedness our society shares has driven the development of advanced tools that allow the modern student to connect from anywhere in the world. High-speed networks change how faculty and students interact, and enable nursing programs to deliver didactic, laboratory, and clinical content to a new generation of nurses.

Using these Web-based environments for the delivery of content can present some challenges. Although there remains skepticism about the quality of the learning experience, research supports its success. This relatively new technology is integrated into mainstream educational arenas and more innovation continues to add new and unique ways to teach and train online.

Unlike Web-supported environments, Web-based environments deliver all of the content at a distance. In the past, distance learning included correspondence schools and television media. Modern distance learning is primarily done using the Internet. Although today it seems the personal computer is the present and future of Web-based environments, technologies such as "Wi-Fi" and "Wi-MAX" suggest a shift to include more portable devices. For example, one large company offers a picture frame that is a computer screen with its own e-mail and IP address. The user could hang it on the wall and experience continuous streaming content located anywhere wireless Internet access is available.

Web-based environments lose the personalization of instructors delivering content in a more intimate environment. This loss comprises the verbal and nonverbal conversations the instructor has with students; and the inability to receive cues regarding the level of understanding or

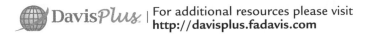

DavisPlus | For additional resources please visit
http://davisplus.fadavis.com

ability to retain content based on comfort, level of alertness, and interest. The advantages to this environment include the freedom to choose the time, location, and type of content delivery. Another positive aspect of Web-based environments is the learner's ability to select the order, type, and the depth of the content delivered. This satisfies some of the qualities of adult learning in that these learners are self-directed and their readiness to learn is affected by their need to know or do something (Lynch, 2002).

LEARNING MANAGEMENT SYSTEMS/WEB-BASED CONTENT MANAGEMENT SYSTEMS

The original Web environments were composed of message boards and other small computer programs usually developed by instructors to enhance instruction of complex concepts and delivery of information. These projects used the term computer-aided instruction (CAI). The pre-Internet systems were developed specifically for on-site classroom use. The program design was a bottom up approach in which the faculty had most input regarding inclusion of content (Morgan, 2003). These programs and message boards were eventually merged into more comprehensive but rudimentary systems. Learning management systems (LMSs) or Web-based content management systems (WBCMSs) were designed to offer massive storage for information accessible to faculty, students, and staff.

There have been four generations of LMSs. The first LMS simply tracked information and testing results. The second generation Web-based systems centralized data into one server, but access was limited and dependent on the user's computer hardware. With more advanced data structures, LMSs used a tiered system with separate collections of databases, programs, and information subdivided and available using multiple computer platforms (Morgan, 2003).

The current generation LMS uses course and degree catalogs, assessment testing, financial aid applications and tracking, messaging capabilities, communication tools, ecommerce, registration systems, and many other support services to maintain the information for faculty, staff, and learners (Woodill, 2007). This fourth generation LMS consolidates the user information for easy archival backup and retrieval.

Meanwhile, Web-based classrooms took a parallel yet similar developmental approach. Primarily asynchronous and discussion-based, these virtual lecture halls initially used e-mail and bulletin-board systems (BBSs) because most learners had access to these tools. These systems used active discussion on various assigned topics as the primary learning method (Morabito, 2009). In 1997, WebCT 1.0, a virtual classroom, was released. The same year, Blackboard, an education development company was founded by Dan Cane and Stephen Gilfus. In 1998, Martin Dougiamas started development of a system later known as Moodle (Dougiamas, 1999). In 2006, Blackboard acquired WebCT. As of the end of 2007, Blackboard reported 4800 installations of its software running in learning, government, and corporate institutions (U.S. Securities and Exchange Commission, 2008).

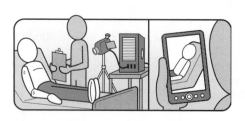

These virtual classrooms have evolved into comprehensive LMSs that include most every form or document needed by staff, faculty, or student. Learners can easily navigate to course content, syllabi, assignment descriptions, supplemental readings, profiles of classmates, archived/scanned documents, and current lectures in multiple formats. More advanced systems include audio and video files, articles, documents, podcasts, and even video podcasts (vodcasts).

Full-time information technology (IT) employees are ideal to design custom systems; however, the expense is enormous and usually left to those colleges that can summon the available funds. Many popular LMSs are easily configured and readily expandable so that even the college with a small budget can afford to use Web-based environments.

If an institution does not have an LMS or the LMS is missing some key items, an inexpensive way to develop a content management system is to use the Web-based software available for personal use. For example, Google offers a document system, a synchronous messaging environment, mail client, calendar, listserv, and many other services that could be configured to develop a Web-based environment for the purpose of delivering education. The faculty also may discuss options for free LMS services with textbook vendors. There are many Web-based collaborative environments to choose from (Box 8.1).

CLASSROOM

The center of a Web-based environment is the classroom. The modern Web-based classroom, known as the forum, has evolved from the computer BBSs first used in the 1980s. These forums have message subject headings called "threads" in which students and faculty communicate. By leaving answers to discussion questions and comments to other students' answers, substantive discussion takes place along with critical reflection. This faculty-to-student and student-to-student interaction is a major tool of distance learning. LMSs, such as Blackboard and Web-CT, began as Web-based classroom environments.

Social networks are poised to become the new classroom. These are online forums that offer applications that add functionality through the addition of simulation, personal

---

BOX 8.1
FREE COLLABORATIVE DOCUMENT MANAGEMENT

http://docs.google.com—Free service for storing, editing, or retrieving word processing documents, slide presentations, and spreadsheets. Share with friends or colleagues. Decide if you want the shared individual to edit the file or view only.

http://www.writeboard.com—Create a word processing document that others can view or edit. With this Web site, the collaborators can edit the whiteboard document, or make general comments that are not part of the text. It can be set up to contact all collaborators if there is a change made to the document.

http://www.officelive.com—A Web-based version of the popular Microsoft Office software. Still in development, this Web site will allow you to store up to 5 gigabytes (gb) of information and share files for collaboration with up to 100 users with no software needed to install.

TECHNOLOGY TIP 8.1

Keep all your reference files in an online collaborative document management system for easy access when you are away from your primary computer. No more need to carry a flash drive or a compact disk (CD) with you when you are on the go.

configurability, and storage and sharing of media files. The user can select which people have permission to view his or her pages or add to the conversation. The user also can customize the content, share opinions about the subject matter, and add to the content.

Although social networks are becoming popular with the public, most schools are using standardized or customized LMSs as their virtual classrooms, or as a communications and storage tool to supplement the on-site classroom experience. Many ideas and concepts are continually added transforming the modern LMS into more of a social networking tool.

Organize

An important part of the Web-based classroom is organization. Too much on-screen confusion often leads to a poor learning experience. Most LMSs will categorize messages and threads in chronological order. The user may be able to expand the thread for a better view of each message and its contributors, or collapse the thread for a better overview of the discussion. Most LMSs have many different tools used to organize and direct the flow of discussion. Although each Web-based classroom is unique, it contains many of the same functions and options as a personal e-mail account. These include the ability to reply, forward, and delete messages.

Web-based classroom environments are divided into forums. These forums include but are not limited to a general/main area, a chat area, and separate forums for each lesson, week, or day. Some LMSs have private forums assigned to each student for private conversations with the instructor. In some systems, a virtual mailbox serves this purpose. When a message is left by faculty or a student, it is flagged as "new" or "unread." This assists the user to see and continue where they may have finished in the last session. These new message flags also show how popular a topic may be, or can notify everyone when a new subject or important announcement is added.

Along with a forum for each topic, the instructor will want to have an area for general small talk and nonclass-related activities. This is a place where students may wish each other happy holidays, or plan events that are unrelated to the coursework. Users may want to share individual information about what is important in their lives. For example, during hurricane Katrina, a learner in one educational program communicated about her difficulties accessing the course room during a natural disaster. She was able to give her fellow classmates situational information about the storm and updated contact information. Many students felt a special connection to her, even offering assistance. An area for announcements also may be helpful.

The instructor can include an area where students can download and view important files, such as the syllabus and the college handbook. Students and faculty sometimes need the flexibility to look up something while away from their main computers. Being able to access a syllabus from an airport or hotel is convenient, and helps keep the student and faculty operational.

TECHNOLOGY TIP 8.2

It is a good idea to separate each lesson into its own forum. When a discussion is complete, the class starts with a fresh slate in a new area, and the overall lesson is much more organized for retrieval at a later time.

The ability to control colors and fonts helps a great deal with organization. Colors can be used to categorize items within a forum for easier reading. A different color for each respondent or the capacity to highlight a concept can be of great help for learning.

Communicate

Communication is the basis for successful interchange within the Web-based classroom environment. Words must be chosen carefully to ensure a peaceful, happy, and engaged room. In addition to the importance of content, even the way things are said can cause mixed emotions and responses. For example, using ALL CAPS to express a point might be interpreted as yelling. A nonresponse to a student can be interpreted as a slight. There are many small ways of enhancing communication. In addition to basic Internet netiquette, guidelines can include a limitation of message reply lengths, number of messages left to individuals in each forum, content pertaining to the forum subject, and organization of reply messages.

Some instructors will require students to make a substantive post to a general discussion question, and a substantive reply to one or two other students' answers. This is a way to add depth and increase critical reflection of each lesson point. A disadvantage can be forced discussion that does not offer new learning concepts. By putting too much weight on grading substantive replies, the student may be less encouraged and engaged because replying becomes more of a chore than a desire. Another way to encourage substantive discussion is to require that each discussion question answer include a value statement, research, references, or a word count.

Everyone is well aware that text does not contain facial expression, body language, or voice inflection. This can lead to misunderstanding between students and facilitators and create unneeded tension. Emoticons are small pictures that are included within message text to communicate an emotion or concept. These are useful to delineate sarcasm from seriousness, or humor from anger (see Table 8.1).

There are other ways to communicate from within the Web-based classroom. One technique is through the use of PowerPoint with audio narrative. This can be available as a link within the forum that will open a viewer in the student's home browser. PowerPoint presentations are created to timed slideshows that are put to audio. This allows the instructor to communicate content with sufficient visuals to allow for an online lecture.

TECHNOLOGY TIP 8.3

As a classroom guideline, request the students leave one reply message and address each individual by name within the message. Suggest that the student use a different color for each respondent. This is more personalized, adds to the student's feeling of connectedness, and helps develop an internal concept and memory of a student he or she may have never met.

TECHNOLOGY TIP 8.4

Some LMSs have "push" technology, which means forum messages are immediately sent to a user device: home computer, cell phone, or other e-mail system. This encourages a whole new level of student and faculty involvement.

TABLE 8.1	
Common Emoticons	
:)	Happy
:))	Laughing
:(	Sad
:((	Crying
;)	Winking
:-/	Confused
:D	Big grin
:-O	Surprised
Common Chat/Text "Netlingo"	
?	I have a question
AAMOF	As a matter of fact
BC	Because
BRB	Be right back
EOD	End of discussion
EOM	End of message
IDK	I don't know
IMHO	In my humble opinion
JK	Just kidding
LOL	Laughing out loud
NRN	No reply necessary
QQ	Quick question
TIA	Thanks in advance
YW	You're welcome

TECHNOLOGY TIP 8.5

If you are using a system that does not offer emoticons, you can make your own using different punctuation items. For example, a smile :), shock :o, perturbed : / to name a few. There also is generally accepted shorthand that is sometimes used (see Table 8.1).

Audio and video files have become portable enough in a Web-based environment to readily share within the electronic classroom. Often high-resolution pictures or audio can be shared between students and by the instructor to enhance a teaching point. If a student, for example, asks a question about what pneumonia may sound like during a pulmonary examination, the instructor can share an audio file that will realistically sound like what the student may be hearing in a clinical setting. Often these items can be transferred to portable devices, such as MP3 players or cell phones, for further reference.

Other items that typically can be imbedded in the Web-based classroom environment include hyperlinks that enable an immediate reference to a specific Web site. These can be included within the text so the student can choose which links to follow. This concept works well for vocabulary words that might be unknown to some students. While reading about cardiomyopathy, for example, the word might be underlined and colored blue to signify that the student can click on the word for an expanded definition.

Another way to communicate within the Web-based classroom is to schedule a Webinar. This is a synchronous scheduled Web-based meeting in which a presenter can discuss content with a limited amount of students in "real time." Students can download software or PowerPoint presentations to watch while the content is being delivered. In some cases, electronic meeting systems (EMSs) can be used to complement the presentations by offering various collaborative tools that allow for categorizing, brainstorming, or polling, for better audience interactivity.

Engage

Paramount to any Web-based environment is engagement. As with other types of learning, the student must be interested and motivated to obtain the best results. Often discussion questions are used as motivation to stimulate a learner's curiosity. Other means of motivation come through debate and disagreement.

There are many different ways to engage students. After they are engaged, the fear of any instructor is loss of interest. Difficulty navigating the Web-based environment or time delay to get information can cause disengagement. Watching commercials on television is much less engaging than switching to a commercial-free channel. If there are large delays in getting information, the student may be less engaged, and the additional substantive posts become laborious. Offering a variety of media can encourage student engagement. Assignments that may include sharing pictures or video can add interest to any classroom discussion.

Part of engaging students successfully is ensuring their involvement in the learning process. In a Web-based environment, there is a high level of interactivity, which can be used to the student's advantage. Polls and sharing icons can be used to send the content to other students or friends at social networking sites. The students' ability to rate the content can alert others to items of interest while allowing the students the ability to share their opinions.

Evaluate

Important for all learning goals is evaluation of the student. Using many different techniques, the instructor can determine if the student is reaching these objectives. Prelearning assessments, done at the beginning of the course, can collect baseline information about how knowledgeable the student is, and where she or he has strengths and deficits. This information can be used to change or modify his or her personal objectives. Care must be taken to not change the core learning objectives too much, or this becomes a regulatory problem for the program.

Any preprogram assessment can include virtual meetings, placement examinations, surveys, measurable exercises, and evaluation of the student's previous work. Along with this assessment, the faculty also can consider determining the student's learning style, which will be invaluable when individualizing the coursework. Research suggests that assessing the learning styles of each student allows the faculty and institution to incorporate different and emerging technologies into their courses (Saeed, Yang, & Sinnappan, 2009). Incorporating learning strategies are positively correlated with learning results (Wang, Peng, Huang, Hou, & Wang, 2008) (see Evidence-Based Practice Box 8.1).

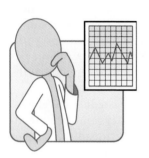

During the educational process in the Web-based environment, continuous student feedback is helpful to identify difficulties or concerns. These assessments allow the instructor to make modifications to upcoming coursework or offer supplemental material before the end of class to help meet the final objectives (O'Neil, Fisher, & Newbold, 2009). Assessment techniques in the course room can include strategies, such as journaling, diaries, or discussion questions.

EVIDENCE-BASED PRACTICE BOX 8.1

Relationships Between Learning Results and Characteristics of Distance Learning

Issue: Do Characteristics of Distance Learning Correlate in Better Learning Results?

Psychological characteristics of distance learning including motivation, learning strategy, and self-efficacy were compared with learning results.

Study Findings

There is an interest in studying some of the psychological characteristics that appear to make distance learning more successful. These characteristics were found to have a positive predictable relationship on the effects of learning results.

Nursing Implications

- When instructing distance learners it is important to identify a student's learning attributes before the beginning of a course and incorporate strategies to improve motivation and self-efficacy.
- Identify learning strategies that will allow students to be successful in a distance learning environment for better overall advisement.
- Review successful learning strategies for online nursing faculty to help them better understand how to modify facilitation techniques to enhance successful learning (Wang, Peng, Huang, Hou, & Wang, 2008).

Substantive discussion is a form of continuous student feedback. This allows for immediate assessment of the student's level of knowledge and understanding. It also permits evaluation of the student's critical thinking skills. Discussion encourages debate, which allows the instructor to push students closer to the learning goals by challenging their basic opinions and knowledge of conceptual ideas.

Many programs use a nationally recognized standardized test system called the REACH examination by Evolve (formally the Health Education Systems, Inc.). Although some schools use this for testing the readiness of students to graduate and take the National Council Licensure Examinations-Practical Nurse and Registered Nurse (NCLEX-PN, -RN), or American Academy of Nurse Practitioners (AANP)/American Nurses Credentialing Center (ANCC) examinations, others will have the assessment done at several points in the program to follow student progress. This test can be done from home with an available log-in name and password. The company administering the test also offers remediation plans along with statistics on the students' strong and weak areas. There have been many studies to support the predictability and validity of this test. Higher test scores positively correlate with better test results on the NCLEX examination (Morris & Hancock, 2008). Some experts, however, have expressed concern about using this test as the only evaluation tool for success, and they encourage the use of additional indicators when concerning the student's readiness to graduate (Spurlock & Hunt, 2008). (See Evidence-Based Practice Box 8.2.)

EVIDENCE-BASED PRACTICE BOX 8.2

Using the Health Education Systems, Inc. (HESI) Examination to Predict NCLEX-RN Outcomes and the Usage of These Outcomes to Support Progression Policies for Testing Failures

Issue: Does the HESI Examination Positively Predict NCLEX-RN Passage When Used as Part of a Progression Policy in Which the Student Is Able to Retest Multiple Times?

When a nursing program was not able to successfully increase its NCLEX-RN passing rate by developing a progression policy, they did further research to see if using the progression policy positively correlated with increased pass rates on the NCLEX-RN examination.

Study Findings

Analysis of the study found that there was no positive or negative correlation in NCLEX-RN examination scores when students were allowed to retake the HESI examination to improve their scores.

Nursing Implications

- Using the online HESI (now the REACH examination) as a progression tool to graduate is not supported by the current study.
- Nursing departments should consider other factors besides HESI score to graduate students.
- Repeating the HESI test more than once may not be helpful to the student.
- There appear to be other factors that need further study to determine other independent variables that affect a student's performance on the NCLEX-RN examination (Spurlock & Hunt, 2008).

CLINICAL ROTATIONS

Web-based environments can enhance a student's clinical experiences. Although clinical learning in an online environment can pose challenges, there are many advantages. Nothing may replace standing at the bedside for a clinical rotation, however, Web-based environments can be used to supplement, and in some cases, improve clinical learning. A great example is Ann Myers Medical Center, a place in a Web-based environment called Second Life, where students can simulate a day in nursing life within the safe confines of their computers. Web-based clinical environments can include teaching modules, clinical tracking programs, synchronous and asynchronous discussion forums, and videoconferencing. Many of these tools can be used in combination to provide an educational clinical experience.

Communications in Clinical Rotations

The didactic portion of any nursing program can be modified, reconstructed, and delivered in a Web-based environment. But the challenge is that the nursing student will still need to spend time in the psychomotor domain learning the tasks and skills needed to be a nurse. In a Web-based environment, communication between the faculty, preceptor, agency, and student are critical to this task.

Although nursing faculty members know how to communicate with students, many clinics and hospitals have their own communications methods and electronic health records. During the clinical experience, students should be able to continue to communicate with their classmates and faculty as they have done in their didactic classrooms. Students also should continue to have a private area where they can spend asynchronous time with their instructor discussing their clinical experiences and problems that may arise.

This is where LMSs become the lifeline for both the student and faculty. The forums in LMSs allow the students to talk with instructors and classmates regarding their clinical experiences. If this is not available, e-mail, text messaging, and phone calls can be a good substitute but do not offer the group experience. Care must be taken at all times, however, to protect the privacy of the student and the patient's information he or she may be discussing.

A great way to help the student build contextual relationships with the clinical rotation in a Web-based environment is to have each student answer two questions in a separate forum specifically for each clinical week. These two questions should be open-ended and encourage further query. Questions might include: What one experience stands out above the rest this week? What one task do you enjoy most about the clinical shift? What disease process would you like to learn more about?

Faculty Communicating With Faculty

Communication between faculty members is paramount to a strong clinical experience. Each instructor may have their own styles, but discussion about student performance or concerns can ensure patient safety and address significant clinical issues early in the process. An area where several faculty members could discuss a clinical issue with a student is ideal as this yields a collaborative response to a student's questions or problems.

A LMS can offer an area or forum in which faculty can discuss student issues with each other. These areas can store and archive correspondence between faculty for a potential future need. In addition, an e-mail listserv is a good communications medium for faculty. A listserv uses a major service to keep a list of e-mail addresses for a specific group. In this case, it may be a list of faculty members. Whenever someone wants to send a message to the group, he or she sends an e-mail to a specific listserv address. All members on the list receive the message and have the option of replying to that message, which goes out to the list again. An advantage to using a listserv environment is that correspondence is "pushed" to the receiver. Pushing information is the process of the message being sent to the user, instead of the user needing to log on to see new or incoming messages. With this tool, privacy can become a concern and therefore this may not be an ideal tool.

A listserv also can offer a forum for faculty to share new journal articles, interesting experiences, and reports regarding clinical outcomes, and how this may relate to specific student situations. If a clinical problem develops, it is a good idea to keep an archive of communications between faculty and the student about this problem. A permanent record helps further disciplinary actions if problems continue to occur, or if litigation is likely.

Communication With Preceptor and Agency

Direct and open communication with the preceptor and agency should be available to the faculty and to the student. This can be difficult as each agency may have differing policies on how office communication is used. Although much of this could be done through e-mail, faculty should be careful about archiving these for the record, and abide by any privacy policies for the school and the clinic institution.

If e-mail is used for faculty to preceptor or agency communication, consider adding a school legal department approved signature line that specifies that the communications are private with suggestions of how to proceed if they were received in error. An example may say, "This is a private and confidential communication. If you have received this in error, please destroy/delete. This communication should not be forwarded, posted, or copied for any purpose without permission of the original sender. This communication may be protected under the HIPAA or FERPA act."

Communication With Student and Client

Faculty communication is paramount to a good clinical experience. The faculty acts as a mentor and role model in the nursing students learning process. The instructor is there to listen to the student's clinical experiences and offer his or her own experiences and opinions that may move that student toward his or her learning goals. The channels of communication become critical in the clinical process for the student and the instructor. In addition, there may be times when the instructor will need to communicate with the client. For example, if there is a specific referral source or piece of information that the instructor has offered to the client, he or she can communicate this directly. Recently in a clinical setting, a patient asked if the

---

TECHNOLOGY TIP 8.6

Consider having the student contact you at a class-dedicated e-mail. Set the e-mail service to page your phone or send all e-mails to your personal digital assistant (PDA). You can then shut off this function when you are not available, and turn it on when you are willing to receive student messages.

nurse practitioner student's instructor was knowledgeable about acupuncture services. The instructor was able to give the client a referral to an acupuncturist in the general area.

In a Web-based environment, access to communications tools with the faculty allows the student much more flexibility in contacting faculty. Using an LMS, the student can leave a private communication with the faculty. Furthermore, many of these systems are set up for synchronous communication, which enables the student to check his or her chat client to see if the instructor is flagged as being "online".

There are a number of other Web-based tools that can be used for student and faculty communication. Some depend on the student's or the instructor's availability of Internet access and computer. Many cell phones now have instant or text messaging capability. Plus, many laptops now use cellular modems to obtain high-speed Internet access at any location that has cell phone access. Again, privacy issues and agency policies may need to be addressed, especially if any type of videoconferencing software is used.

Instant messaging programs have become mainstream and are bundled with new computers. Several free and pay services offer instant messaging clients. There are many free programs that work with different instant messaging programs and services. Trillian Astra offers the ability to interface several different instant messaging programs into one for ease of compatibility (visit www.cnet.com for more information). The faculty and student may agree to use text messaging on their cell phones, or perhaps even videoconferencing.

Videoconferencing software, such as Skype or Windows Meeting Space gives the faculty and student ability to discuss issues in a synchronous environment using microphones and Web cameras for a more immersive experience. Provided the student have Internet access at the clinical site with a Web camera available, the instructor can see and hear the student and address many issues that may not be possible by forms of text or voice communication alone.

With all these synchronous communications tools, the faculty must consider their hours of availability as these tools allow immediate access. Palloff and Pratt (2003) discuss where this availability can lead to disturbances at inconvenient times. For example, an instructor offered his or her cell phone number with the statement, "text me any time to get a hold of me". The instructor received a text message at 3 a.m. concerning an assignment due the next day. Clear boundaries must be set for when and where it is and is not alright to contact the instructor. The faculty also must consider having the means of turning off their equipment if they do not wish to be bothered.

There may be a case in which the instructor will need to discuss a case with a client. Particularly in the graduate nursing programs in which the instructor is a nurse practitioner who is involved with the client's care along with the student, communication with client about his or her care, patient education, or referrals beyond the student's knowledge may be essential. A teleconferencing setup could be considered, however, do not forget that phone communication can be a great tool.

TECHNOLOGY TIP 8.7

Many LMSs offer a guest or limited log-in that may be used by the preceptor or agency for communication with faculty and the student. For preceptors who wish close involvement with faculty, this would be a great option.

Preclinical Assessment/Study

Before a clinical rotation starts, it is important to measure a student's knowledge level and ability. At this time a set of clinical goals can be established and developed. This can be done as a collaborative or individual assignment. Doing a preclinical assessment in a Web-based environment means using online tools to help measure a student's knowledge and preparedness.

A preclinical assessment and statement of objectives will enable the student to be better prepared for his or her clinical situation and allow the instructor to identify preclinical areas that may need more study, or that may be of concern regarding student or patient safety.

Using available online collaborative document systems, students can create a working document that both students and faculty can have access to and edit in real time (Fig. 8.1). Another good tool for this purpose is Elluminate. This is a virtual synchronous classroom in which a moderator can maintain and make changes to a document and share the information with the students by sharing the moderator's monitor.

For another option, LMSs often have a polling or quiz option that will allow the student to answer questions with a report sent to the instructor either divided by each individual student, or as a summary for the class.

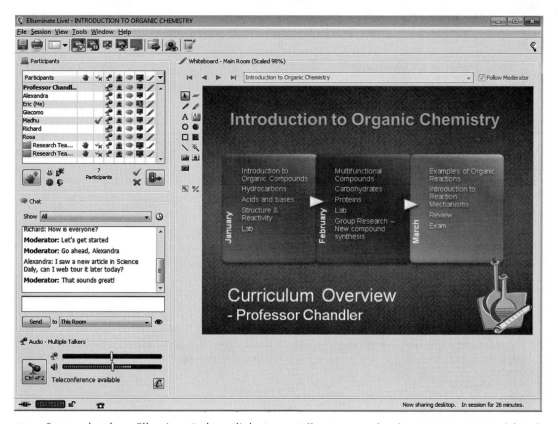

Figure 8.1 Screen shot from Elluminate's demo link. *Source: Elluminate; used with permission. Retrieved from https:// sas.elluminate.com/site/external/jwsdetect/meeting.jnlp?sid=345&password=M.AD379BCB0A40D3D8C33C6B16A84C0B& username=Test*

If this is not available in your LMS, Survey Monkey or a voting program through a listserv may be an option. Faculty can develop a form in most modern word processing or portable document format (PDF) programs, which can be e-mailed and completed by the student before the clinical rotation begins.

Clinical Quizzes and Testing

Online quizzes can be used to test students on didactic information that they may need in the clinical environment. Whether testing is done as open-ended essay questions or multiple-choice quizzes, this can be a valuable learning tool for the student. Being online, there is little control in monitoring a student's truthfulness in taking a quiz. Even "open-book" testing encourages learning, and in some cases can be more successful at teaching than "closed-book" testing.

Many LMSs offer the ability to build quizzes that can be graded automatically, allowing the student instant feedback on how he or she performed. Quizzes also can be set up so if the wrong answer is selected, a rationale why this answer is incorrect further aids the student in selecting the correct option.

Preclinical quizzes help the student remember issues; particularly safety related items that will help enforce a safe clinical environment. This can cover clinical content or required readings. Often the instructor can pull statistics to look for deficiencies between students and trends regarding wrong answers on specific questions (Figs. 8.2 and 8.3).

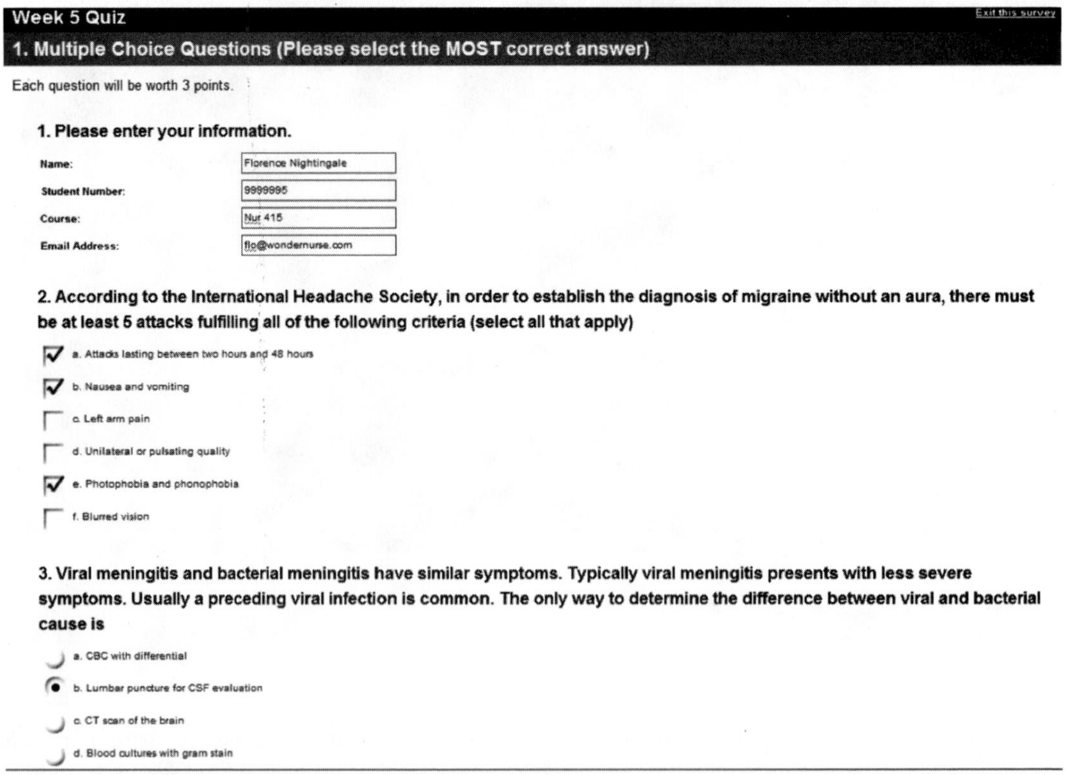

Figure 8.2   Sample quiz developed in Surveymonkey. *Source: SurveyMonkey; used with permission.*

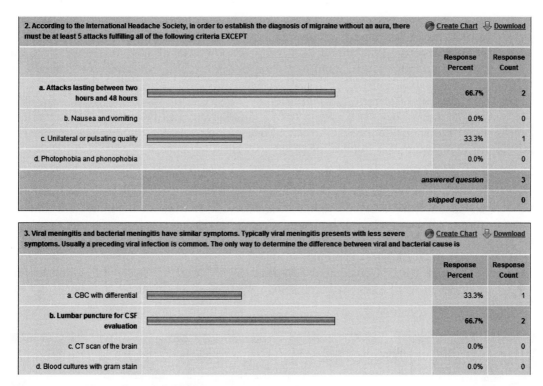

Figure 8.3 Test results from SurveyMonkey. *Source: SurveyMonkey; used with permission.*

Document Management

An important part of the clinical rotation is the monotonous task of keeping records regarding the clinical experience. A Web-based environment offers the ability to maintain and organize clinical records in an efficient manner and enables rapid access by students, faculty, and administrators.

Many LMSs have the ability to keep some documentation. Unfortunately, much of the required information for clinical rotations usually is not available unless the system has been customized specifically for nursing. Several companies offer Internet-based, clinical rotation tracking systems. Some Web-based systems include: www.typhongroup.com and www.e-value.net, which enable nursing and nurse practitioner students to track clinical time and experiences that can be customized for school and regulatory needs (Figs. 8.4 and 8.5). In

TECHNOLOGY TIP 8.8

There are several online survey clients that can be used to develop quizzes. For example, www.surveymonkey.com can be set up to put a quiz on as a survey in which the students can be identified by school number, or can remain anonymous. Usually a "screen shot" can be e-mailed to the instructor to ensure that the student completed the assignment.

addition, these systems offer portfolio building utilities that can keep statistics on the patient type, demographic, illness, and clinical skills accomplished. This is a vital tool for the student to use even after graduation as an aid to job placement. The ability to quantify the amount and type of patient or skill performed in the clinical setting gives the student increased marketability (Fig. 8.6).

Documents also can be stored as word processing or spreadsheet files on a document management system or on a centralized computer for ease of retrieval. These are much more readable than handwritten information, but in some cases is a disadvantage as they may lack a "wet signature" as proof of the student's clinical attendance.

Online Postconference

The postclinical conference is important because it allows for critical reflection. Critical reflection enhances learning and supports the development of critical thinking skills. This reflection also gives the students time to contemplate new questions and identify which goals they are close to accomplishing.

Although postclinical conferences historically have taken place at the clinical site in a borrowed room with a hastened atmosphere, Web-based postclinical conferences can be more

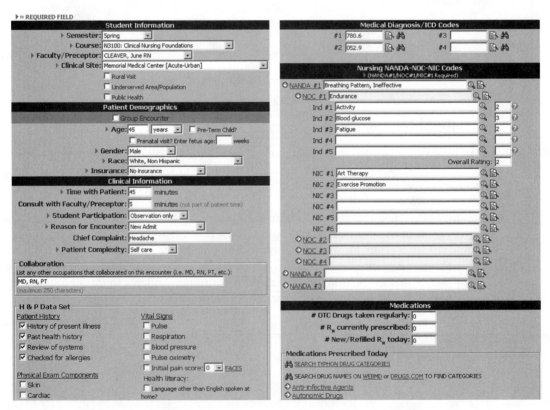

Figure 8.4 Typhon Group demo site. *Source: Typhon Group demo site; used with permission. Retrieved from http://www.typhongroup.com/products/nsst/nsst2.gif*

STUDENT SPREADSHEET
Totals by student for a variety of case log items. Press 'Apply Filters' to generate the report.

FILTER YOUR RESULTS WITH ANY OF THE FOLLOWING (Leave blank for all):

Date Range: From [____] To [____] mm/dd/yy
Grad. Class: Month [--All--] Year [--All--]
Specialty: [--All--]
Semester: [--All--]
Course: [--All--]
Clinical Site: [--All--] ○ MORE
Faculty/Preceptor: [--All--] ○ MORE

[Apply Filters] [Clear Filters] 📄 View/Export Results to Excel

Click a student row to **highlight**/un-highlight that row.

FILTERS: NONE

Name	Class	Specialty	Total Cases Entered	Total Unique Patients	Total Days w/Cases	Total Patient Hrs	Total Consult Hrs	Avg Case Load/Day	Avg Minutes/Patient	Rural Visits	Underserved	Public Health	Group Encounters	Prenatal	0-3 mo	4-6 mo	7-12 mo	13-18 mo	19-23 mo	<2
Beesly, Pam	12/11	BSN	21	21	18	36.4	24.0	1	104	2	6	1	1	3 1.3	0 0.0	0 0.0	0 0.0	0 0.0	0 0.0	0
Halpert, Jim	05/11	BSN	23	23	16	56.8	15.6	1	148	0	1	1	0	1 0.4	0 0.0	0 0.0	0 0.0	0 0.0	0 0.0	0
Hudson, Stanley	12/11	BSN-X	54	41	39	57.6	4.0	1	64	0	6	0	0	3 1.2	1 0.0	0 0.0	0 0.0	0 0.0	0 0.0	1
Lapin, Phyllis	05/11	BSN	11	11	10	9.5	3.0	1	52	0	0	0	0	0 0.0	0 0.0	1 0.2	0 0.0	0 0.0	0 0.0	1
Levinson, Jan	12/11	BSN	36	36	27	53.1	17.9	1	88	0	1	1	0	0 0.0	0 0.0	0 0.0	0 0.0	0 0.0	0 0.0	0
Malone, Kevin	12/11	BSN	17	17	9	25.5	3.7	1	90	0	0	3	0	1 0.7	0 0.0	0 0.0	0 0.0	0 0.0	0 0.0	0
Martin, Angela	05/11	BSN-X	41	41	22	69.0	12.0	1	101	0	41	0	0	1 0.3	0 0.0	0 0.0	0 0.0	0 0.0	0 0.0	0
Martinez, Oscar	05/11	BSN-X	11	11	11	20.7	6.5	1	113	0	0	2	0	0 0.0	0 0.0	0 0.0	0 0.0	0 0.0	0 0.0	0
Palmer, Meredith	05/11	BSN-X	11	11	10	38.0	6.5	1	207	0	0	0	0	0 0.0	0 0.0	0 0.0	0 0.0	0 0.0	0 0.0	0
Schrute, Dwight	05/11	BSN-X	13	13	11	23.7	8.5	1	109	0	0	5	0	1 0.4	0 0.0	0 0.0	0 0.0	0 0.0	0 0.0	0
TOTALS:			238	225	173	390.3	101.6	1	108	2	55	13	1	10 4.3	1 0.0	1 0.2	0 0.0	0 0.0	0 0.0	2
AVERAGES:			24	23	17	39.0	10.2	1	108	0	6	1	0	1 0.4	0 0.0	0 0.0	0 0.0	0 0.0	0 0.0	0

N/A = None chosen or left blank

Figure 8.5 Typhon Group demo site. *Source: Typhon Group demo site; used with permission. Retrieved from http://www.typhongroup.com/products/nsst/nsst8.gif*

enhanced and pleasant experiences. These conferences offer a richer learning environment where deep and personal reflection can take place with the use of technology.

Synchronous communication can offer spontaneity to this postclinical experience by capturing the students while their memories are fresh. These meetings can take place by chat client, an online videoconference, or a virtual environment. One nursing program used a virtual environment called Second Life, to have a postclinical conference. Students created avatars (visual character representations of themselves), and met at a specified place in cyberspace to discuss their conference experiences. Both students and faculty found this fulfilling and continued to meet regularly (Schmidt & Stewart, 2009).

TECHNOLOGY TIP 8.9

With the immediacy of cell phones, a photo can document a student's clinical attendance at a clinical site. If this is done, consider taking a photo with the preceptor and a "date" stamp or sheet indicating the date of the clinical day.

TECHNOLOGY TIP 8.10

There are many free chat and listserv clients out there with the ability to use a virtual conference. In some cases, because of multiple computer platforms, clients and computers may be incompatible with each other. Look for a chat client that is compatible with many different environments to avoid problems communicating with students.

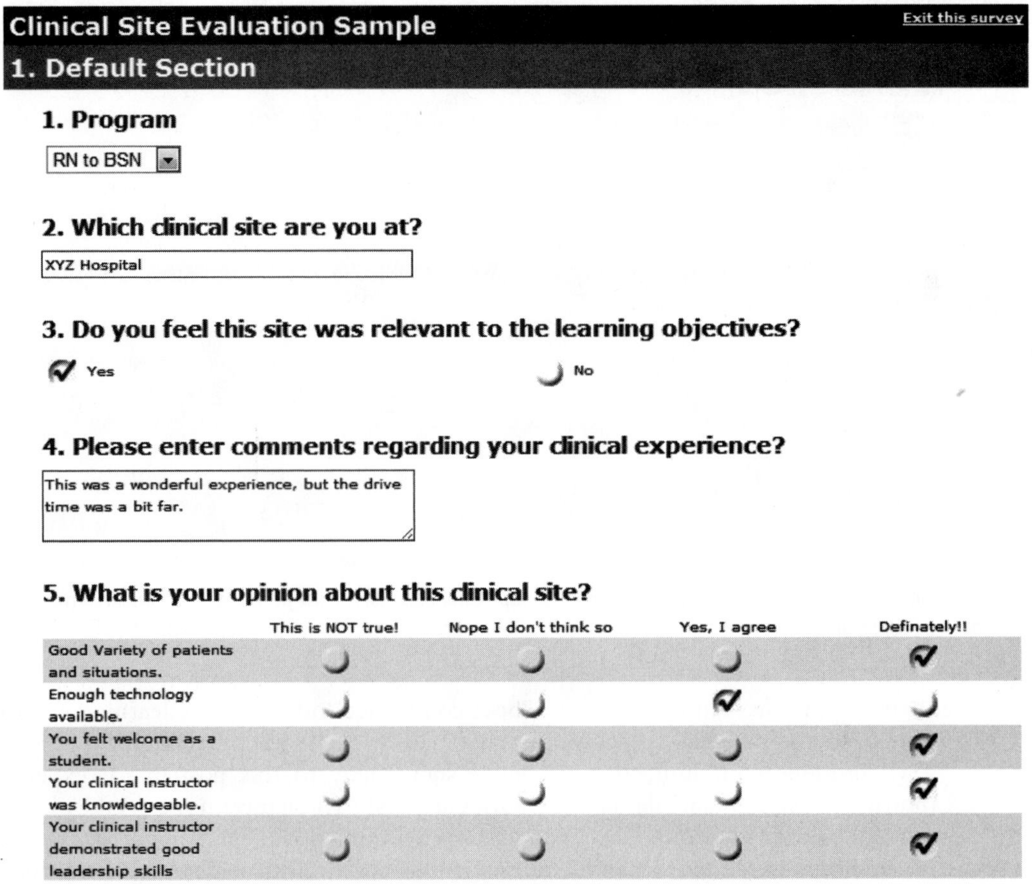

Clinical Site Evaluation Sample Exit this survey

1. Default Section

1. Program

RN to BSN

2. Which clinical site are you at?

XYZ Hospital

3. Do you feel this site was relevant to the learning objectives?

✓ Yes No

4. Please enter comments regarding your clinical experience?

This was a wonderful experience, but the drive time was a bit far.

5. What is your opinion about this clinical site?

	This is NOT true!	Nope I don't think so	Yes, I agree	Definately!!
Good Variety of patients and situations.				✓
Enough technology available.			✓	
You felt welcome as a student.				✓
Your clinical instructor was knowledgeable.				✓
Your clinical instructor demonstrated good leadership skills				✓

Figure 8.6 Survey developed by author in SurveyMonkey. *Source: SurveyMonkey; used with permission.*

Asynchronous environments also can use virtual classroom forums or listserv environments to critically reflect. Although this may be more convenient to the student, it allows his or her memories to fade a bit in the process unless he or she is encouraged to reflect soon after the experience is complete. One strategy is to create a postclinical journal in which students jot (or type) down their memorable experiences, situations, and questions for the purpose of class discussion. This also could be incorporated into a student's personal blog. (See Box 8.2 for information about HIPAA guidelines.)

Postclinical Assessment, Papers, and Projects

The postclinical assessment should include an evaluation of the agency, preceptor, and student, and experience. This often is a requirement of many accreditation agencies, and is important to the faculty to be able to distinguish those locations or preceptors that may not be supportive of the student's learning experience. The results should be anonymous and may only be available to the agency as a general summary to protect the privacy of

> **BOX 8.2**
> **ABOUT "HIPAA"**
>
> The Health Insurance Portability and Accountability Act (HIPAA) enacted in 1993 demands that the health-care professional not disclose private health information without consent of the patient. The student and instructor must be sure that any information regarding the clinical experience remains confidential. This may even include situations in which the client is identifiable based on situation or symptoms even when a name or other identifying information is not mentioned. If medical information is scanned, copied, or shared with other students, it must be clear that the information is being used for learning purposes and must not be shared outside this group or Web-based environment. Furthermore, the syllabus and other course materials should always offer reminders to the student concerning confidentiality. Especially in the Web-based environment, because the user is alone, it is easy to forget how many people are reading and watching.

the student and the school. Although some Web-based clinical tracking programs offer this to students and faculty, the ability to export the data into a spreadsheet format will enable statistic analysis among other uses for the data.

Clinical papers can help the student focus on specific areas for more in-depth study. The preclinical assessment can be a starting point to determine paper subject matter. A student also could choose a particularly interesting clinical case to study. This supports increased motivation and its success with adult learners, who will tend to learn better when they can establish how this pertains to them. Consider offering this as a team or group assignment using an online collaborative whiteboard to complete.

Projects also can be assigned to enhance learning and critical thinking in a clinical rotation. Using a Web-based environment, the assignment could be modified to include development of a slide or other online presentation as part of the grade. An example of this is a PowerPoint presentation of a patient case presented in the forum discussing the history, medications, and diagnosis to include answers to various discussion questions, which will encourage further class participation.

LABORATORY COURSES

Although didactic skills may be easily taught in many different environments, laboratory skills have challenges to Web-based environments. As many new technologies are available to meet some of these challenges, there are still barriers that considerably limit the laboratory content.

TECHNOLOGY TIP 8.11

If using an online survey program, a link can be given to preceptor, student, and agency to use for the survey. This may offer a higher response rate instead of on a piece of paper, which can be lost or forgotten. This link can be given, texted, or e-mailed to the agency, preceptor, and/or student.

The purpose of the laboratory class is to allow the student to experiment with items and equipment in a safe environment in which technical support is present. For example, a nursing student may attend a laboratory class during which they have an opportunity to prime IV tubing and operate an IV pump in a nonclinical setting. Laboratories in which the student works with equipment only can be available in a Web-based environment if that student either has the equipment where he or she has access to the Internet, or he or she is able to control the equipment remotely.

Does the student who does not receive the same hands-on experience at a distance walk away with the same knowledge and abilities? Several studies that looked specifically to the performance of Web-based students and campus students have suggested comparable performance in both writing laboratory reports and final examination scores (Abdel-Salam, Kauffman, & Crossman, 2006; Ogot, Elliott, & Glumac, 2003) (see Evidence Based Practice Box 8.3). Elliott and Kukula (2007) found that success in a Web-based laboratory class was possible, but highly dependent on the students' computer competence in interfacing with the various materials.

Although students may have comparable scores in meeting the objectives of a laboratory class, this may not equate in their ability to move these skills to the psychomotor domain to be able to care for patients in a clinical setting. For example, learning to start an IV line using a Web-based simulation may allow the student to capture and understand the steps, but it does not allow for learning the feel of needle insertion and threading.

There are several alternatives in developing laboratories for Web-environments. One is to schedule concentrated on-campus workshops for on-site instruction. An alternative is to offer distance laboratories using online interactive experience using a combination of multimedia video-based lessons, or computer simulations. This may not offer a "hands-on"

EVIDENCE-BASED PRACTICE BOX 8.3

Lack of Hands-on Experience in a Remotely Delivered Laboratory Course

Issue: Does the Lack of Hands-on Experience in a Remotely Delivered Laboratory Course Adversely Affect Student Learning?

The study compares the scores from laboratory writing reports and a final examination between on-campus and distance learning students in a fluid mechanics laboratory.

Study Findings

The study suggested that students who attended a laboratory at a distance had the same learning outcomes as those who went through an on-campus class. The results showed that the students who attended at a distance and who had no hands-on experience in the class statistically performed as well or better in laboratory writing performance and technical comprehension.

Nursing Implications

- Laboratory classes can be successfully delivered in Web-based environments.
- Despite the high level of kinesthetic learning that takes place, nursing students could learn procedures successfully without hands-on experience.
- Multimedia, including video, is a valid method of displaying laboratory-based techniques and skills (Abdel-Salam, Kauffman, & Crossman, 2006).

experience and the instructor or program designer should consider encouraging students to seek these experiences within their own communities.

Simulations are an alternative for Web-based environments as long as the equipment is transferable to this environment and the learning objectives do not require as much psychomotor skills using equipment that is not available to the student off site.

Preparation and Communicating During the Laboratory

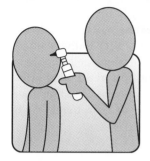

The entire concept of a laboratory is to be able to enhance psychomotor learning by practicing skills and theories in a controlled environment for the purposes of learning. In a Web-based environment, some imagination is required as the psychomotor domain is displayed and simulated instead of directly being used. Offering experiences to as many of the senses as possible makes the need for video, sound, three-dimensional (3-D) enhancement and manipulation an integral part of the laboratory.

Laboratories can be done in a synchronous or asynchronous format. Synchronous laboratories enable the instructor to be available at the time of the laboratory, which can be important to address specific questions vital to the learning process. When doing synchronous laboratories in Web-based environments, it is critical to ensure that all technical issues are addressed well before the scheduled laboratory time. This entails the student to have the ability to connect to the laboratory server before the start of class. Technical issues are difficult to address and in some cases may take new software or hardware for proper operation.

Many conference programs are available with the ability to run synchronous laboratories. A successful laboratory will allow the instructor/moderator to share his or her desktop with the group, operate a Web camera, and send and receive various audio and video files.

One such service available for this purpose is Elluminate. This software/server allows the facilitator to set up a synchronous time when a group of people can meet for a class or session. It offers a collaborating and social network environment and helps to put controls in place so that a moderator can work with a large group of people in a controlled environment.

Common technical problems include camera or microphone problems. Often there can be feedback difficulties because microphones are not set correctly or not turned off when a student is done speaking. If the moderator of the group has the power to control the individual student microphones and other functions, the class can proceed smoothly.

Using 3-D Modeling and Technology

Most Web-based clinical content is two dimensional. This can be difficult when learning 3-D processes, such as anatomy. 3-D modeling uses a process of scanning an object into a computer to build a 3-D image, which can be manipulated in a Web-based environment. Rotation, enlargement, enhancement, and labeling parts of this image can all be done on the screen for the purpose of immersing the student in a more realistic experience without the need for cadaver laboratories and models. Being able to manipulate the image is a critical feature, but being able to hold it in one's hand is much more immersive. This offers challenges to those with a large need for kinesthetic learning. This also is a great use to those who are specifically learning minor surgical procedures, such as joint injection, central or peripherally inserted central catheter (PICC) line placement, or wound debridement.

Bringing life to a 3-D environment involves powerful computers and math. With the current microprocessors becoming more advanced, we are seeing more 3-D modeling and rendering widely available. Web-based environments offer the ability to see a 3-D image, manipulate it in a virtual space, and make changes to the image. A recent study of a biology class comparing students learning from two-dimensional (2-D) renderings versus 3-D renderings demonstrated students who were exposed to more advanced forms of imaging performed better in testing than their 2-D counterparts (Hilbelink, 2009) (see Evidence Based Practice Box 8.4).

Many companies offer external Web sites that use 3-D imaging technology to include virtual manipulation of bones, muscle, organs, and other anatomical structures individually or as a whole. These applications are available for viewing and rotating on some cell phones.

As this technology may teach knowledge, it is limited in developing critical thinking skills. True immersion in virtual worlds continues to evolve in game development. As simulation laboratories seem to be a growing phenomenon for schools, they are far from home use in Web-based environments for the distance learner.

Computer-Based Simulation and Virtual Environments

Virtual environments have their roots in the original "role-playing" games (RPGs). The first RPGs used shields, boards, and dice to simulate real-time outcomes. When networks became more sophisticated, text-based multiplayer networks developed. As computers and telecommunications advanced, these worlds became more complex. Perhaps the most famous at this time are World of Warcraft (www.worldofwarcraft.com) and Second Life (www.secondlife.com). These environments are known as multiuser virtual environments (MUVEs). Although they are used for entertainment, there are many researchers investigating their use for

---

EVIDENCE-BASED PRACTICE BOX 8.4

Measurement of the Effectiveness of Incorporating 3-D Imaging in an Online Anatomy Course

Issue: Do Students Who Use 3-D Anatomy Renderings Perform Better Than Their 2-D Counterparts?

This study analyzed the scores on a practical examination given to two cohorts of students, one cohort using 2-D images to learn anatomy, and the other using 3-D images. Both laboratories were delivered by distance learning methods.

Study Findings

The results showed that the distance learning students who were able to use 3-D images statistically outperformed their counterparts.

Nursing Implications

- 3-D image viewing and manipulation has a clear advantage in teaching physical characteristics in a Web-based environment.
- Further investigation is needed to determine if delivery of skills and other kinesthetic nursing functions can be successfully taught with 3-D technologies.
- There appears to be importance in using spatial relationships to enhance the learning process (Hilbelink, 2009).

simulation in education. These simulations can effectively replace clinical experiences and bridge the gap between the classroom and clinical practice (Vergara, Caudell, Goldsmith, & Alverson, 2008). (See Evidence Based Practice Box 8.5.)

Simulation offers the student an experience solving real-world problems using a computer. In these Web-based environments, simulations can be anything from typing in a series of instructions to obtain a goal or find a problem, to using computer peripherals as tools to mimic the mechanism of a syringe or ventilator setting. A simulation can be goal oriented, or it can be a virtual environment where there may not be a specific or obvious objective.

The goal of any simulation is its realism to an actual process or environment. The realism of a simulation or environment designates it as a partially immersive or fully immersive environment. These computer-based simulations usually require some type of logic engine or program so the computer is able to adjust the framework of the simulations based on your decisions or actions taken or not taken. For example, in a computer flight simulator the computer is constantly watching the controls (i.e., a joystick, keyboard, or specialized control devices) to see what the user does at any moment. Using preset constants and preloaded statistics, such as weather, plane type, weight, thrust, etc., the simulator makes decisions about altitude and airspeed.

To make a simulation more effective, special headgear and glasses can be used for greater immersion. In a Web-based environment with the student logging in from home, this type of immersion is difficult to achieve because much of it is dependent on the availability of specialized hardware or high-speed Internet. It is likely that this will be possible in the near future.

Fully immersive virtual environments use computer technology to trick a user's senses into thinking he or she actually is in a simulated world. This uses a combination of real props (i.e., chairs, tables, and equipment), large computer screens, and surround sound. Unfortunately some of these simulations offer linear scenarios that may not always have significant

---

EVIDENCE-BASED PRACTICE BOX 8.5

The Use of Problem-Based Learning Strategies in Immersive Simulation

Issue: Success of Knowledge Driven Design of a Virtual Patient Simulation.

This case study described the development and usage of a virtual patient to create immersive scenarios for enhancement of problem-based learning in multiuser virtual environments.

Study Findings

Several studies completed by the research team in the development of this multiuser virtual simulation showed knowledge-driven development yielded positive learning outcomes and could successfully be used for distributive medical learning.

Nursing Implications

- It is important that experienced nurses are involved in development of any problem-based virtual learning environments.
- Virtual learning environments can be used to teach nursing through a problem-based approach.
- Virtual environments can be used to teach a large number of students effectively (Vergara, Caudell, Goldsmith, & Alverson, 2008).

flexibility unless the simulator is someone operating the controls in anticipation of the student's actions. Depending upon the area of learning, these can be made quite realistic. Unfortunately the technology and cost is prohibitive for Web-based use.

Task-specific simulations offer a menu of choices for a given situation. For example, an Advanced Cardiac Life Support simulation may give a patient scenario, and then ask the user to select the action or actions he or she wishes to perform. These may include giving oxygen, playing the patient on a monitor, defibrillating, administering multiple medications, or performing cardiopulmonary resuscitation (CPR) (Fig. 8.7). There may be several correct answers, and they may not need to be done in a specific order. This adds to the complexity that the computer simulation requires interpreting the actions and showing the results to the user.

Other virtual environments may not have a specific patient or goal. These environments are set up so the user is interacting as if he or she was at the clinical site. There is no direction but merely a "sandbox" in which he or she begins. The student can select the tasks needed and complete them in any order at any time. Choices may include viewing the student's assignment, perusing the charts or Kardex, preparing medication, or completing discharge and admission paperwork. This uses immersive learning to support a constructivist environment.

Although items can be built into the scenarios, it is difficult to mimic the daily fusion that can occur on any hospital or clinic floor. These virtual environments can work toward developing organizational skills and gives students a better understanding of needed tasks and basic problem-solving techniques needed in their clinical rotations.

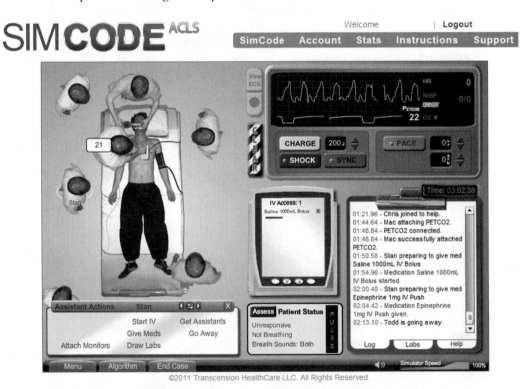

Figure 8.7 *Source: From SimCode ACLS™ (http://www.simcodeacls.com), used with permission from Transcension HealthCare LLC.*

ADMINISTRATIVE ISSUES AND CONSIDERATIONS

There are some administrative issues that should be considered before implementing a complete Web-based environment. The school should develop specific policies that address issues unique to Web-based degree programs. Gellman-Danley and Fetzner (1998) describe seven different policy areas to address including: academic, fiscal, geographic, governance, labor-management, legal, and student support services.

Having a strategic plan, developing policies, and cultivating a well-built software infrastructure are just some of the considerations in a Web-based environment. Strong planning to include administrators and faculty often will lead to a more successful implementation. In addition to regulatory requirements from educational accreditation groups, the administrator also must consider guidelines from nursing accreditation agencies and state boards of nursing.

Organize a Web-Based Environment

The first step to organizing a Web-based environment is to develop a strategic plan for implementation. It is critical to develop a strong technology infrastructure that is able to support this process. With commercially prepared software and companies that specialize in installation and support, LMSs have become easier to implement. Expect that staff will be needed for local support as well.

Part of the strategic plan should include development time lines and goal objectives for implementation. Administrators can work collaboratively with faculty and instructional designers to decide the specific program offerings including media activities, technology used, and data communication requirements. Often faculty input is critical because of their valuable work experience and unique understanding of the needs of the students. Faculty involvement also can decrease or prevent conflict during the implementation. An inclusive committee should be used to help with the decision-making process (Palloff & Pratt, 2001).

Development of the curriculum and design of the learning environment is another area that can cause faculty conflict. Questions about how the faculty will be paid, and whether the developed product is owned by the individual or by the school, are some of the issues at hand. Intellectual property rights are more difficult because some of the development may occur on an individual's home computer. Considering many of the servers are stored on university or vendor property, most property rights belong to the school.

Communicate

Communication between administration and faculty is a key to a successful Web-based environment. Many schools set up faculty forums or develop e-mail lists solely for this purpose. Decisions must be made on which faculty to include in the communication, and how to ensure a communication was received. Many LMSs have faculty pages or forums in place for this reason. Announcements can be placed within the log-in pages to communicate news about the college or the school.

Faculty meetings can be replaced by virtual environments, online forums, or perhaps even podcasts, which can be viewed at the faculty's leisure. Other forms of communication include instant messaging, text messaging, phone conference calls, and videoconferencing. Much of the technology used to deliver education to the students also can be considered for improving faculty communication.

Critical success to the implementation of the Web-based environment is appropriate faculty training. Time and resources for training and support must be included in the strategic plan and the fiscal budget. Without this critical training, a Web-based environment could be a potential disaster. One such program being developed by the National League for Nursing is the "Living Book." These are found as part of a nursing faculty development program entirely available online to assist with faculty development. One of these online courses is specifically for nurse educators using Web-based environments (Fig. 8.8).

The National League for Nursing also is partnering with Indiana State University School of Nursing to deliver a certificate program in how to teach and learn in a Web-based environment. This course is designed to assist nurses to develop the skills they need to develop Web-based content specific to nursing. Find out more at http://nursing.iupui.edu/continuing/courses/teachingwebc1.shtml

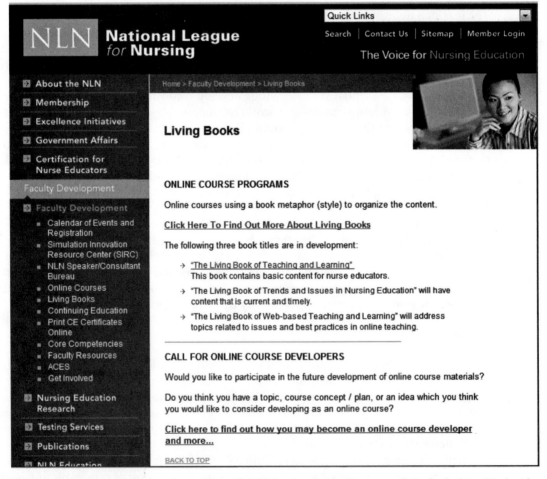

Figure 8.8 *Source: Living Books: http://www.nln.org/facultydevelopment/onlinecourses/livingbooks.htm. Used with permission from the National League for Nursing, New York, NY.*

Technical support for students and faculty requires full-time IT staff that can be contacted and immediately available. Although not all programs have 24-hour support, it may be an important service to invest in given the nature of Web-based environments and schedules. This will ensure both student and faculty satisfaction, and will allow the school to identify critical errors, which rapidly could bring down the environment.

Engage

Finally, engaging the faculty in teaching the course is as important as engaging the students. Faculty who are engaged and eager to develop and discuss substantive information gathered from the assignments and the readings will inspire the students to do extra work to enhance their learning process.

Ensuring that faculty work loads are appropriate and rewarding faculty for additional work needed within the curriculum and infrastructure also will help engage them in the course and the program. Surveys that include questions about time requirements for facilitation and assignment correction may help illuminate what is an appropriate faculty and student load. LMSs often can track the amount of time a faculty member is logged into the system, although this may not be truly accurate of the total time commitment, and should not be used as a sole indicator of faculty participation.

ASSESSMENT AND ACCREDITATION

Accreditation is the basis for monitoring the quality of distance educations programs. These agencies review programs on strict criteria and determine if they are eligible to receive federal financial aid funds. They also grant degrees that include standardized curriculum across the country. This helps employers and licensing agencies in selecting candidates knowing that they have met the requirements set by a regional or national regulatory agency.

Standards for E-Learning

Standards for e-learning fall into several different categories. The technology standards are developed by various engineering organizations to define the electronic and communications infrastructure, which may include specific communications, storage, and equipment standards. This also could include how individual data records are stored, or which encryption algorithm may be used to send confidential information across the Internet.

Educational standards are set by various organizations to improve the quality of the online educational experience. The Sloan Consortium (www.sloan-c.org) is a group of organizations and institutions committed to improving the quality of Web-based education. They offer conferences, publications, and workshops aimed at offering best practices and innovative approaches to enhance online education. Other organizations offer services to improve the quality of Web-based environments. Many of these organizations are used by institutions on a voluntary basis. For example, Quality Matters (www.qualitymatters.org) is an organization that offers a faculty-centered, peer-review–based process to certify the quality of an online program.

The other standards for e-learning are set by the accreditation agencies. Two forms of accreditation for colleges are institutional and specialized accreditation. Institutional accreditation is performed by national associations of colleges and schools. Each may be specific to a region or a particular type of school (i.e., vocational, religious). Specialized accreditation is program specific. There are a couple of nursing associations that perform accreditation specific to nursing programs.

According to the Council for Higher Education Accreditation (CHEA), there are seven key areas that are evaluated. These include: Institutional Mission, Organizational Structure, Available Resources, Curriculum and Instruction, Faculty Support, Student Support, and Student Outcomes (2002). The accreditation agencies want to ensure that the student and faculty have the available resources they need to learn. These include library, textbook, and faculty access. The faculty also must have resources to be able to instruct. Some issues including faculty expectations and student loads need to be evaluated differently in a Web-based environment.

The mission and structure must be integrated into the overall school's structure and include sufficient oversight to ensure the quality of the educational program. This includes institutional policies and procedures that are followed and reviewed regularly.

Curriculum and instruction must be appropriate and comparable to on-campus programs with similar course and degree offerings. Furthermore, the schools are expected to collect information on student outcomes to compare with national benchmarks within the same areas of study.

Standards Specific to Nursing

In addition to the accreditation needs required by the school as a learning institution, nursing programs in Web-based environments face additional regulatory review by nursing organizations as well. Two of the most used accrediting bodies are the Commission on Collegiate Nursing Education (CCNE) and the National League for Nursing Accrediting Commission (NLNAC). Both agencies have specific policies in place for distance education.

NLNAC (2008) provides guidance for all distance learning programs within one policy in its 2008 accreditation manual. This policy includes eight critical elements that should be in all distance education programs for nursing. These are similar to the CHEA recommendations and include: congruence with institutional mission, instructional design methods of the courses, competence and preparation of the faculty, accessibility and quality of support services, current and relevant offerings, appropriate faculty and student interactions, and ongoing evaluation and assessment of student learning. In addition, with each standard listed in the manual, there are separate standards included for those programs engaged in distance education.

In comparison, CCNE (2009) incorporates its standards within the overall accreditation standards for the institution. Throughout the accreditation manual it mentions distance education, but keeps it inclusive with other educational offerings. A statement in its manual acknowledges that education has become innovative, and it wishes to encourage this innovation as long as it benefits the student.

Assessment and Data Collection

As part of the requirements for accreditation, regulatory agencies expect each school to evaluate their program for learning outcomes. Processes must be in place to collect aggregate student data for this process. These outcomes are reviewed and may impact whether the program continues to obtain accreditation.

Data collected for this process can include but is not limited to NCLEX-RN, AANP, or ANCC passing rates, student satisfaction surveys, graduation rates, and employment rates. Programs are expected to collect data on passing rates even in states that may not require national certification or testing. Programs are encouraged to collect additional data that may support other aspects of the program including the mission and goals of the school.

In addition to student data collection, the faculty members also should be surveyed to ensure that their work is congruent with the mission and goals of the program. Other important information could include job satisfaction, software navigation issues, and availability of faculty support and services.

In a Web-based environment, many of these surveys and statistics can be collected using various online survey tools. In addition, structured query language (SQL) databases can be maintained so the faculty, administration, and regulatory agencies cannot only access the data, but can sort it into various aggregate groupings for further analysis. Statistical feedback evaluating response rates and e-mailing student and faculty automatically in the data collection process will help to increase response rates and maintain much more accurate data.

Data Analysis and Reporting

Data Analysis can be done compared with other regional and national programs. If there are deficiencies in the program, this may indicate areas of program improvement. Regulatory agencies wish to ensure that there is a system in place for identifying areas of weakness, and setting up a plan of improvement for any deficits that are identified.

These agencies also look to ensure that any formal complaints are addressed within the program and modifications are made if needed depending upon the specific complaint or problem.

Although regulatory agencies do not usually require reporting of the data unless requested, distance education programs can report the data and use it to compare with national standards and programs. Some state agencies will use the reported data to determine the effectiveness of the educational program. In some cases this data may be published and compared with regional programs. Nursing boards sometimes will use this reportable information to determine if a program is having internal problems that may compromise patient safety.

EMERGING TECHNOLOGIES

As we strive to understand how nursing education should be delivered in an online environment, new technologies are emerging that show new opportunities. Some of these technologies include blogs, social bookmarks, podcasting, vodcasting wikis, social networking, collaborative online documents, and waves. Many of these show promise to enhance and perhaps confuse all of us about what future nursing education will be like.

Blogs are Web pages kept by individuals to chronicle various daily and weekly activities. These are pages that anyone can navigate to, make comments on, and follow to keep up with the individual author. These sites are good for publishing knowledge and offering critical reflection and analysis that can be collectively shared (Yang, 2009). This process helps with building contextual knowledge and relationships while sharing them collectively within the community of interest.

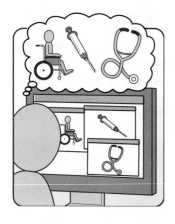

Wikis are collections of Web pages that are linked together and collectively authored. This is similar to a living encyclopedia of knowledge that allows the learner the ability to quickly find useful knowledge and contribute as needed.

Social bookmarks are personalized collections of Web links categorized into useful groups and accessible to anyone who is looking to consolidate and share resources. These allow learners and faculty to share their favorite links with others easily to anyone with a computer and Internet access.

Vodcasting and podcasting is the recording of video and audio for publication and playback on portable media players. This is useful to share information to use at times and locations that may be helpful to the learner. These video or audio clips can include lectures, study groups, meetings, or even audio notes to assist the learner in critical reflection and better knowledge retrieval.

Collaborative online documents allow the sharing of Word, spreadsheet, and presentation documents for review and revision. Learners can build a document simultaneously in a collaborative process without being in the same city or country. During the editing process, each contributor's entries are identified by a different text color in the document. This collaborative process enhances group and team learning while allowing faculty the ability to track individual contributions to a group assignment.

Another technology coming soon developed by Google is the Wave. This is a complex social e-mailing environment that allows synchronous sharing of a collaborative e-mail across two or more individuals. The goal is to offer one Web-based tool that merges social networking, wikis, e-mail, and instant messaging (*Google Wave,* 2009). Although its potential use could make significant changes to online education, this technology is still in its infancy.

Social Networking is the newest online tool to become popular. This allows individuals to have their own Web pages and collections of friends they allow to view them. They can share photos, thoughts, music, and even various games and applications. This certainly could be used as a home class or course page for communicating and sharing information between class or course members.

Although these technologies may be great ways of storing and retrieving information, it is not evident yet as to which learners may benefit from which Web-based environments. One thing that is clear is that faculty members need to have a better understanding of the learning styles within their classes to find which of these tools may be most optimal in each case to deliver critical education (Saeed, Yang, & Sinnappan, 2009). Matching the learning style with the technology could enhance the overall student outcomes.

CONCLUSION

Web-based environments are new and exciting, and continue to become more advanced as our infrastructure and technology becomes better. When it seems that we have reached the limit of possible tools that can be used for delivering learning at a distance, exciting concepts come to market. Portability and bandwidth will likely be the technology that will continue to change Web-based environments. Simulations and virtual environments will become more immersive. Certainly the personal use of the 3-D cameras also will offer new ways of learning.

By understanding Web-based environments, and using the most current concepts for delivery of curriculum content, we can improve learning, and create a nurse who is able to provide safe and effective care.

REFERENCES

Abdel-Salam, T., Kauffman, P. J., & Crossman, G. (2006). Does the lack of hands-on experience in a remotely delivered laboratory course affect student learning? *European Journal of Engineering Education, 31*(6), 747–756.

CHEA Institute for Research and Study of Accreditation. (2002). *Accreditation and assuring quality in distance learning.* Washington, DC: Council for Higher Education Accreditation.

Commission on Collegiate Nursing Education. (2009). *Standards of accreditation of baccalaureate and graduate degree nursing programs.* Washington, DC: Commission on Collegiate Nursing Education.

Dougiamas, M. (1999). Developing tools to foster online educational dialogue. In K. Martin, N. Stanley, & N. Davison (Eds.), *Proceedings of the 8th annual teaching learning forum,* (pp. 119–123). Perth, Australia: University of Western Australia.

Elliott, S. J., & Kukula, E. (2007, November 1). The challenges associated with laboratory-based distance education. *Educause Quarterly, 30*(1), 37–42. Retrieved from http://www.educause.edu/EDUCAUSE+Quarterly/EDUCAUSEQuarterlyMagazineVolum/TheChallengesAssociatedwithLab/157441

Gellman-Danley, B., & Fetzner, M. J. (1998, Spring). Asking the really tough questions: Policy issues for distance learning. Online Journal of Distance Learning Adminiatration, 1(1). Retrieved from http://www.westga.edu/~distance/danley11.html

Google Wave. (2009, December 23). Retrieved from http://en.wikipedia.org/w/index.php?title=Google_Wave&oldid=333570186

Hilbelink, J. (2009). A measure of the effectiveness of incorporating 3-D human anatomy into an online undergraduate laboratory. *British Journal of Educational Technology, 40*(4), 664–672.

Lynch, M. (2002). *The online educator: Guide to creating the virtual classroom.* New York, NY: Rutledge Falmer.

Morabito, M. G. (2009). *CALCampus: Origins.* Retrieved from http://www.calcampus.com/calc.htm

Morgan, G. (2003, May 20). *Course management systems in the history and the future of higher education.* Retrieved from http://net.educause.edu/ir/library/pdf/ers0302/rs/ers030210.pdf

Morris, T., & Hancock, D. (2008). Program exit examinations in nursing education: Using a value added assessment as a measure of the impact of a new curriculum. *Educational Research Quarterly, 32*(2), 19–29.

National League for Nursing Accrediting Commission. (2008). *Accreditation manual 2008 edition.* New York, NY: National League for Nursing Accrediting Commission.

Ogot, M., Elliott, G., & Glumac, N. (2003). An assessment of in-person and remotely operated laboratories. *Journal of Engineering Education, 92,* 57–63.

O'Neil, C. A., Fisher, C. A., & Newbold, S. K. (2009). *Developing online nursing environments in nursing education.* New York, NY: Springer Publishing Company.

Palloff, R. M., & Pratt, K. (2001). *Lessons from the cyberspace classroom.* San Francisco, CA: Jossey-Bass.

Palloff, R. M., & Pratt, K. (2003). *The virtual student.* San Francisco, CA: Jossey-Bass.

Saeed, N., Yang, Y., & Sinnappan, S. (2009). Emerging web technologies in higher education: A case of incorporating blogs, podcasts and social bookmarks in a web programming course based on students' learning styles and technology preferences. *Educational Technology & Society, 12*(4), 98–109.

Schmidt, B., & Stewart, S. (2009). Implementing the virtual reality learning environment: Second life. *Nurse Educator, 34*(4), 152–155.

Spurlock, D. R., & Hunt, L. A. (2008). A study of the usefulness of the HESI exit exam in predicting NCLEX-RN failure. *Journal of Nursing Education, 47*(4), 157–166.

United States Securities and Exchange Commission. (2008). *Form 10K: Blackboard, Inc. Annual Filing.* Washington, DC.

Vergara, V., Caudell, T., Goldsmith, T., & Alverson, D. (2008). *Knowledge-driven design of virtual patient simulations.* Retrieved from http://www.innovateonline.info/index.php?view=article&id=579

Wang, Y., Peng, H., Huang, R., Hou, Y., & Wang, J. (2008). Characteristics of distance learning: Research on relationships of learning motivation, learning strategy, self-efficacy, attribution and learning results. *Open Learning, 23*(1), 17–28.

Woodill, G. (2007, April 23). *The evolution of learning management systems.* Retrieved from http://www.hrreporter.com

Yang, S.H. (2009). Using blogs to enhance critical reflection and community of practice. *Educational Technology & Society, 12*(2), 11–21.

Chapter 9

E-Learning Assessment

Beth Starnes-Vottero, PhD, RN, CNE

The first time I incorporated an online examination for a hybrid course, I focused on details, such as time limits for responses, using standardized questions, and providing the rationale for each correct and incorrect answer. I felt good about how the examination was set up in the learning management system (LMS). The students were given instructions on how to access the examination with a defined time frame for completing the test. On the day of the examination, I watched as the results started coming in, using the management system to analyze how the 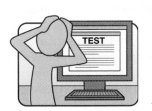 *students responded to each of the questions. I was surprised to see that three of the best students did not attempt to take the examination. During the next class, I was bombarded with questions. First, I realized that I didn't activate the results for viewing by the students. They had no idea how they performed on the test. Second, I didn't take into account that although I lived in the central time zone, the home for LMS was at the main campus, which was in the eastern time zone. Students attempted to take the examination between 11 p.m. and 12 a.m. only to find that the examination timed out! Now I pay close attention to not only the examination itself, but also to how I set it up.*

Assessment is an ongoing process that involves planning, discussion, reflection, analyzing, and making improvements based on data collected about a learning objective. The e-learning environment affords unique opportunities to assess students' learning. Educational technology offers tools and techniques for assessment that yields data to inform what educators know about learning mastery and the effectiveness of their teaching (Buzzetto-More & Alade, 2006). Each interaction in the online format provides rich information about understanding of the content. This chapter provides an overview of fully constrained (i.e., online examinations/quizzes) to least constrained (i.e., projects, papers) e-assessment methods to incorporate into an online course.

The online environment presents opportunities for authentic assessment of students' learning; where individuality, teamwork, collaboration, and communication abilities are assessed through a variety of methods (Seok, 2008). Within the e-learning environment, it is impossible for students to sit quietly in the back of an online course, passively waiting until they are called upon to speak. Participation becomes a requirement; the challenge is to make it significant to learning. Educators are faced with the need to effectively extract meaningful information about student learning. Assessment requires attention to detail, knowledge of the LMS being used, and expertise in the subject content. A variety of techniques are available to assess students' learning; from embedded tools in the management system to instructor-created, course-based methods. Selection of an appropriate assessment instrument results from an analysis of the objectives for the course, the type of course, level of the course, and type of learners.

Learning objectives drive selection of assessment tools. Because objectives are based on verbs that demonstrate learning, the type of verb guides the selection of appropriate assessment techniques to support learning outcomes. For example, if students are required to "identify" a concept, then a multiple-choice format allowing the student to select from choices is a viable option. If "describe" is used, the instructor might want to use a shortanswer or paper to demonstrate a student's learning. Best practice in education dictates that the alignment between the objective and assessment method is essential for demonstrating achievement of learning outcomes (Anderson et al., 2001). For further understanding, a basic list of common verbs with suggestions for electronic assessment methods can be found on Davis Plus.

The type of course involves an analysis of course content. Think of the various types of courses available at your institution. Not every course is conducive to every assessment method and it is up to the educator to select appropriate methods to demonstrate knowledge. For instance, a beginning Fundamentals of Nursing course presents certain challenges that differ from an exit-level nursing course. Initially, students in the Fundamentals course would not be required to demonstrate aseptic technique for Foley catheter insertion until they acquired a basic understanding of aseptic technique. Instead, assessment of learning using an online format could include viewing streaming videos of nursing tasks then selecting the steps in an aseptic task that were appropriate versus inappropriate. Another means of assessment could require students to complete a basic competency test before demonstration of learning in front of an instructor. Streaming videos, compact disks (CDs), and other formats that provide actual scenarios of tasks increase basic knowledge of the steps required to complete the action. As an alternative, in an exit-level course, a discussion format provides a rich understanding of students' learning. Of course this is not the only tool, a variety of assessment methods described both above and throughout this chapter can be employed to assess e-learning.

The level of the course and type of learner contribute to the selection of assessment tools. Undergraduate students with a basic understanding of concepts should be tested differently than graduate level students who use the concepts in their daily practice. The graduate student might be asked to take the concept and provide a deeper analysis or to create a new way to look at the concept. The creation of something new requires assessing various aspects of knowledge and may require more than a multiple-choice format. Rather, the use of projects, papers, discussions, or concept maps enhances the opportunity to demonstrate desired learning.

One caveat is worthy of note; regardless of the student's level, if the assessment requires taking a concept out of the known context, then basic knowledge of the context should be assessed first. For example, teaching a diabetic patient how to care for his or her feet is a basic nursing function and is a new function for the undergraduate student nurse. A graduate nursing student might take the concept of teaching diabetic foot care and apply it to a homeless shelter, a Hispanic culture, or might include research on educational effectiveness.

In this case, assessment of basic concepts related to the context would be essential. This example demonstrates how the different level requires a basic understanding of the context although the concepts are familiar.

BASIC TECHNOLOGY REQUIREMENTS

Before initiating an online course, certain technical requirements must be detailed for all users. Most LMSs provide a browser check to be completed before accessing and entering the course in a LMS. The browser check is an analysis of the computer accessing the course to ensure that certain aspects of the course can be run effectively. Providing students' access to free downloads that support the system encourages consistency in computer capabilities. The browser check is designed to identify certain computer issues, it is essential that the student is given appropriate tools to remedy any issues. It is not the time to find out that your computer does not have the technical abilities to support the course tools when an attempt to access an examination results in an error message. It is essential that students download the most current or recent software application or plug-in to use course assessment tools. Free tools required for most systems can be found in Box 9.1 and see Technology Tip 9.1 for a resource of clear steps to ensure that the user has the most recent and required plug-ins and downloads.

ASSESSMENT METHODS

Innovations in technology for e-assessment build the foundation from which high-quality formative assessments can emerge, allowing alignment between intended learning, instruction, and

---

BOX 9.1
DOWNLOADS

Basic Required Downloads

Java	http://java.com/en/download/index.jsp

File Compression

Winzip	http://www.winzip.com/index.htm

Audio and Media Players

Real Player	http://www.real.com/
Windows Media Player	http://www.microsoft.com/windows/windowsmedia/player/10/default.aspx
Apple Quick Time	http://www.apple.com/quicktime/download/
Adobe Flash Player	http://get.adobe.com/flashplayer/
Adobe Shockwave	http://get.adobe.com/shockwave/
Apple iTunes	http://www.apple.com/itunes/download/

File Readers and Viewers

Adobe Acrobat Reader	http://get.adobe.com/reader/
Microsoft Office Compatibility Pack 2007 File Format	http://www.microsoft.com/downloads/details.aspx?FamilyId=941b3470-3ae9-4aee-8f43-c6bb74cd1466&displaylang=en

TECHNOLOGY TIP 9.1

An example of clear steps to ensure that the user has the most recent and required plug-ins and downloads can be viewed at http://otel.uis.edu/Portal/browsertest/index.asp. Consider sharing this link with students or creating a Web-link page that they can access anytime.

e-assessment (Krathwohl, 2002; Scalise & Gifford, 2006). LMSs incorporate a variety of basic tools to support assessment of students' learning; assorted types of examination questions (alternate format items), the ability to import standardized examination questions from textbook publishers, live chat functions, threading of discussions, whiteboards, and drop-box capabilities. Other tools available to the instructor include the ability to exchange assignments created with Microsoft Word, PowerPoint, flash presentations, and Web sites. To augment testing, computer-aided enhancements include sound, graphics, animation, and video that can be incorporated into the test item. It must be noted that some research suggests that any features added to a test that are not essential to the variable being tested can pose a potential threat to validity (Van der Linden, 2002). Another cautionary note for those who choose to use enhancements, some technology can load slowly or not at all based on the type of Internet connection. Dial-up connections typically experience such issues. To remedy the problem, requiring students to take the assessment at a known location with broadband, dedicated service line (DSL), or T1 capabilities such as a school computer laboratory or library, increases the odds that the enhancements will load and play without problems. See Table 9.1 for objective verbs with associated e-assessment strategies.

TABLE 9.1

Objective Verbs With Associated E-Assessment Strategies

Cognitive Process	Alternative Verbs	E-Assessment
Remember • Recognizing • Recalling	Identify Retrieve	Examination/Quiz questions

Understand
• Interpreting
• Exemplifying
• Classifying
• Summarizing
• Inferring
• Comparing
• Explaining
	Clarify, paraphrase, represent,
	   translate
	Illustrate
	Categorize
	Abstract, generalize
	Conclude, extrapolate, predict
	Contrast, map, match
		Examination questions
		Short answer
		Essay
		Discussion questions
		Concept map (see Davis Plus for
		   online Concept Map Creator)

Apply • Executing • Implementing	Carry out, use	Discussion questions Essay Presentation Simulation

TABLE 9.1—cont'd

Objective Verbs With Associated E-Assessment Strategies

Cognitive Process	Alternative Verbs	E-Assessment
Analyze • Differentiating • Organizing • Attributing	Discriminate, distinguish, focus, select, find coherence, integrate, outline, structure, deconstruct	Discussion questions Essay Presentation Simulation Case Study Paper/Project
Evaluate • Checking • Critiquing	Coordinate, detect, monitor, test, judge	Discussion questions Essay Presentation Simulation Case Study Paper/Project Note: There must be criteria to evaluate self or peers on the above assessment.
Create • Generating • Planning • Producing	Hypothesize, design, construct	Paper/Project Presentation Simulation Case Study Note: Incorporate criteria to create something new within the assignment.

Adapted from Anderson, L. W., Krathwohl, D. R., Airasian, P. W., Cruikshank, K. A., Mayer, R. E., Pintrich, P. R., et al. (Eds.). (2001). *A taxonomy for learning, teaching, and assessing: A revision of Bloom's taxonomy of educational objectives.* New York, NY: Addison Wesley Longman, Inc.

Rubrics

Clearly linking assignment criteria to course objectives using scoring rubrics provide students with an understanding of assignment expectations (Buzzetto-More & Alade, 2006; Nitko, 2004). Rubrics provide the basis for students to gauge the level of effort required to achieve certain criteria or standards of performance. Rubrics also make the life of the instructor easier by clearly delineating performance requirements to meet levels of criteria. This can eliminate some questions by students on why a certain score was given. Rubrics are used for assignments that involve students' participation for evaluation, such as papers, projects, oral presentations, simulations, case studies, discussion threads, and class participation. Davis Plus provides a rubric for assessment of a discussion assignment. A variety of Web sites are available to assist in rubric development (Technology Tip 9.2).

Designing the rubric requires an analysis of the objective for which the assignment is designed to demonstrate achievement. The instructor determines point distribution for each level within a specific area depending on quality subsets. For example, a writing assignment has an overall point allocation. Within the paper, subsets can include grammar/format, introduction, content, flow, concept development, and conclusion. Each subset is allotted a certain amount of points. The rubric provides the student with the criteria for evaluating each subset. Although rubrics help with accountability, they are only a part of assisting with assessment. Scoring rubrics should be explained in detail, including criteria explanation.

A variety of other tools are available for use to assess a student's learning. The following provides an overview of e-assessment functions.

Examinations

One of the most conventional methods for evaluating a student's learning is the examination. The traditional examination can be delivered through an online platform in a LMS using simple steps. Instructors can use two methods for developing the online examination; they can be created in a Microsoft Word document and uploaded into the course or questions can be created within a LMS using the available tools. For those who prefer creating questions within a Microsoft Word document, a few extra steps must be taken. To standardize the language between Microsoft Word and a LMS, a conversion method must be applied. The most widely used technology to enable the upload of questions is shareable content object reference model (SCORM). Similar to how a digital video disc (DVD) regulates the speed of the spinning disc and presentation of data regardless of the type of movie, SCORM allows standardization of material for upload onto a LMS. Developed by the U.S. Department of Defense, SCORM is available free of charge through its Web site at http://www.adlnet.gov/scorm/.

One of the most desirable benefits of creating questions in Word is the ability to create a test question "bank". Storing multiple questions allows the educator to upload the questions desired for the examination. As described in the Security section below, the educator then has the ability to scramble the test questions so that no two tests are alike.

A variety of question formats are available for use within a LMS. Table 9.2 provides an overview of question types found in most pre-established LMSs. The tool permits the instructor to select the appropriate question type from the available list. Once selected, the system guides the user to determine settings for the assessment. Key features can include:

- Amount of time allotted for the question or for the examination as a whole.
- Correct response grade weight (i.e., alphanumerical, numerical, percentage, or grade).
- Availability of the examination (start and stop times and date).
- Whether the student can view the grade after each question, after the entire examination is completed, or after everyone has completed the examination.
- Ability to insert rationales for each response.
- Students view specifications for the examination.

TABLE 9.2

Question Types

Multiple Choice	Presents users with a question followed by a list of choices. One choice may be selected.
True or False	Presents users with a statement that they must determine to be either true or false.
Multiple Select	Presents users with a question followed by a list of choices. Multiple selections are allowed.
Ordering	Presents users with a list of items to be placed in the correct sequence.
Matching	Presents users with a list of items and definitions to be matched.
Fill in the Blank	Presents a question as text and blank spaces where the user must enter the correct phrase for each blank space.
Short Answer	Presents users with a question followed by a single-line answer box. Responses must be manually graded.
Offline Item	Presents users with a question to be completed offline (no answer field appears). Responses are manually graded.
Essay	Presents users with a question followed by a multiline answer box. Responses must be manually graded.
Click on Graphics	Presents users with a graphic, requiring a click on a specific part of the picture.
Drag and Drop	Presents the users with a list of responses that must be moved into a type of format such as an ordered list, words into a paragraph, or other representation.
Reordering	Presents the users with a series of statements or pictures requiring the appropriate sequence.
Construction	Requires the user to construct a graph or other representation. The use of concept maps is a form of construction.

The most constrained questions require the student to select one response from alternatives as represented by the conventional multiple-choice or true/false items. Other less constrained test items include clicking on the correct part of a graphic (hot spot), drag and drop or move items, reorder a series of statements or pictures, or construct a graph or other representation (Scalise & Gifford, 2006). Computer adaptive testing (CAT) alters how the questions flow contingent upon how the student responds to the previous question. As questions are correctly answered, the difficulty increases for the next question. When answered incorrectly, the difficulty level decreases. This form of delivery provides excellent data regarding competency on the content but is not available for all platforms. To note, when using this method the educator must have a "bank" of hierarchal questions to allow for adaptability of questions.

One of the more frustrating complications for students and instructors alike with online examinations is being "kicked off" while taking an examination. The same issues also are noted by students while composing discussion question responses. This occurs as the computer program identifies inactivity as nonproductive time and closes the program. To remedy the issue, a free program is available at http://www.stayaliveonline.com/. The Stay Alive program sends an automated message every few minutes to your computer allowing it to stay connected during periods of inactivity. The computer does not discriminate between the user performing tasks and the automated messages resulting in sustained connectivity.

The beauty of using an e-assessment platform is the instant analysis of data from examinations. Educators have access to a variety of functions that provides a breakdown of data, streamlining the grading process. Based on how the instructor sets the functions, most systems will calculate the individual and class grades for the examination, provide a statistical report on each test item, and give an overall analysis of the class as a whole. The data can be used to discriminate test items, providing insights into the validity of each question to measure intended learning. Viewing of grades is similar to an Excel spreadsheet with many platforms allowing the exportation of data into an Excel spreadsheet that can be saved to a hard drive. Basic descriptive statistics such as the mean, median, and mode is available and an analysis of each individual question. The information can then be used to determine areas of weakness in test item construction for future use.

Standardized Examinations. Many systems also allow the instructor to select questions from other sources, including the ability to select questions from other assessments, browse and search pre-established textbook question banks, or copying and pasting from text files. Many textbooks come with prepackaged standardized assessment questions suitable for use in an online class. Most packaged examinations provide rationales for the correct and incorrect responses and reference pages for students to review areas of weakness. There are several benefits to using the prepackaged examinations but one main point stands clear, the questions have already been analyzed for consistency and validated through multiple iterations. Other benefits include ease of use, time saved from test item creation, and rationales with page numbers already included.

Security. Although not always realistic, the best method for ensuring honesty is to have a dedicated testing computer area with a proctor for the examination. For those courses where face-to-face (f-2-f) meetings are impossible, several methods are proposed that can deter cheating. Randomization of questions, a standard function of most LMSs allows a setting where the same questions are given to each student but in a different order. Randomizing delivery of test questions detracts from memorizing the order of responses to the questions. To go a step further, a test bank can be used to extract questions at random, decreasing the chances of having the same test questions in the same order. Although time-consuming to create a test bank with questions at similar levels, the odds that students can cheat on the examination are much lower. The result is different tests for each student.

Timing the examination can detract from cheating by setting the amount of time the student has to answer each test question. For example, allotting 1 minute for each question decreases the chance that a student taking the examination from home will have time to search for the answer.

> *I time my tests to give the students 1 minute per question. I also tell them that they can use their textbooks. I figure that since they aren't in front of me taking the examination I might as well be upfront about their using the text. This way they still have to know the subject content and be familiar with the concepts before beginning the examination. They dislike these examinations during the course, afterward they tell me that they feel they are held to high standards and really know the course concepts. I started using this method in another course where they are to take a 5-question quiz over the content of the next lecture. They are given 30 seconds per question. I tell you what; they come to class prepared to discuss the content!*

Discussions

Discussion questions are an effective method for creating a collaborative learning experience. The sharing of information and experiences related to the topic of discussion requires students to participate by commenting or providing additional examples or references that support arguments or rationalize a point. Online discussion forums used as an assessment method must have clearly stated standards or criteria for assessment. For students to actively engage and effectively regulate learning, explicit criteria should include at minimum the number of posts required per week, length of the post, content of the message, and appropriate use of discussion forums. The criteria must be detailed during the first class meeting, outlining expectations for participating in discussions. In addition to the standards for participation, what happens when the student does not participate or becomes disruptive also must be clearly detailed. It is important to note that the clearer the requirements for the assessment are, the less likely the educator will encounter issues that detract from learning.

To sustain momentum in an online discussion format, visibility of the instructor is imperative. Guiding discussions, facilitating learning, and maintaining a level of watchfulness ensures that students are aware that their posts are being read and evaluated. When the instructor does not "appear" in the classroom, students begin to wander off topic, are less likely to adhere to guidelines, and exert less effort toward learning (Seok, 2008). To the end of authentic assessment, it is fully upon the instructor to develop, monitor, provide feedback, and evaluate course discussions for evidence of learning.

Two approaches for assessing discussion content include holistic and analytical scoring. Holistic methods involve scoring the discussion as a whole based on established criteria to assign scores based on tone, structure, and content comprehension. The analytical method uses individual criterion with allocation of points and a scoring matrix. Benefits include clarity in student's strengths and weaknesses. Disadvantages are overlooking the quality of posts and communication of ideas (Hazari, 2004). A combination of holistic and analytic methods can be incorporated into a course rubric to provide a well-rounded view of student learning. An example of a rubric for scoring a response to a discussion assignment can be accessed on Davis Plus.

Essays/Papers

Essays and papers comprise the gold standard for assessing higher levels of cognitive functions. Best practices for good feedback encompass seven principles to ensure appropriate

responses for student learning. Evidence Based Practice Box 9.1 outlines the seven principles and provides strategy suggestions for incorporation into an online course for feedback
of written work. It is essential that clear expectations for performance with standards and
criteria for evaluating student's work must be detailed before initiating the assignment.
Students with knowledge of how their work will be graded, including the criteria and standards by which their work is evaluated, will perform better. Evolving research identifies
that knowledge of criteria is not enough. Discussion of the criteria and inclusion of an
exemplar of performance is necessary for students to fully comprehend assessment (Milne,
Heinrich, & Morrison, 2008; Nicol & MacFarlane-Dick, 2006). Depending on the educator's comfort with the assignment, examples of similar work at different levels of quality
provide excellent clarification of performance levels. Be sure to obtain consent from
students before using work as examples!

EVIDENCE-BASED PRACTICE BOX 9.1

Best Practices for Assessment

Nicol and MacFarlane-Dick (2006) synthesized available literature on formative
assessment and learning, developing the following best practices for assessment:
- Helps clarify what good performance is.
  - Have explicit goals, criteria, and expected standards.
  - Provide exemplars of performance.
  - Provide criteria sheets.
  - Reflect on standards in class.
  - Have students mark each other's work based on defined criteria.
  - Negotiate assessment criteria between instructor and student.
- Facilitates the development of self-assessment (reflection) in learning.
  - Teach students how to judge their own work.
  - Request what kind of feedback students would like.
  - Have students identify strengths and weaknesses in work before handing in.
  - Have students reflect on achievements to select portfolio work.
  - Encourage students to reflect back on progress for future work.
- Delivers high-quality information to students about their learning.
  - Provide feedback based on criteria.
  - Pay attention to number of criteria.
  - Provide timely feedback.
  - Give advice for correcting work not just strengths/weaknesses.
  - Limit feedback to specific and meaningful instances.
  - Prioritize areas for improvement.
  - Provide online feedback so that students can access as often as they want.
- Encourages teacher and peer dialogue around learning.
  - Use dialogue rather than one-way communication.
  - Encourage peer dialogue that enhances student's self-control over learning.
  - Use 1-minute papers.
  - Review feedback with peers.
  - Find useful feedback and discuss in class.
  - Encourage descriptive peer feedback in relation to criteria.
  - Assign group projects with discussion of standards and criteria before assignment.

EVIDENCE-BASED PRACTICE BOX 9.1—cont'd

- Encourages positive motivational beliefs and self-esteem.
  - Communicate clearly that feedback is not on the individual, rather on the performance.
  - Provide feedback and request comments from students before releasing grades.
  - Allow time to rewrite pieces of work to change student expectations of learning.
  - Automate testing with feedback/rationales.
  - Work through iterations using drafts and revisions.
- Provides opportunities to close the gap between current and desired performance.
  - Provide feedback on work in progress.
  - Allow iterations and drafts.
  - Give two-stage assignments: feedback on stage one improves performance on stage two.
  - Use instructor model strategies.
  - Provide action points with normal feedback.
- Provides information to teachers that can be used to help shape the teaching.
  - Have students request feedback they would like.
  - Have students identify where they have difficulties.
  - Have students identify "a question worth asking" for the next class.

Drop Box. A variety of tools for submission of written work are available. E-mail attachments from students are a common method for receiving assignments. The attachment is downloaded and saved as a document into the instructor's computer, graded, then sent as an attachment back to the student. Most LMSs have assignment drop-box features that allow uploading of the paper by the student into the system. The instructor then opens the drop box, selects the assignment, and opens the document for grading. The drop-box function places the submissions in order of received (time and date) rather than by alphabetical order. An additional benefit of both the e-mail and drop-box methods is the placement of a time stamp on the submission. Both the student and the instructor have the time and date of submission, ensuring compliance with deadlines.

Track Changes. Formative feedback within the context of the paper provides specific communication of evaluation, a method found more meaningful by students (Orsmond, Merry, & Reiling, 2005). Summary feedback that addresses the work in totality should also accompany the paper. To be effective for learning, summaries should include the strengths and weaknesses as an overall picture of the assessment. Preliminary research suggests that the presence of a grade detracts the student's motivation away from looking at feedback. This suggests that greater gains in student's learning come from returning the assignment with specific and general feedback before displaying the letter grade (Draper, 2009; Milne, Heinrich, & Morrison, 2008). The method allows students to absorb the comments and discuss with the instructor, allowing growth and learning to occur.

Providing feedback on written assignments can be completed using the Track Changes function of Microsoft Word. Gone are the days of writing copious notes on the sides of the paper or at the end. Track changes allow comments and changes to be placed directly into the paper. Students can see exactly what part of the paper or sentence the feedback addresses.

Advantages include the availability of the technology, ease of use for communicating with students, and insertion of content-specific feedback within the assignment. Track Changes allow the instructor to make changes within the paper or provide comments on parts of the text. For more information on Track Changes, see Technology Tip 9.3. Another available tool is the Adobe Acrobat Professional's PDF commenting e-tool. Both allow insertion of comments and feedback directly into the paper.

Electronic Scoring. Evolution of learning technology has resulted in an explosion of innovations for grading e-assessments based on writing. Such technology encompasses scoring, statistical models, and rater analysis. Original tools were premised upon determining the level at which the student wrote the paper, taking into account a one-dimensional scoring method based on grammar and syntax. Newer versions are able to detect variances and subtleties of connections between variables in addition to grammar and syntax allowing another dimension to the scoring of written work. Several writing analysis tools are available with a high level of sophistication. An example of one product with associated research studies that support the use of the tool can be viewed at http://www.ets.org/highered.

Security. An inherent issue in online assessments is the threat of cheating, plagiarism, and sharing of responses. Several free online tools are available to review papers for plagiarism (Technology Tip 9.4). Students also can use the tools to review their papers before submission for accidental or unintentional plagiarism. Another method for increasing security is to require iterations of papers where the assignment is broken into pieces or is submitted at various points during the semester. The method allows insights into the growth of concepts, the development of the paper, and demonstrates how the student cultivated feedback to produce the final submission. To note, the best form of ensuring honesty in paper submission is to clearly outline what plagiarism is and how the university deals with academic dishonesty.

Performance Assessments

The least constrained type of assessment are those activities that include projects, presentations, case studies, portfolios, demonstrations, experiments, diagnoses, teaching, interviews, etc. Presentations can be created using PowerPoint technology and uploaded into a course. The presentation is assessed for content that meets standards for the assignment. Students can submit a written dialogue to accompany the presentation to give a second dimension to

TECHNOLOGY TIP 9.3

A full review of Track Changes, including step-by-step guidelines for using the tool, can be viewed at http://office.microsoft.com/en-us/word/HA012186901033.aspx. Given that many health-care professionals need to edit documents, policies, etc., consider sharing this tool with your students.

TECHNOLOGY TIP 9.4

A repository for plagiarism detection tools can be viewed at http://www.shambles.net/pages/staff/ptools/

the assignment. Of concern is the ability of the student to demonstrate effective presentation techniques. Sophisticated systems can record the student's presentation for viewing by the entire class through Webcam technology. Skype is a free downloadable Webcam technology that allows real time interactions between two geographically divided individuals or groups. The free download is available for Windows, Mac, or phones and can be accessed at http://www.skype.com/download/skype/windows/. Students also may reserve time in an on-campus or at another facility that is equipped with technology to record and share presentations. Selection of this method requires the instructor to take into account the sufficient technology of other learners to view the presentation.

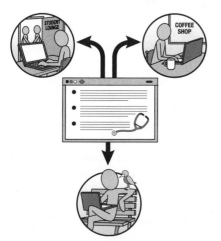

Another way to assess presentations is to require a f-2-f session for presentations. Either way, assessment of learning can be completed in several ways; it can be the sole discretion of the instructor, weighted between the instructor and other students in the class, or arise from peer reviews. When using other student's perceptions of presentations, it is essential that the students are given specific standards with required documentation of evidence to support their assessment. An example peer evaluation form for an assignment where students create a Web site can be viewed on Davis Plus. Using this method, the instructor could identify points that were conveyed and confusing issues from the presentation.

Peer-evaluation techniques are cited by Nicol & MacFarlane-Dick (2006) as a best practice for assessing learning. Whether using peer evaluations for a presentation, performance, or paper, research suggests that students are open to constructive comments from peers, using it as a learning experience more readily than evaluation of the assignment by an instructor. To be effective, peer assessments should be based on criteria for assessment of the particular assignment. Score cards, rubrics, and Likert scales based on specific areas of content with an area for feedback provide guidelines for peer assessments.

Simulations/Case Studies

Simulations and case studies are not only instructional techniques; they also are assessment activities gaining popularity. Both require students to analyze situations, evaluate situations, make judgments, and formulate solutions, all critical thinking skills (Buzzetto-More & Alade, 2006). Simulations require students to provide a scenario or background with manipulation of content, demonstrating application of knowledge. For example, students in a Leadership/Management course can be given an assignment where they create a unit in a hospital. The assignment can include work-flow analysis where the simulation shows how a nurse moves through the unit during a typical workday. The assignment can include both current and proposed changes to provide an evaluation of productivity based on unit structures and possible changes. Technology using simulation can provide a representation of how the work flow looks with current and proposed changes. As technology evolves, simulation as an assessment also matures. It will be interesting to see where this method goes in the future.

Case studies can incorporate actual experiences and completely made-up scenarios. The case study assessment involves providing a situation either complete with nursing functions or with the absence of interventions. Complete case studies provide information on how a nurse performed in a specific situation. Assessment of learning incorporates how a student evaluates the nurse's performance based on criteria for learning. For example, the case study might detail interventions provided by a nurse for a heart failure patient, complete with subjective and objective assessment findings. The student is required to evaluate the interventions for appropriateness or suggest additional interventions. On the other hand, case studies that provide information only on the context, requiring the student to prescribe nursing functions, is another way to assess learning. For example, providing basic information on a patient with a kidney stone then requiring the student to identify not only additional information they need as well as prescribing nursing interventions for the patient is another way to use case study assessments. Both techniques can be applied to individuals or groups depending on instructor preferences.

Portfolios

Portfolios are a project-based activity allowing student's flexibility in demonstrating knowledge. The electronic portfolio is a student directed selection of items to illustrate how they achieved learning objectives. For example, to demonstrate achievement of a course objective a student can select parts of a PowerPoint presentation, portions of an online discussion, and an essay to provide a well-rounded argument. The instructor determines the structure of the portfolio including specific learning objectives. It becomes the responsibility of the student to select those course artifacts that demonstrate mastery of the objective (Buzzetto-More & Alade, 2006). To constrain the volume and type of submissions, the instructor may decide on a limit to the volume for submission. This technique requires the student to concentrate on the objective and to become selective in the type of work to be included in the portfolio.

CONCLUSION

The evolution of e-learning significantly affects the variety of e-assessment methods available to educators. The variety of available tools gives the educator the means to assess learning through a multiple method approach. As new research emerges on learning and assessing, the body of knowledge for assessment grows and matures. The creativity of the educator regarding ways of assessing learning also is affected as evidenced by the growth of innovations in assessment modalities. Accountability for producing evidence of outcomes only reinforces the need to examine current assessment activities. The landscape of e-assessment is constantly changing, producing exciting new possibilities for providing evidence of learning outcomes.

TECHNOLOGY TIP 9.5

A wealth of information and examples of e-portfolios can be viewed online at http://electronicportfolios.org/portfolios.html

REFERENCES

Anderson, L. W., Krathwohl, D. R., Airasian, P. W., Cruikshank, K. A., Mayer, R. E., Pintrich, P. R., et al. (Eds.). (2001). *A taxonomy for learning, teaching, and assessing: A revision of Bloom's taxonomy of educational objectives.* New York, NY: Addison Wesley Longman, Inc.

Buzzetto-More, N. A., & Alade, A. J. (2006). Best practices in e-assessment. *Journal of Information Technology Education, 5,* 251–268.

Draper, S. W. (2009). What are learners actually regulating when given feedback? *British Journal of Educational Technology, 40*(2), 306–315.

Hazari, S. (2004, Winter). Strategy for assessment of online course discussions. *Journal of Information Systems Education, 15*(4), 349–355.

Krathwohl, D. R. (2002). A revision of Bloom's taxonomy: An overview. *Theory Into Practice, 41*(4), 212–218.

Milne, J. Heinrich, E., & Morrison, D. (2008). Technological support for assignment assessment: A New Zealand higher education survey. *Australasian Journal of Educational Technology, 24*(5), 487–504.

Nicol, D. J., & MacFarlane-Dick, D. (2006). Formative assessment and self-regulated learning: A model and seven principles of good feedback practice. *Studies in Higher Education, 31*(2), 199–218.

Nitko, A. J. (2004). *Educational assessment outcomes.* Columbus, OH: Pearson Merrill Prentice Hall.

Orsmond, P., Merry, S., & Reiling, K. (2005). Biology student's utilization of tutor's formative feedback: A qualitative interview study. *Assessment & Evaluation in Higher Education, 30*(4), 369–386.

Scalise, K. & Gifford, B. (2006, June). Computer-based assessment in e-learning: A framework for constructing "intermediate constraint" questions and tasks for technology platforms. *The Journal of Technology, Learning, and Assessment, 4*(6). Retrieved from http://www.jtla.org

Seok, S. (2008). Teaching aspects of e-learning. *International Journal on E-Learning, 7*(4), 725–741.

Van der Linden, B. A. (2002). On complexity in CBT. In C. Mills, M. Potenza, J. Fremer, & W. Ward (Eds.), *Computer-based testing* (pp. 89–102). Mahwah, NJ: Lawrence Erlbaum Associates, Publishers.

Chapter 10

Learners' Special Needs and Considerations

Maria Lauer, MSN, PhD(c), RN, APN-C, CNE

Creating learning experiences that accommodate students with special needs is an essential concern for the nurse educator. Accessible accommodations have benefits to all students in the e-learning environment. In an associate's-degree, hybrid-nursing program, instructors set up the online learning management system (LMS) with lectures, videos, and pictures. Labels were placed on all pictures and audio-voice clips to the pictures. Learners also were provided with links to resources associated with the pictures. In addition, learners had the ability to have written transcripts of all lectures, videos, and graphics contained in the course room. The course room also was designed to comply with accessibility regulations. The freshman class provided verbal and written feedback that this technique has really helped them to learn the vernacular and reinforce what they were learning in class and clinical. This is the fundamental nature of creating a universal design (UD) for learning; that is, courses designed for all learning styles and all learning abilities.

E-learning courses, if properly designed, can offer autonomy and liberation related to the Internet's power to be accessible virtually anywhere at any time. E-learning offers many opportunities for learners particularly for those learners who have special challenges. Incorporated in this chapter are factors associated with creating learning environments that are global and include all populations regardless of location, socioeconomic status, or disability. This chapter also includes strategic planning for implementation of global learning communities that are accessible and economically sound. Specific interventions for meeting the needs of those with physical disabilities, learning disabilities (LDs), and learners who consider English as a second language (ESL) or English as a foreign language (EFL) will be discussed.

When designing online courses, particular attention should be given to accessibility and creating an environment that is respectful of physical limitations and multiple intelligences. Implementing the principles of UD online means anticipating the learning needs and abilities of all students (see Box 10.1). Rather than exclude a segment of the population that stands to gain the most from e-learning, students with special learning needs can benefit from online learning because it offers independence and freedom unavailable through traditional didactic courses.

DavisPlus | For additional resources please visit
http://davisplus.fadavis.com

BOX 10.1
SEVEN PRINCIPLES OF UNIVERSAL DESIGN

The principles of UD easily can be applied to the e-learning environment (http://www.design.ncsu.edu:8120/cud/univ_design/princ_overview.htm). The complete principles and guidelines can be accessed on Davis Plus. Below is an overview of the principles and their definitions:

1. Equitable use: The design is useful to people with diverse abilities.
2. Flexibility in use: The design accommodates a wide range of individual preferences and abilities.
3. Simple and intuitive use: Use of the design is easy to understand, regardless of the user's experience, knowledge, language skills, or current concentration level.
4. Perceptible information: The design communicates necessary information effectively to the user, regardless of ambient conditions or the user's sensory abilities.
5. Tolerance for error: The design minimizes hazards and the adverse consequences of accidental or unintended actions.
6. Low-physical effort: The design can be used efficiently and comfortably with minimum fatigue.
7. Size and space for approach and use: Appropriate size and space is provided for approach, reach, manipulation, and use regardless of user's body size, posture, or mobility.

THEORIES FOR LEARNERS WITH SPECIAL CONSIDERATIONS

As nurse educators, we can best assist students who are academically challenged by implementing adult pedagogies that emphasize all forms of intelligence. Chapter 2 provides an in-depth review of theories that are associated with student-centered learning environments and how they are implemented in the e-learning environment. Specific to learners with special needs is the Theory of Multiple Intelligence (Gardner, 1983). The Theory of Multiple Intelligence (Gardner, 1983) is particularly applicable to teaching academically challenged students because Gardner's focus is on special populations and individuals with LDs.

Central to Gardner's Theory of Multiple Intelligence is that there are at least nine types of intelligence. The nine types of intelligence include: naturalist, musical, logical-mathematical, existential, interpersonal, bodily, kinesthetic, linguistic, intrapersonal, and spatial. All individuals have varying degrees of each type of intelligence; however, each individual has areas in which he or she excels.

The educational experience can be enhanced greatly for learners with special considerations by determining the areas in which the learner excels. Educators also can tailor learning activities that meet the needs of the majority of the students and create a universally designed course room. Educators can accomplish this goal by assessing the learner's individual learning style or preference. Tools that measure areas of multiple intelligences include the Memletics Learning Style inventory. The Memletics assessments can be accessed online at: http://www.memletics.com/manual/learning-styles.asp. Multiple intelligence inventories can provide the educator and learner with valuable input regarding learning styles, learning preferences, and learning needs. There also are many useful tools for the nurse educator to use online. The reference list for this chapter has specific tools listed that can be easily implemented in the online course room.

TECHNOLOGY TIP 10.1

Use of an electronic learning styles inventory enables the educator tracking options. The Memletics learning styles inventory (http://www.learning-styles-online.com/inventory/) will assist the educator in meeting various learning needs that are specific to the student population. In addition, assignments can be created to allow learners to meet learning objectives in a variety of ways. For example, a learner may be permitted to use presentation, poster, blog, or paper to meet assignment criteria on the grading rubric.

"THE DIGITAL DIVIDE"

While computer ownership and Internet use continues to grow, underserved individuals and communities still struggle to become literate in the e-learning environment. This digital divide is defined as those who are separated from technologies because they cannot afford the technology and/or who have low literacy skills necessary to use current technologies. It is vital that the educator address the digital divide in the e-learning environment by strategically creating learning experiences that are mindful of both cost and literacy levels so as not to exclude learners who may not have high literacy skills or the economic resources available to afford the opportunities being presented in the course room.

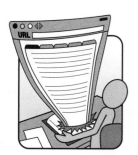

Economic concerns can be a barrier to quality education. Fortunately, there are many cost saving measures that the educator can employ to reduce expenses for the learner without compromising the quality of the education. Measures for reducing costs include using the companion Web site that comes with textbook adoptions, piloting new technologies before purchase, obtaining grant monies for technology integration, and creating universal designs for learning (UDLs). By far, the greatest savings will be realized by creating an environment that is universally designed.

The concept of UD is not new; in fact, the building industry has been incorporating UDs into structures since 1998 (International Code Council, 1998). The International Code law (1998) mandates that buildings be planned to feature designs that are accessible to persons with physical disabilities. Buildings that incorporate UD benefit all individuals are thus considered "universal." An example of UD would be doors that open automatically. Whereas automatic doors were originally designed for those in wheelchairs, those using a stroller or shopping cart also attain access.

Similarly, the concept of UDLs can be used in the e-learning environment to create both a cost effective and nondiscriminatory course room online. Educators can accomplish this goal by creating a learning environment that is intuitive and self-explanatory. For example, the design of the course room is such that all links are labeled, text features can be modified, and the site is easy to navigate regardless of the user's experience. A well-designed learning environment also takes into consideration those who have a physical disability.

APPLICATION OF UNIVERSAL DESIGN IN THE EDUCATIONAL SETTING

Another way to plan learning experiences that are cost effective is to incorporate all learning resources that accompany the adopted textbook for the course including companion Web-site materials into the curriculum. Companion Web sites are economical because they are free with textbook adoption. Not only are companion Web sites economical, they also are educationally sound because the materials are congruent with the learning objectives stated in the textbook and chosen by faculty.

One example of maximizing the use of companion Web sites was that of a nursing instructor from a university. The instructor was given the challenge of incorporating e-learning into two associate's degree-nursing programs. The two programs had limited financial resources for technology, and were not able to afford an LMS. The instructor implemented all learning resources from the companion Web site and added lectures, quizzes, videos, and discussion boards to the Web site. Learners and instructors communicated through the e-mail features of the companion Web sites. With the assistance of the publisher's technical support team, all Web sites the students and faculty used were placed on the companion Web site creating a congruent site. The goal of having an online course was realized at no cost to the university.

The uses of electronic textbooks are becoming more widely available and help to create a UD that is particularly useful in online courses. Electronic textbooks are in digital format and may include audiovisual, graphics, Web resources, and ancillary materials for the educator and learners. Learners who do not read well with printed textbooks have reported greater retention and a meaningful learning experience due to the interactivity components of the electronic textbook and the ability to customize the learning environment based on their individual preferences.

Addressing Literacy and the Digital Divide

Before the start of the online course, the educator will need to determine the literacy level of the learner and the comfort level with the online learning format. To do this, the educator will find assessment tools useful in identifying learners who may need remediation before entering the course room. Many schools have developed an online readiness assessment that the student can complete before entering the online course.

One such tool is the Readiness Index for Learning Online (RILO) (2004) was developed for students as a self-assessment for taking online courses. The RILO is an interactive quiz that the learner completes independently. The quiz helps the student identify areas that need

---

TECHNOLOGY TIP 10.2

Check teaching and learning materials for UD at http://udlselfcheck.cast.org/check.php. This site also offers many suggestions for increasing accessibility, information of physical and LDs, and current research and best practices in UDL.

TECHNOLOGY TIP 10.3

Consider using the companion Web site as the portal for entry to all coursework. For example, learners can access e-mail, lectures, and discussion boards; check the status of grades; and communicate with peers and instructors. The advantage to creating one access point for all online activities is that learners and faculties only need to access one site for all applications. Another benefit to this approach is that it is easier for instructors to track learners' online activities.

remediation. Remediation will ensure that the learner is able to fully immerse in the learning experience. Another tool that is useful to identify learning needs and for subsequent remediation is the Pretest for Attitudes Toward Computers in Health Care (PATCH) self-assessment examination (Kaminski, 2006). The PATCH results include resources for remediation that the learner can address independently.

GLOBAL LEARNING INITIATIVES

Global learning initiatives also are geared toward narrowing the digital divide. Online learning is central to global learning because online education is accessible and affordable. The dream of creating a global learning environment that can be accessed by learners from all over the world has become a reality because of the Internet and online classrooms. When educators are designing courses in the global learning environment the focus needs to be on economic, sociocultural, and language barriers. Particular issues include working with learners whose primary language many not be English, learners who speak ESL, or learners who speak more than two languages and EFL. Thus, the educator must find ways in which to communicate with learners who may not all be speaking the same language.

Adding a translator to an online course is an easy way to accomplish the task of assisting learners to communicate. The Google Translator can be added to any online course by simply copying and pasting a widget to the Web-site template. Widgets are tools that are created in online code known as hypertext markup language (HTML). This code allows the user to add applications to Web sites by copying and pasting the HTML code to the Web site. Examples of widgets include translators, screen readers, and text-to-speech tools.

Once the translator widget is installed, participants will be able to communicate in their native languages. Another useful tool is the addition of an audio dictionary. Google has a widget that will allow a dictionary to be installed to the Web site. This dictionary is made available in most languages and includes the audio feature. In addition, many published textbooks have online ancillary features that include an audio dictionary. The audio

TECHNOLOGY TIP 10.4

Consider mandating that learners take a readiness for online learning assessment as a prerequisite to entering the course room, then award the learner with a certificate at the completion of the assessment. The certificate can be used to document competencies and verify completion. One Web site that provides surveys for free is Penn State University Online: http://psuonline.pdx.edu/info.php?page=5. In addition to the readiness quiz, there also is a computer skills questionnaire and a learning styles inventory assessment.

TECHNOLOGY TIP 10.5

Widgets also are called "gadgets" and "pageflakes" but more commonly "widget." Http://www.widgetbox.com is a great site for those who would like to try to make their own and also has "prefabricated" widgets. Another key site for the online educator is http://teacher.pageflakes.com. In addition, Google and Yahoo have translators, dictionaries, and Web-page screen readers. Http://www.Google.com has "gadgets" and http://www.widgets.Yahoo.com has widgets that are relatively easy to install. Simply copy and paste the HTML code into the Web page.

dictionary is particularly useful for those trying to learn English because words can be heard by the learner, seen in print, and used in context, which promotes reinforcement for language acquisition.

Application of Global Learning in the Educational Setting

Global learning can bring quality education to Third-World countries. An example of a recent educational experience was that of a group of nursing students from Haiti. The

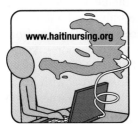

Haiti Nursing Foundation (HNF) was committed to supporting the educational needs of the nursing school and implementing online learning. Administrators from a nursing school in Haiti and a dean and e-learning specialist from a Minnesota nursing school embraced the concept of global learning and teaching by collaborating with the nursing school in Haiti to teach the pharmacology course to nursing students. The director of the Haiti nursing program and the e-learning specialist designed a curriculum online that could be taught to students in both schools.

Course and anecdotal evaluations revealed that both groups of learners rated the educational experience as very rewarding because they felt a special connection and valued the interactions with their online classmates. The learners from Haiti especially enjoyed working and accessing all the resources available to them online. This combined effort included the support of a national publisher that allowed use of the LMS and access of the Internet via satellites. To date, students from each program still "visit" with each other online. In addition, during spring and summer breaks, student and faculty groups from the Minnesota school travels to Haiti to work with their "sister" school to support the mission and integrate current technologies.

In the United States, President Barack Obama has increased funding for broadband access in rural areas of America to address global learning. The American College Initiative (2009) is an initiative aimed at increasing the number of college graduates in America by 2020. Online learning is a central aspect to meeting the goals because of the flexible nature of the online venue and that a teacher at one college can teach across the country. In fact, President Barack Obama stated he would provide funding to institutions that develop online courses that will eventually be free to all Americans regardless of sex, race, creed, color, or disability.

SELECTED CHALLENGES

Disability is common. According to the Disability Status report, 12.8% of Americans age 21 to 64 are classified as disabled (Erickson & Lee, 2008). E-learning technologies have enhanced the learning experiences of students with disabilities and helped to shape the way educators design curriculums. The same technologies can help all learners, especially those

TECHNOLOGY TIP 10.6

There has been an increase in interest and funding to implement global learning in higher education. Consider sponsoring a school abroad or in this country and using the HNF as a model for increasing your school's global community. For more information on the HNF, please visit: http://haitinursing.org

learners who are academically challenged. Academic challenges include LDs, physical disabilities, and those individuals who are learning the English language. Eliminating barriers in curriculum design is a vital aspect of curriculum and course design. One major benefit for the educator is that the educator can reach and engage more learners. To learners, the benefits are endless.

Common Types of Learning Disabilities

Not all disabilities are apparent. LDs can be difficult for both the learner and educator to detect. The educator will benefit from an understanding of the most common types of LDs. This understanding will lead to interventions that can be implemented for learners who are classified with LDs. In addition, the educator will need to know laws that apply to students with physical disabilities and LDs, how to implement interventions that comply with government regulations, and how to evaluate learners who are classified with LDs. Laws and government regulations that apply to students with disabilities will be covered later in this chapter. We will first examine the types of LDs and what specific interventions are necessary for the stated disability.

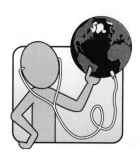

There are many types and forms of LDs. LDs discussed in the chapter include dyslexia, auditory processing disorder, and visual processing disorder. Although attention-deficit hyperactivity disorder (ADHD) is considered a medical disorder by the National Institute of Mental Health (1998), it is discussed in this section because learners with ADHD have difficulties in the postsecondary educational setting. Individuals with ADHD are characterized by lack of ability to focus for long periods and thus become easily distracted. For this reason, an individual with ADHD will benefit greatly from the use of text-to-speech software capable of reading words to the learner. Learners with ADHD also do well with less distraction and may wear headphones to block out external noise. When designing learning experiences online, the educator can incorporate these same interventions by minimizing the distractions and creating a simple design that will be easy to follow.

Dyslexic learners have difficulty with the written word and have difficulty reading and writing as a result. Dyslexic learners tend to do well with online courses because learners can make use of software applications that can read aloud to the learner, known as screen readers. Specific course designs would include pages that are compatible with screen readers. Other interventions for dyslexic individuals are to keep fonts consistent and avoid animations or distracting sounds or flashing texts. These types of designs can succeed at distracting the dyslexic individual.

Individuals with auditory processing also may have trouble with reading and writing and will therefore benefit from online courses because these individuals can make use of various software applications. How individuals differ with auditory processing delays is that sounds are difficult to discern. To this end, the educator should use caution in selecting audiovisual content for the online course or provide transcripts of the audiovisuals as an alternative. Video and speech transcript software, such as Adobe CS4 speech transcription can be used in conjunction with media players to easily convert video to text for sight and auditory processing impairments.

Much like individuals with auditory processing delays, those with visual processing delays may have difficulty discerning words in audiovisual presentations; however, individuals with visual processing delays also may have difficulty with maps, charts, symbols, and pictures.

Providing clear descriptions of all graphic material on the Web site will assist the learner who is sight impaired or has auditory processing delays because the electronic readers will detect labels thereby assisting the learner to comprehend the material contained in the graphic being presented.

Table 10.1 summarizes the various learning needs and common difficulties that may present to these learners and suggests tools for learning.

Applications for Learning Disabilities in the Educational Setting

As stated earlier, UDs can meet the learning needs of most individuals. Individuals that are diagnosed with LD also will benefit from having an individual development plan (IDP) that is based on their specific LD and customized to meet their learning needs. The IDP may

TABLE 10.1		
Learning Needs and Common Difficulties With Suggested Tools for Learning		
Learning Need	**Learning Difficulties**	**Tools for Learning**
ADHD	Lack of ability to focus Difficulty acquiring and retaining information	Vary learning materials PowerPoint Videos Gaming/activities Webquest
Dyslexia	Difficulty with the written word Often will reverse order of words	Audio glossary Record lectures Concept mapping

Hearing Impaired	Difficulty discerning audio
	    materials
		Recorders
		Microphones for speakers
		PowerPoint with speaker notes
		Videos with closed caption
		Transcripts for audiovisual
		    materials

Auditory Processing
    Delays
	Difficulty with reading and
	    writing
		PowerPoint with speaker notes
		Record lectures
		Gaming
		Videos

Visual Processing
    Disorders
	Vision normal; however,
	    difficulty processing and
	    making sense of information
	    taken in through the eyes
		Spacing out letters and using
		    larger print reading materials
		Highlighting important
		    information
		Recording lectures
		Use transcripts for all graphics
		    and pictures

TECHNOLOGY TIP 10.7

Internet browsers allow the viewer to customize the Web page. In addition, a course developer can create a "site-customization page" that provides options for viewers of the Web site or course. Customizations for fonts, color, background, and displaying graphics can be altered for ease of viewing and preferences can be set for individual learning needs.

include suggestions, such as allowing additional time on unit assignments and postings or receiving verbal explanation of assignments. Other useful interventions include providing alternate formats for textbooks including electronic and audio-taped books. It is helpful to give advanced copies of the syllabus and course requirements to the learner so that an IDP can be tailored to not only the individual but the course requirements as well.

Assessment of LDs in the postsecondary educational setting differs from early educational assessment in that the school is responsible for identifying students with disability by testing and then providing a plan and services for those students. At the college level, the student must identify him- or herself to the school and provide documentation to support the need for special accommodations or requests. Many students are not willing to disclose information regarding a LD because they feel they are or will be discriminated against. While the educator is not responsible for identifying the learner with special needs, it would be prudent to be knowledgeable about the testing process and provide resources for students with LD.

There are various LD assessment tests online that the educator can recommend to students suspected of having a LD. There are Web sites entirely dedicated to individuals with LDs and many provide self-assessment quizzes and resources for students with LDs. The companion disc lists several of the Web sites, books, and assessment tests that the learner can use to identify his or her LD. In general, an educator may see a learner who is adept at practical skills; however, the learner does not do well on objective testing. Once a learner is able to identify his or her LD, much can be done to assist the student in achieving his or her learning goals.

Physical Disabilities

Physical disabilities included in this chapter are those individuals with sight, hearing, and mobility issues. Individuals who have difficulty with sight include those individuals who wear corrective lenses, are color blind, or have varying degrees of sight impairment. One advantage for individuals with sight impairment is that a screen reader can read course-room and Web-site content. Two examples of software, include JAWS and Kurzweil, which can be downloaded to the learners' computers. In addition, Web Anywhere, a Web accessible sight-reader maintained by Washington University can be accessed via the Internet at http://webanywhere.cs.washington.edu/wa.php. Web Anywhere can be used by the student when he or she is using a computer that is not equipped with a site reader. Sight-readers greatly enhance the learning experience for those with sight impairment; however, the course room would need to be compatible with this technology. Course designs should include allowing the user to customize the fonts and color backgrounds of the Web page. Textbooks and course materials should be available in digital format, Braille, or audio to accommodate learners with sight impairments.

TECHNOLOGY TIP 10.8

Before the first day of class, consider checking your course room for accessibility using the Web Anywhere site reader at http://webanywhere.cs.washington.edu/wa.php to check for errors in accessibility for low-vision or blind users.

Hearing impairment is one of the most prevalent chronic disabilities in the United States. Approximately 22 million people in the United States (8.2%) have hearing impairments (Vanderheiden & Vanderheiden, 1991). Hearing impairment is also a common disability for nurses; therefore, the nurse educator may encounter hearing-impaired learners in the online setting. In the classroom setting, a hearing-impaired student has the right to use sign language interpreters and use recording devices to improve the learning experience. In the online classroom, hearing-impaired students are able to adjust the sound coming from their computer or simply read the text that is presented in the course. The hearing-impaired students are able to participate in all online discussions because this activity is done through typing. The educator will want to be sure that audiovisual materials are accessible to hearing-impaired individuals. To achieve this goal, the audiovisual material should have an accompanying transcript as an alternate to the visual presentation. In the future, all audiovisuals will have closed captioning or text that is contained in the video much like televisions do today.

For learners with mobility impairments, the online learning environment offers great potential. Here, the learner is able to adapt his or her home environment to enhance the learning experience. The learner with mobility impairment may have an adjustable computer desk and chair to accommodate for his or her physical needs. In addition, adaptive equipment can be attached to the computer for individuals with dexterity impairments. For example, learners who have limited use of their hands can use a microphone that works with speech recognition software allowing the user the ability to execute commands, type, and explore the Internet and course room. Another learner who is in a wheelchair can adjust computer heights to accommodate the use of the chair. Even a quadriplegic can use a sip and puff straw to operate the computer and navigate the Internet and course room. Specific interventions for individuals with physical limitation will vary and will greatly depend on the type and extent of the disability; however, nothing is impossible in the online venue.

English as a Second Language

Many colleges have a minimum acceptable score for learners who consider ESL. Admission standards generally include stipulations that the learner is expected to read, speak, write, and understand the English language fluently. In addition, most colleges also will require

TECHNOLOGY TIP 10.9

There are many online communities offering support, research, and information for hearing-impaired health-care providers. Mentorship programs are available online. One such community is the Association of Medical Professionals with Hearing Losses (AMPHL) mentorship program. AMPHL has many other resources for educators of health-care professionals. Visit http:// www.amphl.org

the Test of English as a Foreign Language (TOEFL) and set a minimum score requirement before the learner may enroll in courses. TOEFL educators who work with learners who are not proficient in English may have difficulty reading assignments and posts from students who are ESL.

The online learning environment offers an advantage to learners who are learning English or ESL. Learners with limited English proficiency (LEPs) can make use of audio dictionaries that pronounce words in English. Another useful tool is the use of an online translator. The online translator is available in most languages and easily can be added to the online course room. One disadvantage that should be noted is that the learner may not learn the English language because he or she becomes too reliant on the technology.

In addition to online translators, there are widgets that will convert an entire Web page to another language. Examples of these translators are available on Davis Plus. Learning and teaching materials should include objectives for increasing comprehension and language acquisition. For example, one practical application would be use the translators to create content-assessment quizzes. The learner would be assigned the self-assessment quiz in his or her native language, then use the translator to covert the quiz to English. The learner then will be able to compare comprehension and increase acquisition through reinforcement.

Strategic Planning for Learners With Special Considerations

Strategic planning for nursing education and e-learning includes adhering to regulations set forth by government, national licensure organizations, state boards of nursing, and accrediting agencies for nursing and education institutions. In addition, there are specific technical standards that must be met for global and e-learning courses. Chapter 4 provides an in-depth review of strategic planning for curriculum development and implementation. This section will focus on meeting the requirements of global learning communities and the specific needs of learners with special considerations.

Laws and Legal Issues

Educational institutions are legally required to comply with all laws for persons with disabilities including the Americans with Disabilities Act, The Rehabilitation Act of 1973, and Section 504, which pertains to postsecondary education. These laws were created to ensure that persons with disabilities have the same access to physical and electronic resources that is afforded to persons without disabilities. The learner also has the right to reasonable accommodations. Failure to make reasonable accommodations is considered discrimination (Helms & Weiler, 1993). An educational institution and the educator can be sued for violations of the law. To this end, it is important for educators to know the laws and create learning environments that comply with these laws and regulations.

By law, it is the student's responsibility to notify the institution of the disability or special needs. Disclosure is voluntary and many learners chose to remain anonymous. The learner may opt not to share information regarding their disabilities for fear of discrimination. In one instance, a minority learner shared that the discrimination for her LD was similar to that she had felt when she experienced racism. The educator can prevent reluctance of disclosure by establishing an environment that promotes trust and encourages disclosure. To establish this rapport, the educator should try to meet with learners individually or provide a means for private interaction early in the course. It is also important that the educator have a working knowledge of laws associated with disabilities.

TECHNOLOGY TIP 10.10

Have a section of the online course devoted to resources for students with academic challenges. This section can include self-assessment tools, Web links, and contact information for on-site and online resources available to learners with special needs.

The Rehabilitation Act of 1973 was the first major legislative effort to mandate that citizens with disabilities had equal rights and that reasonable accommodations be made for persons with special needs. This legislation provides a wide range of services for persons with physical and cognitive disabilities. The Section 504 of the Rehabilitation Act is specific to postsecondary educational institutions that receive federal funding and protects learners from being discriminated against because of disability. According to Section 504, postsecondary educational institutions that receive federal funding may not discriminate against persons with a documented disability.

Section 508 is an amendment to the Rehabilitation Act of 1998 and includes electronic information. According to the amendment, all agencies are required to insure that their electronic and information technology be accessible to people with disabilities. Section 508 was enacted to eliminate barriers in information technology, to make available new opportunities for people with disabilities, and to encourage development of technologies that will help achieve these goals.

Section 508 compliance does not guarantee that all special populations will have accessibility. For instance, when courses are designed using a LMS, such as Blackboard or eCollege, faculty can add course materials easily to the LMS. Courseware products, such as PowerPoint, graphics, animations, and videos may create a challenge to learners with disabilities because of coding issues.

Along with Section 508, there are clear-cut guidelines for designing Web pages that comply with existing regulations. The Web Accessibility Initiative (WAI) created guidelines and categorized the guidelines into three priorities. By law, if an educational institution is developing a course online, the institution must meet the minimum standards outlined in the guidelines. According to the guidelines, if the Web page does not pass all priorities in the guidelines it would exclude one or more groups of learners with disabilities. In essence, the learner would not be able to access the learning environment.

TECHNOLOGY TIP 10.11

Many colleges use a standard format to display variations in how the course room can be viewed. For example, the course room would include options, such as increasing text size, audio podcasts, or color-changing options.

TECHNOLOGY TIP 10.12

Educators can test materials for shareable content object reference model (SCORM) compliance online at: http://www.scorm.com/scorm-solved/test-track/. In addition, the Web Accessibility Initiative (WAI) provides guidelines for educational institutions. The WAI created a checklist that can be used for creating teaching materials. The checklist can be accessed on the WAI's Web site (http://www.webaim.org/standards/508/checklist).

TECHNOLOGIES THAT ASSIST IN CREATING UNIVERSAL DESIGN

Available technologies assist with creating accessibility. In addition, they also help to level the playing field by giving all qualified applicants a chance to succeed. Many operating systems have built-in features to improve usability and accessibility. For example, Windows 7, Windows XP, and Vista have accessibility options, such as magnifiers, narrators, and on-screen keyboards that allow users to optimize the computer for visual, physical, and hearing-impaired individuals. The Mac OS X features are similar to the Windows operating system. In addition to built-in computer operating system designs, there also are similar features in most Web browsers that allow users to customize the viewing content of Internet pages.

Assistive technologies that also can be used in the online learning environment include the use of speech synthesizers, voice-recognition software, and closed-captioning software. Speech synthesizers allow the learner who cannot speak to type his or her thoughts, and an audio file will produce a computer voice. The software will "speak" the text aloud. The opposite would be true of speech-recognition systems. Voice-recognition systems will type the verbal word that is spoken by the learner. Voice-recognition software allows users to take information recorded in the classroom and transfers the information to a Microsoft Word document on their computers.

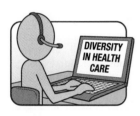

Most voice-recognition software requires the user to train the device by speaking into a microphone on his or her computer; however, newer software is available that does not require voice training. Learners can focus on listening in class, record the lecture, and upload the notes on the computer. Any word-processing software reads the notes. Dragon Naturally Speaking 9 is a software program that does not need voice training and can be used with all common Microsoft applications. Along with transcribing notes, the software will eliminate unnecessary words and punctuate according to natural pauses in the recording. Dragon Natural Speaking 9 also can be used to browse the Internet and works well with e-mail and course-room functions.

The National Centre for Accessible Media (NCAM) is a free tool for creating and exporting caption files. The NCAM MAGpie can be used with media players, including QuickTime and Windows Media Player. Once an educator creates a lecture or presentation MAGpie will add captions and timings to the presentation. MAGpie can convert lectures to video casts or vodcasts with open captioning. Open captioning can be used in the classroom to benefit all learners, but in particular learners with hearing disabilities. There also are services that can arrange closed captioning for fees and pricing is based on the project to be captioned.

Assistive technology is an important piece of the online learning environment. There are many advances in technologies that create UD. One major advance is the inclusion of interactive electronic textbooks. These electronic versions of printed textbook are highly

TECHNOLOGY TIP 10.13

Try implementing the accessibility options on your computer. For MAC users' accessibility options are located in the System Preferences under the Apple menu. After the System Preferences opens, select the Universal Access Preference pane. For Windows operating systems, accessibility features are located in the control panel, select accessibility control panel, or ease of access center.

interactive and appeal to many learning needs thus creating a student-centered solution and the ultimate UD. Another technology that goes along with the interactive textbooks is the netbook. These mini-computers allow users to easily download and navigate electronic versions of their books.

CONCLUSION

In conclusion, strategic planning for online learning should include strategies for helping students who have a variety of learning needs to include physical challenges, language barriers, or socioeconomic restrictions. E-learning offers much promise for achieving the goal of creating global learning communities that can be accessed by all regardless of these limitations.

E-learning offers so many opportunities for learners who have special needs. The advance in technology and the online venue provide intuitive solutions for most problems associated with learning and physical limitations thereby providing those populations with realistic reasonable accommodations. The educator in the online learning environment can facilitate learning for students with physical and learning disabilities because e-learning courses that are universally designed benefit the entire student population and create a sense of autonomy for those who previously have been limited.

REFERENCES

Erickson, W., & Lee, C. (2008). 2007 disability status report: United States. Ithaca, NY: Cornell University Rehabilitation Research and Training Center on Disability Demographics and Statistics. Retrieved from: http://digitalcommons.ilr.cornell.edu/cgi/viewcontent.cgi?article=1256&context=edicollect

Gardner, H. (1983). *Frames of mind: The theory of multiple intelligences.* New York, NY: Basic.

Helms, L. B., & Weiler, L. (1993). Disability discrimination in nursing education: An evaluation of legislation and litigation. *Journal of Professional Nursing, 9*(6), 358–366.

International Code Council (1998). Retrieved from: http://www.iccsafe.org

Kaminski, J. (2006) P.A.T.C.H. Pretest assessment scale for attitudes toward computers in healthcare. Retrieved from http://www.nursing-informatics.com/kwantlen/patch.html

National Institutes of Health (NIH). (1998). Diagnosis and treatment of attention deficit hyperactivity disorder (ADHD). NIH Consensus Statement, Nov 16-18; *16*(2).

Obama, B. (2009). Remarks by the President on the American Graduation Initiative. *Macomb Community College Warren, Michigan* July 14, 2009. Retrieved from http://www.whitehouse.gov/the_press_office/Remarks-by-the-President-on-the-American-Graduation-Initiative-in-Warren-MI/8

Readiness Index for Learning Online. (RILO). (2004). WebCT. Center for Teaching and Lifelong Learning. Retrieved from http://www.webct.com/oriented/ViewContent?contentID=1811174

The Center for Universal Design: Connell, B.R., Jones, M., Mace, R., Mueller, J., Mullick, A., Ostroff, E., Sanford, J., Steinfeld, E., Story, M., & Vanderheiden, G. (1997). *The principles of universal design, version 2.0.* Raleigh, NC: North Carolina State University. Retrieved from http://www.design.ncsu.edu/cud/about_ud/udprinciplestext.htm

Vanderheiden, G. C., & Vanderheiden, K. (1991). Accessible design of consumer products: Guidelines for the design of consumer products to increase their accessibility to people with disabilities or who are aging. Madison, WI: Trace Research & Development Center. Retrieved from http://trace.wisc.edu/docs/consumer_product_guidelines/consumer.htm

Wheeler, L., Reynolds, T., & Russell, J. (2000). *Teaching online: A guide for teachers, facilitators and mentors, RMIT.* Retrieved from http://www.learnlinks.com.au/docs/downloads/online.pdf

Chapter 11

Distance and Distributed Educational Units

Ebony Fisher, PhD(c), MSN, RN

Distance education learning is not a new concept in nursing education. There is much research to indicate that distance education is going to continue to be the way of the future because of the technology driven health-care industry and the technology literate student body. Nursing education units must consider the needs of their students. Students want curriculums that offer flexibility and autonomy.

Nursing education units should be making preparations to meet the needs of adult learners. Adult learners today want curriculums that allow them the flexibility and convenience to achieve their academic goals. According to a report by the SLOAN Consortium (2006), more than 67% of higher education facilities offer distance education courses. Because of this statistical data, trends, and the need to be competitive with other institutions, more schools of nursing are considering, planning, and implementing distance and distributed education into their curriculum (Bitler, 2001). Nursing education units, who are resistant to developing these types of curriculums, will soon find that they are not able to compete in the market (Hawkins, 2003). Distance and distributed learning methods are changing how nursing departments are delivering education and training to their students.

FACULTY SUPPORT

First, before a distance education course can be developed and implemented, there must be support, input, and buy-in from the faculty (Schraeder, Swamidass, & Morrison, 2006). There are many institutions that have had big ideas and plans about starting an online program, but their plans flopped or ended because they had disgruntled faculty members. As with any curriculum idea, faculty should be involved in its development at the very beginning. If not, the idea is sure to fail because all curriculums should be faculty-driven.

Faculty members may be somewhat apprehensive about implementing distance education programs and/or courses for many various reasons. Nursing faculty could possibly be hesitant about implementing an online program and/or course because they do not feel comfortable with technology. Faculty, who teach in distance learning programs, should feel relaxed with e-mailing a student, using course-management tools, such as the chat room, the discussion board, the course grade book, etc. (Levy, 2003; Hazari & Borkowski, 2001). Nursing distance education units should develop a training course for faculty and encourage faculty

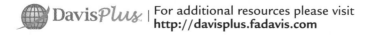 For additional resources please visit
http://davisplus.fadavis.com

members to enroll in continuing education courses and/or program degrees that are offered via online (Hazari & Borkowski, 2001).

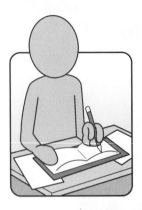

It would be helpful if there were some faculty members who were familiar with online teaching pedagogies. The faculty, who are knowledgeable in online learning, could be instrumental in helping the other faculty members to become up-to-date in online methodologies. Schools of nursing and programs should remember that faculty members do not necessarily have to be proficient in online learning, but they must be enthusiastic to learn about its teaching methodologies, then try online learning and be ready to accept the challenges that it brings, and shift forward. "Distance education requires new ways of thinking about teaching and learning and challenges deeply held assumptions and long-established practices (Bates, 2000)." It may be difficult for nursing faculty members to give up the "control" they once had in the face-to-face (f-2-f) learning environment. With online learning, the instructor is the facilitator in a student-centered learning environment.

PARENT-INSTITUTION SUPPORT

After faculty support is received, nursing education units should ensure that they have their parent institution support. Depending on the type of institution (i.e., public, private, or proprietary), this could be a tedious and long process. It would be helpful if research and a needs assessment were conducted before meeting with your institution's administration and discussing your department's plan to implement distance education into the curriculum. It may be beneficial to conduct a student survey to inquire if current students are interested in the proposed online program and/or course. Administrations often are cautious about investing any monies if there are no students buying in. Survey results that demonstrate students' interest in the proposed program and/or online course may be instrumental in helping administration in making a decision that is within your department's and/or program's favor.

Deans, program chairs, and directors should be ready to discuss the money involved to start the distance education program and/or course. Consideration should be given if the department and/or program will be using grant money to start this venture. Funds are available, from government and private sponsors, for starting online nursing courses and/or programs. Within this budget, there needs to be consideration if adjunct or full-time faculty members will be used, the cost of the course-management system, and cost of technical support and maintenance.

When planning to meet with your administration, it is important that the nursing education unit is ready and prepared for the questions and/or negative commentary administration may have about your idea. Most deans, program chairs, and directors find that preparation

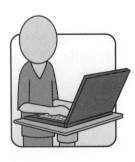

usually is the key that helps them successfully defend their department or program's plan to receive funds and/or approval for a new idea. Many administrators already realize the importance of implementing distance education into curriculum. Allen and Seaman (2003) surveyed university administrators and found that 75% of them felt that distance learning outcomes can be equivalent or be superior to traditional learning.

Nursing deans, program chairs, and/or directors need to make sure that they emphasize that the school or program must move with technology. Technology is all around us. It is important to remind administration that students must be ready for the technology-driven, health-care environment. "All health professionals should be educated to deliver patient-centered care as members of an interdisciplinary team, emphasizing evidence-based practice, quality improvement approaches, and informatics" (Hundert, Wakefield, Bootman, et al., 2003, p. 45). It may be important to demonstrate that students are expected to have computer skills to do computer charting, access electronic health records, and to use information systems and software for dispensing medications. Administrations must realize that students will not do well in the future if they do not have adequate technology skills (Donofrio, 2006).

DISTRIBUTED LEARNING VERSUS DISTANCE LEARNING

You have faculty and administration support and buy-in. What's next? The department and/or program needs to decide what type of instructional models will be used. There are two types: distance learning and distributed education models. Distance learning in the United States has been around since the 19th century (Neal, 1999). The first distance learning program was a mail correspondence education program in the 1800s.

Sometimes distance learning and distributed learning are used interchangeably. Distributed learning allows learners and their instructors the opportunity to learn and teach at different times and geographical locations. This learning could take place online or through other correspondence media (i.e., print, television, videoconferencing, and e-mail). For example, a nursing student could complete his or her studies in another country, through e-mail, Internet, television, or a blend of various strategies. Distributed learning offers nursing programs and their faculty the ability to teach beyond the traditional method (f-2-f) and incorporate multiple teaching delivery methods. This instructional model is commonly known as a blended or a hybrid model. In the blended or hybrid model, faculty may be able to deliver majority of the program and/or course content in the online environment. Two to three f-2-f visits may be required to complete clinical or skills validations.

Developing a hybrid or a blended course may be an excellent way for the department or program to practice online pedagogies and technical skills. This also may be ideal if the nursing faculty is still struggling with "giving up control" in the classroom setting. This method may allow them time to triumph over the challenges that distance learning may bring.

Distance learning allows the adult learners to receive instruction, other than f-2-f, in a geographical location that is different from the instructor (Keegan, 1995). This instruction could be in an asynchronous or synchronous environment. An asynchronous distance learning environment allows the instructor and the learner flexibility to complete teaching and learning activities at a different time and different place. A synchronous distance learning environment allows the instructor and the learner to complete teaching and learning activities at different places, but at the same time.

There are various delivery methods that are used in distance education (Table 11.1). "The intended delivery mode for instruction is a very important consideration in the development of materials based on the planned instructional strategy" (Dick & Carey, 1990). Some of the most popular delivery methods are as follows: Internet-instruction, mail correspondence, video- or television-broadcasted, and videostream.

TYPES OF ONLINE NURSING PROGRAMS

Nursing distance education units need to decide on what types of nursing programs (prelicensure or postlicensure) and/or courses they would desire to implement and use distance or

TABLE 11.1		
Distance Education Delivery Systems		
Types of Delivery Methods	**Definition**	**Helpful Information**
Internet Instruction	An online course management tool allows student to access and participate in classroom assignments.	Considered the most popular method. Various online CMSs that can be used: Blackboard, Angel, and eCollege.
Mail Correspondence	Coursework, evaluation, and material taken are received and sent via postal mail.	May be costly to initially develop this program. Possibility of lost correspondence.
Teleconferencing	Television and video equipment is used to allow students in another geographical area to participate in a class that is conducted in another geographical area (typically on the main campus).	Requires more personnel for production and technical support. Expensive due to increase in personnel and video and television equipment.
Videostream	Video is recorded, from a live lecture, and then streamed over the Internet. Learners have unlimited access to retrieving this recorded video.	Students can access anywhere there is Internet service. Requires personnel for production and technical support.

distributed learning methodologies. After deciding on the types of programs and/or courses to develop, the unit needs to settle upon what types of distance and/or distributed education methodologies will be used. Will this course or program be entirely online? Will course or program have blended delivery options? Will this course or program be an independent study? Will it be broadcasted or televised?

If one were to Google the types of nursing programs that are available online, then one would find that there are hundreds of nursing programs on the Internet. There are programs available for students who are interested in pursuing a degree in nursing (i.e., prelicensure programs) and there are programs for nurses who want to advance their education and training (i.e., postlicensure programs).

Prelicensure Nursing Programs

When one thinks about prelicensure nursing programs, they think about the f-2-f and the brink-and-mortar programs for students. These include practical nursing, registered nursing (i.e., associate and baccalaureate prepared) program, and, sometimes, programs leading to a

TABLE 11.2

Types of Prelicensure Programs

Types of Prelicensure Programs	Average Completion Time	Traditionally: F-2-f, Online, and/or Hybrid
LPN Program	9 months–18 years	F-2-f & hybrid
Diploma Program	2–3 years	F-2-f & hybrid
ADN Program, Generic	18 months–2 years	F-2-f, online, & hybrid
Prelicensure BSN Program, Generic	3–4 years	F-2-f, online, & hybrid
Accelerated BSN Program, Generic (2nd degree)	1–1½ years	F-2-f & hybrid
Prelicensure Master's Program	1½–3 years	F-2-f, online, & hybrid

master's in nursing (Table 11.2). Today, it is not unusual for these programs to include some online coursework into the curriculum. These programs are considered hybrid programs. Nursing students could benefit from taking nonclinical courses online.

Amazingly, there are programs that have been successful and offer their entire curriculum via online. This was unheard of 10 years ago in nursing, but more and more programs are starting to think of innovative ways to meet the needs of the ever changing and technology-driven student body. If a nursing department is considering converting its entire curriculum in an online format, then one must consider how the clinical rotations will be arranged. As with any major curriculum change, the state board of nursing should be contacted. Some state boards of nursing have regulations on concerning prelicensure programs offering courses online. Check with your state board of nursing and its regulations to ensure you are within its guidelines.

If planned appropriately, much of the entire nursing program can be online. There have been programs in recent past that did not consider student-learning outcomes and were not successful. Because of this, some state boards of nursing have shut down those programs. It is important that nursing programs that are interested in having much of their curriculum online have a good plan for tutoring, remediation, advising, and other student services.

There are many boards of nursing and states that will embrace online prelicensure programs. For example, Western Governors University, an online university, recently opened a prelicensure baccalaureate in nursing program. This program is available to students in Texas and California. This program received $11 million in grant monies from the state of California. It is the program and the state of California's goal to address the nursing shortage with this online prelicensure program. According to Governor Arnold Schwarzenegger (2009):

> *This partnership is a great example of our health-care providers, educators, and the state working together to alleviate our nursing shortage and get more Californians to*

work. This new online program is a win-win for California by making nursing programs more accessible to people interested in pursuing this career path and helping to fill critically needed jobs throughout the state (http://www.labor.ca.gov/ pdf/nwsrel09-08.pdf).

Clinical and Clinical Learning Laboratory

The clinical learning laboratories and clinical rotations are important part of learning in nursing education. Of course patient care cannot be done online. At least, not yet! So, nursing departments and/or programs must take careful consideration when developing programs and/or courses with these components. There are some programs that have their students visit campus, once a quarter, to demonstrate and validate laboratory skills. While on campus, these students also will attend their clinical rotations. This usually is done in the last couple of weeks of the semester or quarter.

When planning your distance learning course and/or program, it is important to remember that the clinical learning laboratory and rotations are important to develop psychomotor and critical thinking skills. Many book publishers realize that these are important skills and are developing tools that can be accessed online. These tools include skills videos and clinical case studies. Faculty may consider incorporating these tools and/or objects into their courses.

Simulation, both virtual and high-fidelity, also is important in developing clinical and critical thinking skills. Simulations allow nursing students the ability to role-play realistic clinical scenarios, while demonstrating psychomotor skills, clinical judgment, and subsequently critical thinking ability. Gaming simulations (such as Elsevier's Virtual Clinical Excursion) also can be used in an online environment. Some software programs that allow nursing students the ability to interact with various medias (video, audio, etc.) to discover and solve clinical problems in a virtual setting.

Western Governors University's program provides students with at least four intensive clinical rotations a year. E-line in Texas (http://www.eline.delmar.edu/) allows students to complete clinicals in their hometowns by hiring local preceptors and educators. University of South Dakota partners with long-term care facilities across the nation to help them grow their own registered nurses. These are just a few examples of how distance education programs manage prelicensure clinical learning.

Postlicensure Nursing Programs

The American Association of Colleges of Nursing (AACN) applauded nursing pioneer, Patricia Benner's study that called for all entry-level nurses to be prepared at the baccalaureate level, and for nurses to receive their master's degree upon 10 years after initial licensing

TECHNOLOGY TIP 11.1

Use an Internet search engine to search the various types of prelicensure programs that are available. When searching the Internet, be sure to look at admission guidelines, time to complete the program, and what online courses the program offers.

(http://www.aacn.nche.edu/Media/NewsReleases/2010/carnegie.html). Hospitals across the country are seeking Magnet Status. Magnet Status is awarded to hospitals who have met a rigorous set of criteria provided by the American Nurses' Credentialing Center (ANCC). This organization is a partner of the American Nurses Association (ANA). These hospitals are considered those who have outstanding patient outcomes, which are attributed to advanced nursing education. For a hospital to be awarded this designation, there must be a certain number of nurses who are baccalaureate prepared and higher. Nurses, across the country, are starting to realize that to advance in nursing, advanced education has to be achieved. Because of this there has been a great need for postlicensure nursing programs.

There are various postlicensure nursing programs (Table 11.3). A nursing department and/or program, who is considering offering postlicensure programs and/or courses online or programs, should consider its mission and philosophy. Faculty also should consider the outcomes and competencies, if not already developed, that need to be met. Nursing faculty are encouraged to consider the trends and the research when developing programs. There is much controversy about whether the doctorate of nursing practice (DNP) should be the entry level for nurse practitioners, clinical nursing specialists, and nurse midwives. It may not be a good idea to develop a master's-level, clinical-focus degree if the research is suggesting that by the year 2015, the DNP will be an entry-level degree for these clinical-focused, advanced practice nurses (http://www.aacn.nche.edu/DNP/DNPPositionStatement.htm).

Finally, nursing education units, who are considering offering distance education nursing terminal degrees, need to understand their differences. There are a number of terminal degrees for nurses available. The doctor of philosophy (PhD) and the doctorate of nursing science (DNSc) degrees prepare nurses to be scholars and contribute scholarly research to advance the nursing profession. The DNP degree is considered the clinical instead of research

TABLE 11.3

Types of Postlicensure Programs

Types of Postlicensure Programs	Average Completion Time	Traditionally: F-2-f, Online, and/or Hybrid
Postlicensure BSN Program	1–2 years	F-2-f, online, & hybrid
Master's in Nursing-Clinical Tracks (NP, Midwife, Clinical Nurse Specialist)	1–2 years	F-2-f, online, & hybrid
Master's in Nursing-Nonclinical Tracks (Education, Administration)	1–2 years	F-2-f, online, & hybrid
PhD in Nursing	2–4 years	F-2-f, online, & hybrid
DNP Program	1–2 years	F-2-f, online, & hybrid

focused. The University of Alabama is offering its postlicensure students, who are baccalaureate of master's prepared, the opportunity to earn their doctor of education (EdD) in nursing. This program is considered a hybrid because students are able to complete their studies via online and in the f-2-f environment.

THE STRATEGIC PLAN

Many nursing departments and schools of nursing have excellent ideas, but if a strategic plan is not developed then many of them are just that, ideas. In addition to the strategic plan, there needs to be a time line for developing the online course and/or program. This could be instrumental to the nursing department in getting the idea off of the paper and "on the ground and running."

A time line simply divides each of the major tasks and milestones into pieces. Because time is usually of the essence for most nurse educators, the time line should include a deadline for when each task or milestone should be started and completed.

It is important that all nursing administrators and faculty involved in the development of the distance education program contribute to this time line. A time line for development helps the nursing program to consider required steps to implementation. The time line also highlights the needed resources for success. When developing this time line, the nursing department should estimate how long it will take a task or milestone to be accomplished. Underestimating a milestone and/or task, could cause the nursing department to become behind in its implementation of developing a course and/or program. In return, this could lead to the nursing program overspending funds allocated in the budget. It is better to overestimate, because if there is some time left over then one can start the next milestone or take time to analyze and review the steps taken to meet this milestone and assess if anything was missing.

The next step will be to identify who will be responsible for each milestone and/or task (Table 11.4). The responsible party should have a clear understanding of what is his or her role in completing the task and how long it should take to complete it.

Next, a time line should then be developed and used. Nursing schools need to assess their own departments and parent-institutions to find out if they are distance-learning ready and capable. There needs to be an adequate budget for developing and implementing these programs and/or courses into the curriculum.

Finally, the department needs to consider what instructional delivery method systems and learning management systems to deliver distance and/or distributed curriculums to its students.

COURSE MANAGEMENT SYSTEM

It may be very difficult for a nursing department and/or program to decide on which type of course management system (CMS) to use. CMSs provide a virtual environment for online teaching and instruction. The CMS or virtual learning environment allows faculty to add,

TECHNOLOGY TIP 11.2

Use Google® documents (docs.google.com) to share the timeline among team members. This free service will allow all on the team to see changes and updates in realtime.

TABLE 11.4

Developing a Time Line of Milestones and Tasks

Milestone	Task	Start and Finish Date	Responsible Party
Milestone 1	Speaking with university provost about the possibility of providing an online RN to BSN program.	12/1/2010–12/7/2010	Dean, School of Nursing
Milestone 2	Research various online RN to BSN programs' admission guidelines and report findings to committee.	12/15/2010–1/15/2011	The RN to BSN Program Nursing Faculty 1. Jane Smith RN, PhD 2. James Doe RN, PhD (c) 3. Mary Doe RN, MSN

edit, and/or delete course materials, such as the syllabus, graded assignments, quizzes, and lectures. A number of tools such as chat, threaded discussion board, announcement section, whiteboards, document sharing folder, blogs, calendar, grade books, and e-mail are available by using a CMS. Nursing faculty will have the capability to insert PowerPoint lectures and videos through the online course room.

There are many different brands available for higher learning institutions and their academic programs. Some of the popular CMSs are Blackboard, eCollege, Angel, and Desire to Learn. CMSs differ in the types of tool they offer.

Selecting a CMS may be difficult for the nursing department or program. Faculty members may find one CMS more user friendly than another. The decision also may include the type technical support offered by the CMS.

Check with your institution before researching a CMS. Some institutions may already be under contract with a particular CMS. The nursing department may have little to no input on the selection and will need to use the system that is in place.

If nursing departments and/or programs are interested in only creating a few online courses, it may not cost effective to purchase the rights to use a commercial brand of CMS. There are some free online CMSs that allow nursing faculty to create and/or develop online environments for instruction and learning. For example, Moodle is an example of a free CMS (http://moodle.org/). A program also should consider contacting its textbook publisher because many offer access to a standardized online course shell if the nursing program adopts a particular textbook.

TECHNOLOGY TIP 11.3

Edutool is a free, easy-to-use Web site that offers online tools, which will assist nursing departments and programs in making rational decisions about various distance learning production, such as selecting a CMS. This Web site can be found by accessing http://www.edutools.info/index.jsp?pj=1

ONLINE FACULTY HIRING AND TRAINING

There is a shortage of qualified nursing educators in the United States (LaRocco, 2006). Nursing departments and/or schools are having trouble recruiting qualified faculty to teach nursing students. Nursing education units across the United States are claiming that they had to turn away qualified applicants because of the lack of qualified nurse educators (American Association of Colleges of Nursing, 2009).

Online learning may be instrumental in affecting this nursing shortage (Talbert, 2009). Nursing education units, who use online learning, may be able to recruit qualified faculty that may not be in their geographical area. Online faculty also may be able to maintain their full-time employment in addition to instructing an online course because online learning allows for flexibility. One of the reasons why nurses with advanced education are reluctant to make the transition to full-time nursing faculty is because of the lower salaries. According to Nevada Nurses Association (2004), a master's-prepared, clinical advance practice nurse made an annual salary of $80,697, while the master's prepared nurse educator made an annual salary of $60,831.

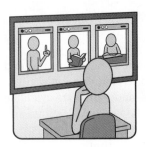

Nursing education units are able to hire qualified adjuncts for a fraction of the salary of a qualified full-time nursing faculty. This may be another incentive for many programs to develop and implement online nursing education. Using online nursing adjuncts could possibly reduce the workload of the nursing education unit's full-time nursing faculty.

Nursing education units should research what other nursing education units are paying their online adjunct faculty. It is important for the nursing unit to offer fair, equitable, and competitive contract salaries to online adjunct nursing faculty. Low salaries could potentially affect the nursing unit's ability to attract qualified and quality online faculty members. Salaries usually consist of the online adjunct faculty member being paid by the semester or quarter credit hour. There are some nursing education units that compensate faculty based on the number of students enrolled in an online course. For example, an adjunct faculty may be contracted to teach online nursing research course. For every student that enrolls in the program, the faculty member will receive $100.

Nursing education units should consider online faculty members' workload. Online faculty workload consists of how much time a faculty spends in the online classroom to get his or her work completed. Research has shown that online faculty may spend more time in the online classroom than the traditional f-2-f classroom because of increased interaction with students (Hartman, Dziuban, & Moskal 2000; Lazarus, 2003). Student enrollment, in each course, should be limited to 20 or less students. This allows the instructor to be able to build community with the learners and to effectively interact with his or her students.

Many nursing education units may question if adjunct faculty are qualified. They may question if the quality of education will be sacrificed because of the use of adjunct nursing faculty. These are all questions that need to be addressed when the nursing education unit is planning on implementing online programs and/or courses into the curriculum (see Appendix C).

Nursing education units must have a recruitment plan and process in place for recruiting nursing adjunct faculty. Hiring online adjunct nursing faculty that are not in the geographical area may propose some concerns for nursing administrators who are comfortable with interviewing prospective faculty members in a f-2-f environment. Nursing education units must develop a process that will help them to recognize quality online adjunct nursing faculty.

Hiring decisions should be made based on the applicant's ability to meet the needs of the institution, support the mission and philosophy of the nursing education unit, and his or her commitment to delivering and providing quality nursing education. It may be helpful for the nursing administrators to inquire about the adjunct's teaching philosophy. The teaching philosophy may provide a reflection of the adjunct's beliefs about teaching and learning. It may also shed light on how the faculty may incorporate teaching strategies into practice.

The nursing education unit may want to develop case studies for the interviewing process. This may provide the nursing education unit with an idea of how potential adjunct faculty may respond in difficult situations that involve students. It also allows for assessment of the potential adjunct's critical thinking skills. It is important for adjuncts to have great critical thinking skills because there is autonomy in the online course room. Online adjuncts need to be quick in making proper judgments and decisions in the online classroom.

It is important to access the potential adjunct faculty member's written communication ability. Nursing education administrators may want to communicate with potential adjunct faculty members via e-mail. This allows the administrator the ability to access the faculty's written communication. The administrator should pay close attention to grammar, spelling, and the applicant's tone.

It is imperative that the nursing education develop a training program for online adjunct nursing faculty and/or full-time faculty with little to no online teaching experience. A training program could be a condition of employment. Nursing education units may have to make the decision if they are going to implement this training program to screen qualified applicants or if it will be considered a part of employee orientation.

The training program could be paid or unpaid. Training programs are usually 1 to 2 weeks in length. It is important for the training program to resemble the instructional environment that the adjunct or the potential adjunct may be instructing. Faculty should have the opportunity to be able to learn about and use the various course tools available in the CMSs. Best practices would be to incorporate other potential adjuncts or adjuncts in the training session. This allows the participants to learn how to build community and interact with other learners.

Providing mentors to new faculty may help with retaining faculty members. New faculty may take comfort in knowing that there is a seasoned faculty member that will be available to answer questions. Mentoring should occur at least for one semester or quarter. After this time, the nursing administrators should access the online faculty to see if more mentoring and/or training is needed.

It is essential for the new faculty to be properly evaluated by students and the nursing administrator each semester and/or quarter. Evaluation could be instrumental in allowing the nursing education unit to assess if the faculty member fits the program and/or department's needs, mission, and philosophy. It allows the nursing education unit the ability to see if the students are receiving quality instruction. It is important for the nursing education unit to share these evaluations with the online faculty each semester and/or quarter. Evaluations are useful in helping the online nursing faculty member to grow and mature in his or her instruction and teaching strategies.

Distance education nursing units may need to develop policies and expectations for their online faculty to safeguard their students and ensure that distance education courses and programs are of quality. It may be useful for distance education nursing units to create policies that address faculty participation, grading, feedback, and faculty's timely response to students' e-mails.

PREDEVELOPED CONTENT VERSUS INSTRUCTOR AUTONOMY

Nursing education units must decide if the proposed online program and/or course will be predeveloped or if the instructor will have autonomy in developing the course content. Full-time nursing faculty may have some concerns with having a course shell and content that is standardized, especially when he or she is used to having instructor autonomy or freedom in his or her f-2-f courses. Nursing faculty may feel that the quality of the instruction may be lowered and that there is no academic freedom or autonomy (Reigle, 2008).

Predeveloped course content may be the way to go for programs that are using the majority of online nursing adjuncts because this may be an incentive for faculty member teaching in the program. New faculty may not feel comfortable with developing, adding, deleting, and/or editing course content. Nursing education units also may struggle with granting online nursing adjuncts the autonomy and freedom of changing the course content each semester and/or quarter. There may be a fear of that the outcomes of the course will not be met because course content could be missing and/or deleted.

The decision to offer predeveloped courses and/or programs or not should belong to the nursing education unit. The unit should consider what is right for the needs of the students and the program. If autonomy is allowed for faculty to edit, develop, and/or add course content, the nursing program should have a plan to monitor and critique the content to ensure that the students' outcomes are being met.

STUDENT SUPPORT SERVICES

Online nursing students should have the same rights and privileges as the brick-and-mortar nursing students. Nursing education units must be careful to include student services into the online learning environment. This should be done before the implementation of the online nursing program and/or course and not after a problem and/or concern has arrived. Nursing education should realize that online learning may be a innovative instructional delivery method, but students' needs are the same regardless of whether the class is online or in a f-2-f environment. Student support services include, but are not limited to: technology support, library services, tutoring and remediation, and academic advising.

Nursing education units who do not consider offering students services may find disgruntled or dissatisfied nursing students. These students may feel that they are being shortchanged in comparison with the traditional-setting nursing student. In return, the lack of student support services may have an extreme effect on program and/or course attrition rates.

When planning student support services, it is important for the nursing education unit to make sure that these services are available for students despite their geographical location. For example, students should be able to access the library without having to travel to campus.

It is imperative for nursing education units to provide an overview, tour, and/or training, to the online learners and the faculty on the various student services that are available. Students and faculty should feel comfortable with being able to locate these services when the need arises.

Students and faculty, alike, should be able to access and use the library. This is especially critical in nursing education because it is of extreme importance for nursing faculty to incorporate and use evidence-based practice into the curriculum. Nursing faculty also should be encouraging nursing students to use evidence-based practice in their academic and professional careers.

The nursing education department must meet with the institution's librarian to determine the resources that will be of extreme importance to its online nursing faculty and students. There are library databases, such as CINAHL, that allow nursing students and faculty to access resources, such as books, journals, and magazines online. The nursing education unit will have to incur a license fee to access this information. Fees will vary according to the vendor.

Libraries can be intimidating to students because of the wealth and abundance of information and resources. It is key that the librarian develops a training module that teaches the nursing students and faculty how to access the online library.

Students should have ongoing technical support. There may be issues with retrieving a document in the CMS. Students should have access to a technician preferably 24/7, especially since the beauty of online learning is being able to access your coursework anytime of the day. Students should be able to e-mail, phone (if possible a toll-free number), and/or instant message (IM) a technician to have technical questions answered.

It also may be helpful to have a frequently answered questions (FAQ) section for current and potential students. Students should be well informed of the computer, hardware, software, and Internet expectations of an online program. An online Web page that addresses Internet connectivity and the minimum hardware and software requirements should be created and visibly displayed on the program's Web page.

Distance nursing education units must plan for the advising of online students. Units should ensure that students have the necessary tools and guidance to be able to make appropriate decisions concerning their academic courses in the program. It is not uncommon for nursing education units to develop and implement nursing advisors in their programs. It may be helpful if the advisor meets with the student at the beginning of the program to develop a plan of study and again when the plan changes. Nursing education units should have a plan in place for online students to meet with their advisors at least once a quarter and/or semester and, if necessary, when needed.

Tutoring and remediation services are some ways in which a nursing education unit can assist its distance education nursing students. These services can be provided by the faculty and/or the nursing education may choose to use an outside vendor who provides these tutoring and remediation services. There are online writing-tutoring services, such as SmartThinking, which are available to distance education students online. The nursing education unit must purchase a license to access and use these services. Unfortunately, there are few, if any, tutoring services that offer to the nursing education unit the right to purchase a license agreement and access tutoring for its distance education nursing students.

CONCLUSION

In summary, distance education learning is not a new concept in nursing education. There is much research to indicate that distance education is going to continue to be the way of the future because of the technology driven health-care industry and the technology literate student body. Nursing education units must consider the needs of their students. Students want curriculums that offer flexibility and autonomy.

Nursing education units who are preparing to meet the need of the students and health-care industry must, by offering distance education courses and/or programs, need to be adequately prepared. There must be a strategic plan that includes the nursing faculty at the beginning to consider the trends and current needs of the nursing profession and the needs of the student body. The strategic plan must meet the parent institution's and the nursing education unit's mission and philosophy.

Nursing education units must remember that distance education students have the same need and concerns as f-2-f students. Care must be taken to ensure that distance education students have the same rights, privileges, pedagogies, and qualified nursing faculty members as their on-campus peers.

REFERENCES

Allen, I. E., & Seaman, J. (2003). *Seizing the opportunity: The quality and extent of online education in the United States, 2002 and 2003.* Needham, MA: The Sloan Consortium. Retrieved from http://www.aln.org/resources/sizing_opportunity.pdf

American Association of Colleges of Nursing. (2009). *Nursing shortage fact sheet.* Retrieved from http://www.aacn.nche.edu/Media/pdf/NrsgShortageFS.pdf

American Association of Colleges of Nursing. (2009). *AACN applauds the Carnegie Report calling for a more highly educated nursing workforce.* Retrieved from https://www.aacn.nche.edu/Media/NewsReleases/2010/carnegie.html

Bates, A. W. (2000). *Managing technological change: Strategies for college and university leaders.* San Francisco: Jossey-Bass.

Bitler, D. (2001). Managing technological changes: Strategies for college and university leaders. *Journal of College Student Development, 42,* 80–82.

California Labor & Workforce Development Agency News Release. (2009). Retrieved from http://www.labor.ca.gov/pdf/nwsrel09-08.pdf

Dick, W., & Carey L. (1990). *The systematic design of instruction.* Glenview, IL: Scott, Foresman.

Donofrio, N. (2006). An engine of innovation. *Diverse Issues in Higher Education, 23,* 45.

Hartman, J., Dziuban, C., & Moskal, P. (2000). Faculty satisfaction in ALNs: A dependent or independent variable? *Journal of Asynchronous Learning Networks, 4*(3), 155–179.

Hawkins, B. (2003). Making a commitment. *EDUCAUSE Review, 38,* 68.

Hazari, S. I., & Borkowski, E. Y (2001). *Looking beyond course development tools: Faculty training issues.* Proceedings of Educause 2001 Conference. Retrieved from http://www.sunilhazari.com/education/documents/educause2001.htm

Hundert, E. M., Wakefield, M., Bootman, J. L., Cassel, C. K., Ching, W., Chow, M. P., et al. (2003). *Institute of Medicine report—Health professions education: A bridge to quality.* Washington, DC: National Academies Press.

Keegan, D. (1995). *Distance education technology for the new millennium: Compressed video teaching.* ZIFF Papiere. Hagen, Germany: Institute for Research into Distance Education.

LaRocco, S. (2006). Who will teach the nurses? *Academe, 92*(3), 38–40. Retrieved from http://www.aaup.org/AAUP/pubsres/academe/2006/MJ/feat/laro.htm

Lazarus, B. D. (2003). Teaching courses online: How much time does it take? *Journal of Asynchronous Learning Networks, 7*(3) 47–53.

Levy, S. (2003). Six factors to consider when planning online distance learning programs in higher education. *Online Journal of Distance Learning Administration, 6*(1), 1–2.

Neal, E. (1999). Distance education: Prospects and problems. *Phi Kappa Phi Journal, 79*(1) 40–43.

Nevada Nurses Association. (2004). Nursing faculty shortage facts and factors. *RNformation, 13(2),* 16.

Reigle, R. (2008). *Teacher autonomy defined in online education* (Online submission). Retrieved from ERIC database (ED503316).

Schraeder, M., Swamidass, P., & Morrison, R. (2006). Employee involvement, attitudes, and reactions to technology changes. *Journal of Leadership & Organizational Studies, 12,* 85–101.

Sloan Consortium (2006). *Making the grade: Online education in the United States, 2006.* Retrieved from http://www.sloanconsortium.org/sites/default/files/Making_the_Grade.pdf

Talbert, J. (2009). Distance education: One solution to the nursing shortage? *Clinical Journal of Oncology Nursing, 13*(3), 269–270.

Technology for the Nursing Curriculum

Chapter 12

Nursing Informatics 101 for Nurse Educators

Cheryl D. Parker, PhD, MSN, RN

During a visit to a client, a faith-based home health organization, I had the privilege of hearing of the experience of one of the ministers using technology.

He told of a patient in their hospice program who was elderly, without many resources, and pretty much alone. During his visit, the patient mentioned that she would like to hear the classic hymns sung again but since she could no longer attend church and did not have a radio, she had no way to do so. The minister told us how he suddenly realized he had his mobile computing device with built-in speakers and a connection to the Internet. He went online, found her favorite hymns, and played them for her. This act brought joy into the life of one whose days were short. He told how he went home, downloaded more music, and provided others with this comfort.

The minister was not a young man, he did not grow up surrounded by technology, but he had learned to see technology as more than a necessary evil, but as another tool to provide caring and comfort. He had truly found the place at the crossroads of caring and technology (Parker, 2009).

Several years ago, I spent 2 years as a nursing instructor in a rural associate's-degree nursing program in Washington state. I experienced the intrinsic rewards of contributing to the education of new generations of nurses but also struggled to balance the number of allowed course and clinical hours with the core knowledge requirements for today's professional nurse. Informatics skills were not high on the list. However, in my experience, nursing educators can be divided into two groups: those whose students are being affected by informatics and those who soon will be. Understanding the basics of how informatics is affecting nursing practice can assist nursing educators with the integration of informatics into future curricula, updating current curricula, and assessing their own skills set.

This chapter will focus on what is important for nurse educators to know to help their students navigate the world of patient care in a technology-rich, health-care environment. To help navigate this chapter, here is a list of important abbreviations (Table 12.1).

DavisPlus | For additional resources please visit
http://davisplus.fadavis.com

TABLE 12.1	
Nursing Informatics Abbreviations	
ADT	Admission, discharge, and transfer system
ARRA	American Recovery and Reinvestment Act
BCMA	Bar-code medication administration
CDS	Clinical decision support
CDSS	Clinical decision support system
CPOE	Computerized physician/provider order entry
EHR	Electronic health record
EHRS	Electronic health record system
eMAR	Electronic medication administration record
EMR	Electronic medical record
HIMSS	Healthcare Information Management Systems Society
HIPAA	Health Insurance Portability and Accountability Act
HRSA	Health Resources and Services Administration of the U.S. Department of Health and Human Services
IN	Informatics nurse
INS	Informatics nurse specialist
PHR	Personal health record
SNLs	Standardized nursing languages
TICC	TIGER Informatics Competency Collaborative
TIGER	Technology Informatics Guiding Educational Reform Initiative

WHAT IS NURSING INFORMATICS AND WHY SHOULD I CARE?

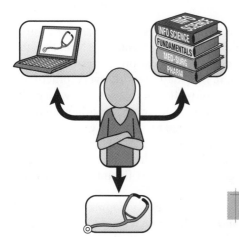

Nursing informatics (NI) was first recognized as a specialty by the American Nurses Association (ANA) in 1992 and first ANA definition was published in 2002 (Bickford, 2007). The ANA definition was updated in 2008 as

"a specialty that integrates nursing science, computer science, and information science to manage and communicate data, information, knowledge, and wisdom in nursing practice" (p. 1). In addition to supporting nursing practice, nursing informatics also supports the decision-making practices of consumers, patients, and other health-care providers (American Nurses Association, 2008).

NURSING INFORMATICS PRACTICE

Unlike other nursing disciplines that are normally classified by job titles or roles, nursing informatics titles have little standardization so the ANA uses functional areas to describe the work of those in NI practice. Functional areas of NI include "administration, leadership, and management; analysis; compliance and integrity management; consultation; coordination, facilitation, and integration; development; educational and professional development; policy development and advocacy; and research and evaluation" (American Nurses Association, 2008, pp. 17–18). The most visible role for nurses involved in informatics is with the design and implementation of the electronic health record system (EHRS) at both inpatient and ambulatory facilities across the country. Many nurses think that implementation of electronic documentation is the only thing that those of us in informatics do on a daily basis. Although that is an important part of what informatics nurses do, it certainly does not include everything. The HIMSS 2009 Informatics Nurse Impact Survey (Healthcare Information and Management Systems Society, 2009b, p. 6) listed the following activities performed by informatics nurses within their organizations:

- User education–93%
- System implementation–89%.
- User support–86%.
- Workflow analysis–84%.
- Getting buy-in from end users–80%.
- System design–79%.
- Selection/placement of devices–70%.
- Quality initiatives–69%.
- System optimization–62%.
- System selection–62%.
- Database management/reporting–53%.

- Data integration–48%.
- Outcomes management–47%.
- Medical device integration–46%.
- Hardware/device support–43%.

The ANA describes two levels of practice in nursing informatics; the informatics nurse specialist (INS) who has studied informatics or a related field at the graduate level and the informatics nurse (IN) who has experience but no graduate education (American Nurses Association, 2008, p. 2). However, the reality is that in today's world, every practicing nurse uses the principles of informatics even if they do not realize it. Every nurse who gathers and uses data from a cardiac or fetal monitor, IV pump, glucometer, or other device is working within the domain of nursing informatics. Every nurse manager or executive who uses a computer to track and report on data also is using nursing informatics skills. Every nursing student who pulls out his or her iPhone or Blackberry to look up the meaning of a laboratory test, information about a drug, or searches the Internet for information for a patient is demonstrating core informatics competencies.

It is not just the INS and the IN who are involved with the development of clinical systems. Clinical nurses, clinical nurse specialists, and nursing management are serving as subject matter experts on committees and work groups that deal with the convergence of technology and nursing practice within their facilities (Saletnik, Niedlinger, & Wilson, 2008). Unfortunately, many of these teams, especially in smaller facilities, may not have nurses experienced in informatics concepts to help guide their decision making.

Given the pervasive nature of informatics on the daily practice of nursing, two basic questions arise, namely what are the informatics competencies needed by all nurses and how do they learn the skills they need to practice in today's technology rich environment?

NURSES AND INFORMATICS – WHERE DO WE STAND TODAY?

Prensky (2001) coined the terms digital natives and digital immigrants to describe students in the U.S. educational system and these terms also can be used to describe practicing nurses today. Digital natives grew up with technology and are "native speakers of the digital language of computers, video games, and the Internet" (p. 1). While digital immigrants may learn the digital language it will never be their primary language. When they need information, digital immigrants will instinctively reach for a book while a digital native will Google the subject on the Internet. If you do not know what Google means in this context, you are definitely a digital immigrant; it means to search the Internet for information using a search engine. It comes from the popular and successful search engine Google; at least it was popular at the time this chapter was written. Things change rapidly in technology. To quote Heidi Klum in *Project Runway:* "One day you're in—the next day you're out," and this is true of popular Internet applications.

Today's practicing nurses come from both groups. However, they are primarily comprised of digital immigrants given that the average age has climbed to 46.8 years and more than 41% of registered nurses (RNs) are more than 50 years old (Health Resources and Services Administration, 2004). Even students in their basic nursing program cannot be assumed to be digital natives as the average age at graduation for RNs during the 5 years before the survey was 29.6 years for the Health Resources and Services Administration of the U.S. Department of Health and Human Services' (HRSA) 2004 survey (American Nurses

Association, 2009). Nursing students within the United States may not be as computer literate as they might think or faculty might assume. In a study by Elder and Koehn (2009), nursing students in entry-level Bachelor of Science in Nursing (BSN) and RN-BSN programs at a Midwestern university indicated that the students lacked many of the computer skills needed to complete college level coursework despite their self-assessment, which indicted they possessed all the necessary skills.

Clearly, the majority of students and practicing nurses are not going to be digital natives for many years to come and therefore may be less comfortable with the use of informatics in their daily practice. In recognition of this situation, nursing leaders from academia, nursing administration, informatics, government, and technology organizations came together in 2004 to form the Technology Informatics Guiding Educational Reform (TIGER) Initiative. The goal of this initiative was to "create a vision for the future of nursing that bridges the quality chasm with information technology, enabling nurses to use informatics in practice and education to provide safer, higher-quality patient care" (The TIGER Initiative, 2007, p. 4). A set of recommendations/action plan for academic institutions, professional nursing organizations, information technology vendors, government/policy makers, health-care delivery organizations, and health information management professionals was developed and published in the summary report entitled *Evidence and Informatics Transforming Nursing: 3-Year Action Steps Toward a 10-Year Vision* (The TIGER Initiative, 2007).

Over the next 2 years, hundreds of professionals volunteered their time to work in nine collaborative teams to work on the action plan outlined in 2007. These collaborative teams included:

- Standards and interoperability.
- National health information technology agenda.
- Informatics competencies.
- Education and faculty development.
- Staff development.
- Usability and clinical application design.
- Virtual demonstration center.
- Leadership development.
- Consumer empowerment and personal health records.

INFORMATICS COMPETENCIES FOR THE PRACTICING NURSE

Based on an extensive literature review, the TIGER Informatics Competency Collaborative (TICC) developed the *TIGER Nursing Informatics Competencies Model* that includes basic computer competencies, information literacy, and information management (Gugerty &

TECHNOLOGY TIP 12.1

The results of this TIGER work are summarized in the 2009 *Collaborating to Integrate Evidence and Informatics into Nursing Practice and Education: An Executive Summary* and can be found at http://www.tigersummit.com/Downloads.html. The two areas that are of interest in this discussion are informatics competencies and education and faculty development.

Delaney, 2009). This is an excellent place for nursing educators to start when developing new informatics focused curricula or when integrating informatics concepts into existing ones.

Basic Computer Competencies

Basic computer competencies allow the nurse to manage essential tools for effective practice. These competencies include:

- Concepts of information and communication technology.
- Using the computer and managing files.
- Word processing.
- Spreadsheets.
- Using databases.
- Presentation software.
- Web browsing and communication.

Information Literacy

The second competency identified by the TIGER initiative is information literacy. The Association of College & Research Libraries (2010, p. para. 1) defined information literacy as "the set of skills needed to find, retrieve, analyze, and use information." After a systematic literature review, Hart (2008) concluded that nurses in the United States are not prepared for evidence-based practice due to the lack of competency in information literacy skills. The TIGER recommendation is that all practicing nurses and graduating nursing students will have the ability to:

1. Determine the nature and extent of the information needed.
2. Access needed information effectively and efficiently.
3. Evaluate information and its sources critically and incorporates selected information into his or her knowledge base and value system.
4. Individually or as a member of a group, use information effectively to accomplish a specific purpose.
5. Evaluate outcomes of the use of information (Gugerty & Delaney, 2009, p. 5).

Information Management

Nelson (2002) created the data-to-wisdom continuum based on the earlier works by Bruce L. Blum, Graves, and Corcoran, and Nelson and Joos. The elements of this continuum are data, information, knowledge, and wisdom. Hebda and Czar (2009, p. 525) define data as the "collection

TECHNOLOGY TIP 12.2

There seems to be a lack of consensus of what skills are needed to demonstrate basic computer competence (Elder & Koehn, 2009). Rather than develop another set of skills, the TICC basic competencies recommendations are based on The European Computer Driving Licence (ECDL) Foundation's (www.ecdl.org) syllabus, which can be found at: http://www.ecdl.org/files/2009/programmes/docs/20090722114405_Equalskills_1.6.pdf

TECHNOLOGY TIP 12.3

Two resources for educators that can assist with assessing learners' information literacy skills include:
1. The commercially available Information Literacy in Technology test can be found at http://www.ilitassessment.com
2. The American Library Association's report, *Information Literacy Competency Standards for Higher Education,* could be used to develop assessment and learning tools. This report contains recommended competencies and performance indicators and outcomes, which can be found at http://www.ala.org/ala/mgrps/divs/acrl/standards/informationliteracycompetency.cfm

of numbers, characters, or facts that are gathered according to some perceived need for analysis and possibly action at a later point in time." Data, on its own, may be meaningless without context. The number 7 means little to a nurse until the context is known. Knowing that a patient's reported pain score is a 7/10 now transforms the data into information. Knowledge is the process of gathering and synthesizing the pertinent information into a concept or idea (Hebda & Czar, 2009). Continuing the pain score example, the nurse uses knowledge to assess other patient parameters, which may lead to a decision to deliver a prn medication. Nursing wisdom is evidenced by using one's values, experience, and knowledge gained by analyzing the information gained from the data to manage or solve patient problems. In our example, the use of nursing wisdom may lead the nurse to suspect that the pain is a symptom of some other problem with the patient and that further assessment is needed.

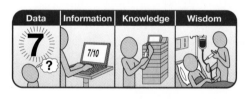

Nurses operate on this continuum every working minute. We are continuously gathering data on our patients then turning it into information and knowledge. These data may come from our physical senses during a patient assessment or the data that a patient provides us, such as a numerical representation of his or her level of pain. Data collected from technology, such as cardiac monitors, fetal monitors, glucometers, oximeters, etc., also may be synthesized into the process.

Information management is a process consisting of (1) collecting data, (2) processing the data, and (3) presenting and communicating the processed data as information or knowledge (Gugerty & Delaney, 2009, p. 7). Nurses have been managing information in a variety of ways over the years, from the patient charts, to scratch pieces of paper, to writing on anything that is available including clothing, bed linen, or on their own arms. While this paper-based system has been in use for many years, it truly did not support the development of knowledge synthesis through research because it was difficult to codify the mountains of data collected. To codify written data, someone has to read the data and assign a code based on a set of criteria that can allow the data to be grouped and analyzed. With the advent of electronic documentation, it is now possible to report on data collected during nursing care. This data forms the basis of evidenced-based care.

The TIGER Informatics Competency Collaborative (TICC) developed the set of clinical information management competencies for nurses (Gugerty & Delaney, 2009) working with hospital information management systems. These competencies have been provided in a useful form on Davis Plus.

Clinical Information Management Competencies

- Identify and maintain a patient record.
- Capture:
  - Data and documentation from external clinical sources.
  - Patient-originated data.
  - Patient health data derived from administrative.
- Interact with financial data and documentation.
- Produce a summary record of care.
- Present ad hoc views of the health record.
- Interact with guidelines and protocols for planning care.
- Manage:
  - Patient demographics.
  - Patient history.
  - Patient and family preferences.
  - Patient advance directives.
  - Consents and authorizations.
  - Allergy, intolerance, and adverse reaction lists.
  - Medication lists.
  - Problem lists.
  - Immunization lists.
  - Patient-specific care and treatment plans.
  - Medication orders as appropriate for scope of practice.
  - Nonmedication patient care orders.
  - Orders for diagnostic tests.
  - Orders for blood products and other biologics.
  - Referrals.
  - Order sets.
  - Medication administration.
  - Immunization administration.
  - Test results.
  - Patient clinical measurements.
  - Clinical documents and notes.
  - Documentation of clinician response to decision support prompts.
- Generate and record patient-specific instructions.
- Manage health information to provide decision support for:
  - Standard assessments.
  - Patient context-driven assessments manage health information to provide decision support for identification of potential problems and trends.
  - Patient and family preferences.
  - Consistent health care.
  - Research protocols relative to individual patient care.
  - Management of patient groups or populations.
  - Epidemiological investigations of clinical health within a population.
  - Notification and response regarding population health issues.
  - Monitoring response notifications regarding a specific patient's health.

- Interact with decision support system for:
  - Standard care plans, guidelines, and protocols.
  - Context-sensitive care plans, guidelines, and protocols.
  - Self-care.
  - Medication and immunization ordering as appropriate for an individual's scope of practice.
  - Drug-interaction checking.
  - Patient-specific dosing and warnings.
  - Medication recommendations.
  - Medication and immunization administration.
  - Nonmedication ordering.
  - Result interpretation.
  - Referral process.
  - Referral recommendations.
  - Safe blood administration.
  - Accurate specimen collection.
  - Alerts for preventive services and wellness.
  - Interact with decision support for notifications and reminders for preventive services and wellness.
- Access health-care guidance.
- Interact with clinical information system (CIS) for:
  - Workflow tasking.
  - Task assignment and routing.
  - Task linking.
  - Task tracking.
- Facilitate:
  - Inter-provider communication.
  - Provider-pharmacy communication.
  - Communications between provider and patient and/or the patient representative.
  - Patient, family, and caregiver education.
  - Communication with medical devices.

The two questions that nursing educators need to ask are (1) how well their course curricula integrate these skills and (2) how well prepared are they to teach these skills? Research indicates that nursing faculty are resistant to including informatics competencies due to their own discomfort (Ornes & Gassert, 2007; Saba & Riley, 1997). Just as it is uncomfortable for our students to learn basic nursing skills, it is uncomfortable for nursing faculty to put themselves in a learner role to master basic informatics skills. However, to be able to provide our students with these necessary competencies, we must do so.

WHAT DO EDUCATORS NEED TO KNOW ABOUT NURSING INFORMATICS CONCEPTS?

Your students are going to a variety of different clinical locations and they may have to work with a variety of different electronic health record systems in various stages of implementation. One facility may have full electronic clinical documentation but only for nursing while another may have for all clinical disciples including physicians. One facility may have electronic medication administration record (eMAR) in the pharmacy but a paper copy for nursing documentation. The following section will work to explain why these differences occur and what you might be able to look forward to in the future.

Electronic Health Record System

Since the passage of the American Recovery and Reinvestment Act (ARRA) of 2009 we are moving to electronic information management within the health-care space in the form of the EHRS. It is critical that all practicing nurses gain an understanding of how an ERHS works and the competencies that are needed to managing information within it.

But you may be asking yourself "just what is an EHRS anyway and how does it compare to the computer patient record (CPR), the electronic medical record (EMR), the electronic health record (EHR) that I've heard of? It is understandable that there may be confusion because there is no true consensus as to the meaning of the various terms among informatics professions quite yet. The term *computer patient record* (CPR) has virtually disappeared from the informatics lexicon in the past several years and for good reason. We really did not need two meanings to the acronym CPR!

In some of the literature, the terms *EHR* and *EMR* have been interchangeable. However, some informatics leaders have asserted that the two terms have very different meanings. Garets and Davis (2006, p. 2) assert that the EMR is "the legal record created in hospitals and ambulatory environments that is the source of data for the EHR" while the EHR is a virtual construct that "represents the ability to easily share medical information among stakeholders and to have a patient's information follow him or her through the various modalities of care engaged by that individual." The Institute of Medicine's (IOM) report on the eight key capabilities of an electronic health record system are:

1. Health information and data. Having immediate access to key information, such as patients' diagnoses, allergies, laboratory test results, and medications, would improve caregivers' ability to make sound clinical decisions in a timely manner.
2. Result management. The ability for all providers participating in the care of a patient in multiple settings to quickly access new and past test results would increase patient safety and the effectiveness of care.
3. Order management. The ability to enter and store orders for prescriptions, tests, and other services in a computer-based system should enhance legibility, reduce duplication, and improve the speed with which orders are executed.
4. Decision support. Using reminders, prompts, and alerts, computerized decision-support systems would help improve compliance with best clinical practices, ensure regular screenings and other preventive practices, identify possible drug interactions, and facilitate diagnoses and treatments.
5. Electronic communication and connectivity. Efficient, secure, and readily accessible communication among providers and patients would improve the continuity of care, increase the timeliness of diagnoses and treatments, and reduce the frequency of adverse events.
6. Patient support. Tools that give patients access to their health records, provide interactive patient education, and help them carry out home-monitoring and self-testing can improve control of chronic conditions, such as diabetes.

7. Administrative processes. Computerized administrative tools, such as scheduling systems, would greatly improve hospitals' and clinics' efficiency and provide more timely service to patients.
8. Reporting and population management. Electronic data storage that employs uniform data standards will enable health-care organizations to respond more quickly to federal, state, and private reporting requirements, including those that support patient safety and disease surveillance (OpenClinical, 2005; Tang, 2003, pp. 7–11).

Regardless of which "nomenclature camp" you subscribe to, as nursing educators, it is important that we understand and convey the concepts to our students so they will understand what they are hearing or reading.

The term *EHRS* has come to indicate the actual software applications that hold the data about the patient. There are three basic components to an EHRS, the financial information system, management information system, and the clinical information system. The financial and management systems include components, such as the admission, transfer, and discharge (ADT) system that contains the patient demographic and insurance information, billing system, contracting system, human resources system, risk management system, and payroll system. The CIS may consist of clinical documentation for all disciples, orders management, pharmacy, laboratory, and radiology systems, closed-loop medication administration, clinical monitoring systems, clinical decision support (CDS), and physician/provider order entry (CPOE). Please notice the term "may consist of" because this is where things become confusing. Each of the components of the CIS is an individual module that, for the most part, can be purchased and implemented in any order depending on the software vendor.

Health-care facilities have had financial and management information systems for years and may have had laboratory, pharmacy, and radiology systems for nearly as long. Some may even had order-entry systems in which physician/provider orders were transcribed into the computer by someone else. Now these facilities are working toward implementation of the entire EMR and to do so, they need to implement the clinical information system modules. This is the most complex part. Where do health-care facilities stand in this journey?

HIMSS Analytics, a division of the Healthcare Information Management Systems Society, has developed a modeling system called the EMR Adoption Model (Healthcare Information and Management Systems Society, 2009a) to track EMR implementation progress at hospitals and health systems but not in ambulatory care clinics. This model can help you determine where your school's clinical facilities are on the implementation continuum and what changes might be needed in your curricula in the future. Figure 12.1 shows the seven stages of EMR adoption as they were at the time of publication; however the percentages are updated every 6 months. The EMR Adoption's Web site (http://www.himssanalytics.org/hc_providers_/emr_adoption.asp) provides the latest percentages and a detailed description of the stages. Talk to an IN or information management leader within the organization and he or she should be able to give you an idea of where the organization is on the adoption model and what changes are coming and when.

It is important to understand that health-care organizations have purchased EHRS systems using one of two approaches; single vendor or best of breed. In the single vendor approach, the facility selected one of the major EHRS vendors that provided an enterprise-wide system and had most if not all, the modules needed by the facility. Many organizations stayed with the vendor who provided their financial information systems.

EMR Adoption Model^{SM}

Stage	Cumulative Capabilities
Stage 7	Complete EMR; CCD transactions to share data; Data warehousing; Data continuity with ED, ambulatory, OP
Stage 6	Physician documentation (structured templates), full CDSS (variance & compliance), full R-PACS
Stage 5	Closed loop medication administration
Stage 4	CPOE, Clinical Decision Support (clinical protocols)
Stage 3	Nursing/clinical documentation (flow sheets), CDSS (error checking), PACS available outside Radiology
Stage 2	CDR, Controlled Medical Vocabulary, CDS, may have Document Imaging; HIE capable
Stage 1	Ancillaries – Lab, Rad, Pharmacy - All Installed
Stage 0	All Three Ancillaries Not Installed

© 2010 HIMSS Analytics™

Figure 12.1   Seven stages of EMR adoption.

Other organizations adopted a best of breed approach and selected various modules of the clinical information system from different vendors. Therefore, their radiology system, also known as a picture archiving and communication system (PACS) might come from one vendor, while their laboratory system might come from another vendor. Niche vendors for clinical specialties, such as emergency services, family birth centers, and home care might be different than the vendor for the medical-surgical units. Why do you need to understand this? So that you can explain to students why these various systems may not "talk" to each other and exchange information when they ask why the emergency department (ED) nurse has to print out the patient's ED chart and send it to the medical-surgical unit so that the nurses there can re-enter all the data into their computer system.

Personal Health Record

If we use the HIMSS's proposed definitions that the EHR is a construct made up of data from EMRs located in various places, then what might be the place of a personal health record (PHR). There are several third-party services, such as Google Health and Microsoft's Health Vault, which are now hosting personal health records. Some insurance companies are doing the same. But what is a PHR? It is the health information that people collect about themselves.

Here is an example of how one might work. An overweight person with diabetes has, on the recommendation of her health-care provider, joined the local gym and Weight Watchers. At the gym, she signs into a computer program that gathers data on her daily exercise. At home, she tracks her diet and weight at Weight Watchers online. What if both systems could send this data to her designed PHR application? In addition, what if her glucometer could upload daily blood sugar data to her PHR as well? Then before her next visit with her provider, she authorizes the data to be sent to the EMR at the clinic.

This is not science fiction but the world in which today's nursing students will be practicing. Are you ready?

EMR's Effect on Nursing Documentation

Over the years, there have been many efforts to standardize nursing documentation using standardized nursing languages (SNLs) such as North American Nursing Diagnosis Association (NANDA), Nursing Interventions Classification (NIC), Nursing Outcomes Classification (NOC), but as long as nursing documentation remained paper-based, the impetus for change was not compelling. However, with the implementation of EMRs and the demand for research to support evidence-based practice, the need for documentation that is easily codifiable will continue.

Although there are understandable concerns that "point-and-click" or template-driven documentation loses the unique patient story (Enhanced Online News, 2009), the need for computer codification of clinical data will continue. Until technologies, such as natural language processing, are available for commercial use in EMR systems, template-based documentation will continue.

Along with electronic documentation comes a different set of rules and practices surrounding the concepts of patient confidentiality and information security. The Health Insurance Portability and Accountability Act (HIPAA) of 1996 was enacted to protect individuals' rights to privacy and confidentiality and assure the security of electronic transfer of personal information.

What does this mean for the education of nursing students? Students need to be taught the basics of computer confidentiality including the need to keep their passwords secure, logging off when leaving a computer terminal, and not leaving patient information displayed for nonauthorized viewing even by other staff members. HIPAA regulations need to be incorporated into curricula and updated when changes which affect nursing practice occur. Many schools are providing this training as self-study online modules. Search the Internet for "HIPAA for nursing students" to find available examples. HIPAA training also may need to be provided at each clinical site so that any organizational specific information or practices are covered.

In my graduate class, a student shared a story regarding the misuse of a social networking site by clinicians who came off of a long shift and posted something about their experiences,

TECHNOLOGY TIP 12.4

Today's educators must be aware of new environments, such as social networking sites including Facebook, MySpace, or nursing-specific sites, such as NurseLinkUp, which may be used to share information and in some cases, too much information.

which is fine. However, there were instances in which patients' names and details of their care were posted. It is important that nursing educators include these types of situation in their discussions of patient privacy.

The most common breach of HIPAA and the EMR is accessing patient records without the need to do so. Looking up health information about family, friends, coworkers, celebrities, and even one's own information outside of the patient-nurse relationship is not acceptable. At many facilities this may lead to immediate termination of employment. We must acculturate students with a sense that if they are not caring for the patient, they must not access the patient's EMR. All nurses must be careful of their practice and truly understand the privacy procedures at their clinical site. Most facilities have verbiage about using patient information for education but just because a student took care of a patient last week does not give him or her the right to access the patient's record this week "just to see how the patient is doing," if it is not part of the student's assigned educational experience.

Students also need to be taught how to best use template documentation. Although the health-care facility may teach the students how to use a particular EHRS, it is important that they understand the basics before they learn to use specific applications. A template-based clinical documentation system may be based on chart-by-exception, may or may not use one or more of the standardized nursing languages, and may include evidence-based practice references. An excellent overview of standardized nursing languages can be found in article by Margaret Rutherford (2008). Students need to become familiar with the two basic forms of documentation; the point-and-click fields and the free-text fields, also

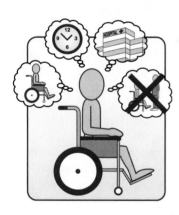

known as comment or narrative fields. These fields allow the user to type-in additional information if using a keyboard or handwrite if using a tablet computer.

One practice that continues to be seen with electronic documentation is the repetition of data documented using templates and then also in the narrative or free-text fields. This double documentation not only wastes time, it can have legal implications. For example, a student or practicing nurse documents a neurological assessment and selects the template block that says the patient is awake, alert, and oriented ×4 (i.e., person, place, time, and events) but then in the free-text field documents that "the patient is awake, alert, and oriented to time, person, and place and is c/o of a headache" there is a problem. This double documentation has created confusion as to whether the patient is oriented ×3 or ×4. Should this EMR entry ever have to be defended in court, it is going to be difficult, if not impossible, to account for the discrepancy.

It is up to nursing educators to become familiar with the changes that electronic documentation has brought to nursing practice. We must update both educational material and, if need be, our own thinking and habits.

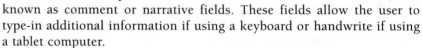

TECHNOLOGY TIP 12.5

Have students conduct a Web search on the following phrases: "HIPAA violation jail" and "nurse fired Facebook." Ask them to discuss their findings.

Closed-Loop Medication Administration

Many nurses confuse bar-code medication administration (BCMA) with a full closed-loop medication administration system when it is only a step in the full process. A closed-loop medication system must automate every step of the medication administration process and to do so it must begin with the medication order. In a truly closed-loop system, the order must be input into the computer by the ordering provider not transcribed by someone else. It includes medication reconciliation and robotic dispensing systems. Finally, it ends with positive patient identification with the clinical information system using bar coding or other technology. Figure 12.2 illustrates the comparison of medication administration without the use of information technology with a closed-loop medication administration process.

A facility may have implemented a completely closed-loop medication administration system or may have only implemented one or two components. The most common component is the implementation of the pharmacy information system from which a paper medication administration record (MAR) is generated for use by the nursing staff to administer medication. The second most common component is BCMA using an electronic MAR (eMAR). Research has shown that errors in medication administration process occur in four areas: prescribing 49%, administration 26%, dispensing 14%, and transcribing 11%. In a closed-loop administration system, evidence-based alerts can provide warnings to clinicians. These alerts include allergies, incomplete or unclear orders, drug-drug/food/age interactions, dosing implications, and violation of the five rights of medication administration at each step of the process thereby reducing the impact of human error.

Medication Administration

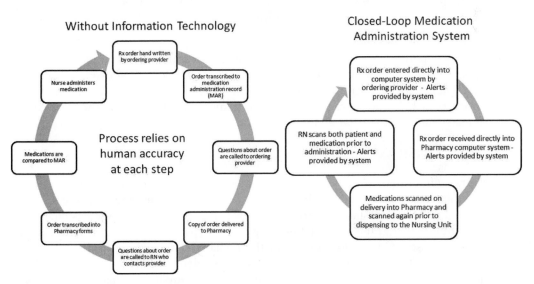

Figure 12.2 The comparison of medication administration without the use of information technology with a closed-loop medication administration process.

It is critical that nursing educators impress upon their students the critical need for following the proper procedures when administrating medications using BCMA just as was done with a paper MAR.

Clinical Decision Support

The Healthcare Information Management Systems Society has defined clinical decision support (CDS) "as a clinical system, application or process that helps health professionals make clinical decisions to enhance patient care" (Healthcare Information and Management Systems Society, p. 1). A clinical decision support system (CDSS) has been simply defined as a computer system that generates patient-specific advice using two or more items of patient data, such as drug, allergy, or laboratory result, with age and/or medication (Wyatt & Spiegelhalter, 1990). The majority of CDSSs have focused on provider workflows, primarily medication ordering.

The systems are only recently becoming available for nursing in part because of the difficulties in identification of nursing knowledge and the needs of a variety of experience levels in the nurses who need the information (Courtney, Alexander, & Demiris, 2008). These systems are designed to provide information, when it is needed, at the point of decision. They can include alerts, providing simple data, such as on drugs or laboratory texts, or best care practices.

Provost and Gray (2007) included an example of a perinatal CDSS results that illustrate how a single entry, "Vaginal bleeding, small," generates a problem list, order list, request for additional information that may affect care, and further documentation requirements:

Data field: Vaginal bleeding
Documentation entry of patient-specific data: Vaginal bleeding, small
CDSS-generated problem list: Bleeding
CDSS-generated order list: Hemorrhage protocol—Venous access, IV hydration, type and screen, blood products consent
CDSS-generated request for additional information: Is patient a Jehovah's Witness?
CDSS-generated documentation requirement: electronic fetal monitoring/contractions assessment (p. 409)

It is important for nursing faculty to help students understand when and how to use the information provided by a CDSS especially as the technology progresses. Therefore, it is crucial that faculty members are conversant with using the systems in place at their clinical sites in order to help the students use these systems correctly. Systems should never replace a nurse's clinical assessment and judgment.

CONCLUSION

Nursing informatics touches almost every part of today's nursing practice and its effect will only grow in the future. Nursing faculty at all levels of nursing education need to make sure that they understand the basics of how information technology has changed and will continue to change the ways that nursing care is delivered and documented. Curricula need to be assessed and updated to reflect these changes. Educators need to assess their own readiness to both use technology and to guide students who must incorporate it into their practice. For those of us who have been practicing nursing for many years, this may be a bit scary but just as we ask our students to grow, so we ourselves must do so as well.

REFERENCES

American Nurses Association. (2008). *Nursing informatics: Scope and standards of practice*. Silver Springs, MD: Nursesbooks.org.

American Nurses Association. (2009). *Background and education*. Retrieved from http://www.nursingworld.org/MainMenuCategories/ThePracticeofProfessionalNursing/workplace/Work-Environment/InfoforNurses/ANAPolicyPapersandBrochures/February2006SurveyInfo/Background.aspx

Association of College & Research Libraries. (2010). *Introduction to information literacy*. Retrieved from http://www.ala.org/ala/mgrps/divs/acrl/issues/infolit/overview/intro/index.cfm

Bickford, C. J. (2007). The specialty practice of nursing informatics. *CIN: Computers, Informatics, Nursing, 25*(6), 364–366.

Courtney, K. L., Alexander, G. L., & Demiris, G. (2008). Information technology from novice to expert: implementation implications. *Journal of Nursing Management, 16*(6), 692–699.

Elder, B. L., & Koehn, M. L. (2009). Assessment tool for nursing student computer competencies. *Nursing Education Perspectives, 30*(3), 148–152.

Enhanced Online News. (2009). http://eon.businesswire.com/news/eon/20091221005228/en/EHR/EMR/Hitech-act Retrieved from http://eon.businesswire.com/portal/site/eon/permalink/?ndmViewId=news_view&newsId=20091221005228&newsLang=en

Garets, D., & Davis, M. (2006). *Electronic medical records vs. electronic health records: Yes, there is a difference—A HIMSS Analytics White Paper*. Retrieved from http://www.himssanalytics.org/docs/WP_EMR_EHR.pdf

Gugerty, B., & Delaney, C. (2009). *TIGER informatics competencies collaborative (TICC) final report*. Retrieved from http://tigercompetencies.pbworks.com/f/TICC_Final.pdf

Hart, M. D. (2008). Informatics competency and development within the US nursing population workforce: A systematic literature review. *CIN: Computers, Informatics, Nursing, 26*(6), 320–329.

Health Resources and Services Administration. (2004). *The registered nurse population: Findings from the 2004 National Sample Survey of Registered Nurses*. Retrieved from http://bhpr.hrsa.gov/healthworkforce/rnsurvey04/

Healthcare Information and Management Systems Society. *Clinical decision support*. Retrieved from http://www.himss.org/ASP/topics_clinicalDecision.asp

Healthcare Information and Management Systems Society. (2009a). *EMR adoption model*. Retrieved from http://www.himssanalytics.org/hc_providers/emr_adoption.asp

Healthcare Information and Management Systems Society. (2009b). *HIMSS 2009 informatics nurse impact survey: Final report*. Retrieved from http://www.himss.org/content/files/HIMSS2009NursingInformaticsImpactSurveyFullResults.pdf

Hebda, T., & Czar, P. (2009). *Handbook of informatics for nurses & healthcare professionals* (4th ed.). Upper Saddle River, NJ: Pearson Prentice Hall.

Nelson, R. (2002). Major theories supporting health care informatics. In S. P. Englebardt & R. Nelson (Eds.), *Health care informatics: An interdisciplinary approach* (pp. 3–27). St. Louis: Mosby.

OpenClinical. (2005). *Electronic medical records, electronic health records*. Retrieved from http://www.openclinical.org/emr.html

Ornes, L. L., & Gassert, C. (2007). Computer competencies in a BSN program. *Journal of Nursing Education, 46*(2), 75–78.

Parker, C. D. (2009). Crossroads of caring and technology. Retrieved from http://www.healthcaregoesmobile.com/content/crossroads-caring-and-technology (Reprinted with permission.)

Prensky, M. (2001). Digital natives, digital immigrants. *On the Horizon, 9*(5). Retrieved from http://www.marcprensky.com/writing/Prensky%20-%20Digital%20Natives,%20Digital%20Immigrants%20-%20Part1.pdf

Provost, C., & Gray, M. (2007). Plugged in: Perinatal clinical decision support system: A documentation tool for patient safety. *Nursing for Women's Health, 11*(4), 407–410.

Rutherford, M. A. (2008). Standardized nursing language: What does it mean for nursing practice? *The Online Journal of Issues in Nursing, 13*(1). Retrieved from www.nursingworld.org/MainMenuCategories/ANAMarketplace/ANAPeriodicals/OJIN/TableofContents/vol132008/No1Jan08/ArticlePreviousTopic/StandardizedNursingLanguage.aspx

Saba, V. K., & Riley, J. B. (1997). Nursing informatics in nursing education. *Student Health & Technology Information, 46,* 185–190.

Saletnik, L. A., Niedlinger, M. K., & Wilson, M. (2008). Nursing resource considerations for implementing an electronic documentation system. *AORN Journal, 87*(3), 585.

Tang, P. (2003). Key capabilities of an electronic health record system: Letter Report *Institute of Medicine Committee on Data Standards for Patient Safety*. Retrieved from http://books.nap.edu/openbook.php?isbn=NI000427

The TIGER Initiative. (2007). *Evidence and informatics transforming nursing: 3-year action steps toward a 10-year vision*. Retrieved from http://www.aacn.nche.edu/Education/pdf/TIGER.pdf

Wyatt, J., & Spiegelhalter, D. (1990). Evaluating medical expert systems: What to test and how? *Medical Informatics 15,* 205–217.

Chapter 13

Informatics Across the Curriculum

Barbara Ihrke, PhD, RN

Students at a particular rural nursing program have to travel for clinicals—most students had to adapt to five or more hospital settings and to five or more electronic clinical systems. The ability to adapt and use multiple clinical systems is now deemed an advantage and thus, important to document in a resume.

Subsequently, the new graduate was pleased with the job offer from his preferred employer. He explained that his ability to use multiple electronic clinical systems assisted during his job search. What was once considered an "unfortunate necessity" is now considered an advantage.

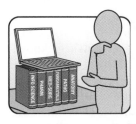

Informatics in nursing education is a contemporary topic of discussion. The question posed is whether a stand-alone nursing informatics course is necessary or could informatics be integrated across the curriculum? Faculty and students have varying opinions regarding the necessity of informatics and the result is a lack of standardization in nursing curricula. After a review of various curriculum plans of study, there appears to be two models: a stand-alone informatics course or the integration of suggested informatics material. Although many curricula do not specifically have an informatics course, the knowledge, skills, and attitudes (KSAs) must be woven throughout the curriculum to meet educational requirements.

WHAT IS INFORMATICS?

Informatics is defined as "the transition of data to information to knowledge to wisdom" (Weiner, 2008, p. ix) and the American Nurses Association (2008) describes nursing informatics as a specialty area that integrates nursing science, computer science, cognitive science, and information science with the goal to improve health care. Although nursing informatics is a specialty, all nurses are expected to meet certain informatics competencies.

Nurses are expected to have certain KSAs regarding informatics and health technology. Understanding informatics and health information technology (IT) must be integrated into nursing education at all levels and in all programs. In 2004, then President Bush signed

Executive Order 13335 (EO) announcing his [President Bush] commitment to the promotion of health information technology to lower costs, reduce medical errors,

DavisPlus | For additional resources please visit
http://davisplus.fadavis.com

improve quality of care, and provide better information for patients and physicians. In particular, the President called for widespread adoption of interoperable electronic health records (EHRs) within 10 years so that health information will follow patients throughout their care in a seamless and secure manner. This means that their medical information is available to the right people at the right time, while remaining protected and secure (Leavitt, 2005).

Although the executive order provided direction for the future of health care, the health-care industry and health-care education must develop standards and guidelines to meet the new challenge.

Informatics competencies have been outlined in the recently published report from the Technology Informatics Guiding Education Reform (TIGER) (2009a). The TIGER model consists of basic computer competencies, information literacy, and information management. Another TIGER report delineates outcomes for each competency (TIGER, 2009c). Nurse educators can use this TIGER Summit report (link found on Davis Plus) to analyze whether their students meet the informatics competencies.

Quality and Safety Education for Nurses

The overall goal for the Quality and Safety Education for Nurses (QSEN) project is to meet the challenge of preparing future nurses who will have the KSAs necessary to continuously improve the quality and safety of the health-care systems within which they work. QSEN defines informatics as using "information and technology to communicate, manage knowledge, mitigate error, and support decision making" (www.qsen.org). Table 13.1 describes the informatics competencies for undergraduate nursing students. A curriculum designed based on these competencies provides undergraduate nurses with the ability to provide excellent, safe health care based on data, knowledge, and information.

Cronenwett, Sherwood, Barnsteiner, Disch, Johnson, Mitchell, Sullivan, and Warren (2007) define informatics competencies. The competencies serve to guide curriculum and provide academic programs guidelines for developing learning outcomes. Didactic, clinical, and simulation experiences will strengthen student learning and achievement of informatics competencies.

TECHNOLOGY TIP 13.1

Information management and informatics competencies are critical for the provision of safe, effective patient care One focus of the QSEN project is the KSA informatics list for prelicensure nursing students found at http://www.qsen.org/ksa_prelicensure.php#infomatics. Have students visit this list at least once in every class to identify how those competencies apply to the content being studied.

TECHNOLOGY TIP 13.2

Have students conduct a Web search on "safety informatics nursing." They will then present to the class the top three reasons for using technology in nursing care. They also will need to share why there may be resistance to incorporating informatics in nursing.

TABLE 13.1

Informatics

Definition: Use information and technology to communicate, manage knowledge, mitigate error, and support decision making.

Knowledge	Skills	Attitudes
Explain why information and technology skills are essential for safe patient care.	Seek education about how information is managed in care settings before providing care. Apply technology and information management tools to support safe processes of care.	Appreciate the necessity for all health professionals to seek lifelong, continuous learning of IT skills.
Identify essential information that must be available in a common database to support patient care. Contrast benefits and limitations of different communication technologies and their effect on safety and quality.	Navigate the EHR. Document and plan patient care in an EHR. Employ communication technologies to coordinate care for patients.	Value technologies that support clinical decision making, error prevention, and care coordination. Protect confidentiality of protected health information in EHRs.
Describe examples of how technology and information management are related to the quality and safety of patient care. Recognize the time, effort, and skill required for computers, databases, and other technologies to become reliable and effective tools for patient care.	Respond appropriately to clinical decision making supports and alerts. Use information management tools to monitor outcomes of care processes. Use high quality electronic sources of health-care information.	Value nurses' involvement in design, selection, implementation, and evaluation of information technologies to support patient care.

Cronenwett, L., Sherwood, G., Barnsteiner, J., Disch, J., Johnson, J., Mitchell, P, Sullivan, D. T., & Warren, J. (2007). Quality and safety education for nurses. *Nursing Outlook, 55*(3), 122-131. Retrieved from http://www.qsen.org/ksas_prelicensure.php#informatics

American Association of Colleges of Nursing and the National League for Nursing

The American Association of Colleges of Nursing (AACN) and The National League for Nursing (NLN) have promoted informatics in nursing curricula and recommend that all graduates of nursing programs have certain data management and information literacy abilities. Graduates must have technical skills, information management skills, and an understanding of the ethical and legal issues related to the use of technology in health care.

American Association of Colleges of Nursing Standards for Bachelor of Science in Nursing

The AACN supports the requirement of baccalaureate graduates of nursing programs to understand information management and to use technology in the delivery of patient care (AACN, 2008). AACN suggest that "course work and clinical experiences will provide the baccalaureate graduate with knowledge and skills to use information management and patient care technologies to delivery safe and effective care" (p. 18). Sample content includes use of patient care technology, analysis of information, application of data for evidence-based practice, and evaluation of online literature and resources. Information literacy is an expected learning outcome for the nursing student graduate.

NLN Position Statement—Preparing the Next Generation of Nurses to Practice in a Technology-Rich Environment: An Informatics Agenda

There are several recommendations in the 2008 NLN position statement on informatics. Key faculty recommendations include faculty development programs, designated informatics champion, integration of informatics across the curriculum, and collaboration with clinical agencies to assist students to develop competencies through hands-on experiences with clinical systems (NLN, 2008). Other proposed recommendations for schools of nursing were adequate resources and funding for faculty development activities and that "all students graduate with up-to-date knowledge and skills in each of the three critical areas: computer literacy, information literacy, and informatics" (p. 5). These recommendations build on reports and position statements from the Institute of Medicine, TIGER Initiative, and the QSEN project and the agenda of the Office of the National Coordinator of Health Information Technology (Decade of Health Information Technology) (NLN, 2008).

INTEGRATION OF INFORMATICS ACROSS THE CURRICULUM: AN EXAMPLE

Nurses must acquire basic computer competencies, information literacy, and information management (including use of an EHR) skills to be competent, safe practitioners (TIGER, 2009a). The three-part model sets the stage for nurse educators to integrate informatics across the curriculum. Each part of the model can be integrated into various courses to meet an overall program outcome of informatics/technology competency. Following is a practical example of integration informatics across the curriculum. Fetter (2007) describes strategies used in one baccalaureate program to improve IT outcomes. TIGER (2009b) describes the "use of informatics competencies, theories, research, and practice examples throughout nursing curriculums" (p. 17). TIGER (2009d) provides curricular examples from schools of nursing.

Basic Computer Skills

Students have basic computer skills when they are admitted into a nursing program (see Box 13.1 and Evidence-Based Practice Box 13.1). The TIGER report lists about 300 basic computer competencies (TIGER, 2009c). Competencies are divided into several board categories: hardware, software, networks, information and communication technologies (ICT) in everyday life, security, law, operating systems, file management, utilities, print management, using the application, the Internet, using the browser, using the Web, Web outputs, electronic communication, using e-mail, and e-mail management.

The difficulty is assessing each student in each of more than 300 basic computer skills. Students are computer savvy (digital native) but may not have simple skills (Prensky, 2001). It is wise to provide students access to computer support—both technical support and software usage support. The educational institution's information/computer/library systems all play an integral role assisting students to access/use/incorporate basic computer skills into every class/course/program.

Integrating Basic Skills at the Program Level

Most students have access to a computer; therefore faculty must require all assignments and reports be done on a computer, submitted electronically via e-mail or a course management system. Specific details of requirements for assignments/work are delineated in syllabi (standardized across the program/within the nursing division).

Documentation standards across the curriculum must be standardized. The use of American Psychological Association's (APA) formatting should be required at the beginning of the program, from the first class and followed through until graduation. Some nursing programs use other formatting policies; the key is to buy in and following through by all faculty. Creating a document citing key concepts and expectations will benefit the student and the faculty.

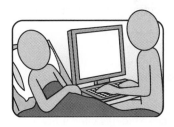

The use of clinical simulation in nursing education is another method to incorporate informatics into the clinical curriculum. Simulation laboratories are no longer "just for practice." Students experience the "real" thing in a simulation setting. High-fidelity mannequins are common in simulation laboratories and provide a near-real clinical situation. Students gain confidence in simulated settings. Documentation of simulated experiences in the EHR provides further acquisition of informatics KSAs.

An integrated learning management system (LMS) is crucial for all programs of nursing. It can be used to support a course (i.e., blended, online, and on site—see Chapters 6–8), to facilitate online learning through assignments, threaded discussions, and assessments, and to streamline information distribution. Each use of the LMS requires the student to use basic computer skills including but not limited to file management, use of the Internet, electronic communication, and using applications (TIGER, 2009c).

TECHNOLOGY TIP 13.3

Faculty must possess computer skills and model them in the classroom. A variety of electronic teaching strategies is available and can be incorporated into assignments or used to facilitate the teaching/learning process. Wikis, Podcasting, Skyping, Simulation, and other e-learning programs are available to faculty. Increase use by faculty of IT will increase student use of IT.

BOX 13.1

TIPS FOR THE DEAN AND/OR DIRECTOR

- Request each faculty to describe how basic computer skills are used in the nursing program.
- Comply and compare the responses to the list of basic computer skills recommended by TIGER.
- Brainstorm how to incorporate basic computer skills into the program.
- Encourage each faculty to add assignments and assessments requiring the use of basic computer skills.
- Host a brown bag luncheon to discuss success and devise methods to overcome obstacles.

EVIDENCE-BASED PRACTICE BOX 13.1

Graduating Nurses' Self-evaluation of Information Technology Competencies

Issue: What Are the Technology Skills Held by Nursing Students?

The 42 students who participated in an IT research study were asked to assess their use and skills of 43 technology skills.

Study Findings

Several recommendations for improving informatics understanding, adoption, and usage were offered. Using Internet resources and word processing tools were some of the strengths. However, there was a significant deficit in valuing electronic documentation and using these tools in client care.

Nursing Implications

- Faculty are the key factor in integrating informatics.
- Faculty should role model the use and appreciation of informatics.
- Structured experiences and simulation usage could enhance overall informatics competencies.
- Although students used IT systems during clinical experiences, students cited a need for more experiences, more advanced system usage, and less redundancy (Fetter, 2009, p. 87).

Integrating Basic Skills at the Course Level

Nursing programs with a stand-alone nursing informatics course will include many of the basic computer skills in the curriculum, whereas nursing programs with an integrated approach to informatics have to map the content over several courses. A wide variety of assignments that require the use of various software applications, discussion of ethical behaviors and regulatory requirements in specified courses, diligence in providing students with a wide variety of clinical settings/information system requirements will help ensure/document student acquisition of basic computer skills.

Although students come with some basic computer skills, two critical computer skills they frequently lack are knowledge and understanding of computer security and laws/regulations related to the use of computers. It should be noted that "[t]he baccalaureate program prepares the graduate to uphold ethical standards related to data security, regulatory requirements, confidentiality, and clients' right to privacy" (AACN, 2008, p. 19). Thus, understanding and incorporating skills relating to password security, data security, virus protection, and copyright regulations/laws into nursing curriculum is essential for safe computer practices by student nurses (TIGER, 2009c).

- **Beginner student:** Learn to access online literature, evaluate it, and use it with proper documentation. Identify components of academic integrity in writing and student work. Discuss and document knowledge of copyright issues, Health Insurance Portability and Accountability Act (HIPAA) regulations, and privacy of patient information. Require use of a LMS. Practice using an EHR in class on a handheld computer or a Smartphone (i.e., nTrack by Skyscape; see Figure 13.1).

- **Advanced beginner student:** Use literature in decision making in planning care. Become familiar with the simulation lab. Begin to use electronic medical records (EMRs) in the clinical/simulation setting. Document in an electronic environment. Program electronic medical equipment. Review client documents for medication reconciliation. Use word processing, presentation software, publishing software, spreadsheets, and standardized languages (North American Nursing Diagnosis Association [NANDA], Nursing Interventions Classification [NIC], Nursing Outcomes Classification [NOC], etc.).

- **Advanced student:** Evaluate patient care technologies. Gain proficiency in word processing, presentation software, publishing software, spreadsheets, and standardized languages.

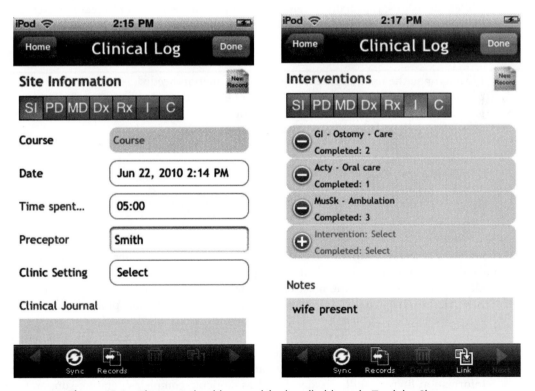

Figure 13.1 Electronic health record for handhelds and nTrack by Skyscape.

Successful complete computerized test taking. Select and evaluate research literature in the development of individualized care of clients. Become an expert in online literature searching. Use technology in communication with interprofessional team. Access health-care databases.

- **Graduating student:** Access and use the Cochrane library. Develop in-depth knowledge in evidence-based practice. Discuss health policy topics and the potential impact of technology. Proficient use of spreadsheets/budgeting. Expertise in research techniques (i.e., literature searching, and analyzation and synthesis of information). Design/redesign work spaces based on ergonomic principles. Participate in telehealth, e-health, and telenursing activities and simulations.

While developing the above mentioned knowledge and skills, students will use technologies ethically, will value technologies and their use in the delivery of safe patient care, and will recognize the nurse's role in information management. Nurses are part of the solution of designing and implementing technology solutions in the care of clients (i.e., development of students' attitudes toward technology in health care).

Information Literacy

Information literacy is the second part of the TIGER model. "Information literacy is the ability to identify information needed for a specific purpose, locate pertinent information, evaluate the information, and apply it correctly" (TIGER, 2009a, p. 5). Every nursing student and practicing nurse must have the skills necessary to use information to make clinical decisions; especially because clinical practice is based on research-based evidence. Information literacy skills must be learned during the basic nursing education program. The TIGER report delineates five information literacy competencies for graduating nursing students:

1. Determine the nature and extent of the information needed.
2. Access needed information effectively and efficiently.
3. Evaluate information and its sources critically and incorporate selected information into his or her knowledge base and value system.
4. Individually or as a member of a group, use information effectively to accomplish a specific purpose.
5. Evaluate outcomes of the use of information (TIGER, 2009c).

ACQUIRING INFORMATION LITERACY AT THE PROGRAM/ COURSE LEVELS

Students in the first nursing course are required to perform a literature search using online databases. Guidance in identification of appropriate information is provided. Frequently, the identification process is the most crucial and time-consuming but once completed, it provides the roadmap to locating relevant information. The library professional staff provides support to students in face-to-face (f-2-f) and online formats.

From the first course to the last course, proper documentation of sources is emphasized and required. The APA book is required of all students. Faculty discusses and decides which items are required (on the title page) and standardization of expectations is encouraged. Information literacy skills are developed as students complete literature-supported clinical paperwork, use best practices during clinical experiences, and educate their clients. Each process requires skills in gathering, evaluating, and disseminating information to nurses, patients, nurse educators, and other students.

Encourage students to submit their papers to a plagiarism checking Web site. Students worry about potentially inadvertently plagiarizing. Providing tools to students for self-regulation will support their creativity while protecting academic integrity.

As students progress in the curriculum, information literacy skills are acquired in through various assignments and required activities. Senior students develop an evidence-based research project based on current literature and best practices. They acquire/use the five required information literacy skills in the development of their research projects. Each project is presented orally to a group of practicing nurses who frequently take the findings and implement changes in their practice settings.

Another model for integrating informatics across the curriculum is cited by Curran (2008). Virtual cases, handheld devices, EHR, and point-of-care technologies are described and methods of integration suggested.

Web sites, such as the Health Information Technology (http://healthit.ahrq.gov), the Agency for Healthcare Research and Quality (http://www.ahrq.gov), and Health Resources and Services Administration (http://www.hrsa.gov) and their related Web links provide students with a wealth of information regarding information literacy. Assignments that require students to "surf" the Internet for health information, technology support systems, and best practices will assist students to become information literate.

INFORMATION MANAGEMENT

Clinical information systems/EHRs are used in health-care settings and their use is quickly becoming the norm. Because nurses document in EHRs, students must be oriented to a variety of these tools. "Information management is a process consisting of 1) collecting data, 2) processing data, and 3) presenting and communicating the processed data as information or knowledge" (TIGER, 2009a, p. 7).

Some of the information management competencies include using the EHR to capture patient information, obtain consent, manage medication administration and documentation, provide decision support for patient care, and facilitate interprofessional communication (TIGER, 2009c). Intentional faculty and program initiatives can assist students to acquire information management competencies.

PRACTICING INFORMATION MANAGEMENT AT THE PROGRAM/ COURSE LEVELS

Frequent access to the simulation laboratory will provide students opportunities to acquire information management skills. A medication administration system with bar coding will provide genuine experience for students. Documenting in an EHR adds to the realistic workplace environment. Organizing interprofessional learning opportunities will facilitate communication skills between the interdisciplinary team.

Clinical experiences offered in a variety of work settings and a variety of institutions will afford students the opportunity to document in numerous EHRSs. Adaptability will assist students to easily integrate into new clinical settings.

TECHNOLOGY TIP 13.4

Create an Interprofessional Facebook group for your nursing students. Invite members of other health professions (i.e., two physicians, two respiratory therapists, two social workers, and two occupational therapists, etc.) to join the group. Then invite your students. Have the students pose certain questions that will facilitate discussion about how best to manage Interprofessional communication. Be sure to create a "closed" or "secret" group in Facebook to ensure you control who is in the group. Also note that you do not need to "friend" the participants of your group.

Introduction to clinical decision support (CDS) systems affords the students a realistic view of work patterns and work situations. Features of a CDS system include a "knowledge base, a program for combining that knowledge with patient-specific information, and a communication mechanism" (Berner, 2009). Accuracy and continuity are benefits of using a clinical CDS system. Early introduction of CDS in the educational arena promotes the ability to provide safe and cost-effective care. Appreciating the value of the CDS in the provision of care by student nurses requires knowledge and use of the systems.

Although CDS systems will increase patient safety and decrease health care costs, there is not yet a standard language for data and thus, frequently systems do "not talk" to each other. Patient data are not codified the same. If one CDS system codes a heart attack as an MI and another system as a myocardial infarction, and yet another system as a heart attack, the data are not standardized and thus unable to be shared across systems. Student nurses need practice in standardized languages, both nursing standardized languages and medical standardized languages.

Students ability to problem solve during use of information management systems will increase their abilities to critically think while caring for patients in a health-care setting. Beginning students need to practice information management skills in the safety of a simulation setting.

CONCLUSION

Although informatics must be part of every curriculum and clinical experiences, faculty and students must not forget the patient. Benner, Sutphen, Leonard, and Day (2010) emphasize the need to "develop pedagogies that keep students focused on the patient's experiences" (p. 220). Students focused on the "technology of the IV" could ignore the patient. Integrating patient-focused informatics across a curriculum promotes quality patient care, critical thinking students, and a safe work environment.

REFERENCES

American Association of Colleges of Nursing. (2008). *The essentials of baccalaureate education for professional nursing practice.* Washington, DC: Author.

American Nurses Association. (2008). *Nursing informatics: Scope and standards of practice.* Silver Spring, MD: Author.

Benner, P., Sutphen, M., Leonard, V., & Day, L. (2010). *Educating nurses: A call for radical transformation.* San Francisco, CA: Jossey-Bass.

Berner, E. S. (2009, June). *Clinical decision support systems: State of the art* (AHRQ Publication No. 09-0069). Rockville, MD: Agency for Healthcare Research and Quality.

Cronenwett, L., Sherwood, G., Barnsteiner, J., Disch, J., Johnson, J., Mitchell, P., Sullivan, D. T., & Warren, J. (2007). Quality and safety education for nurses. *Nursing Outlook, 55*(3), 122–131.

Curran, C. R. (2008). Faculty development initiatives for integration of informatics competencies and point-of-care technologies in undergraduate nursing education. In E. E. Weiner, *Technology: The interface to nursing educational technologies. Nursing Clinics of North America, 43*(4), pp 523–533.

Fetter, M. S. (2007). Curriculum strategies to improve baccalaureate nursing information technology outcomes. *Journal of Nursing Education, 48*(2), 78–85.

Fetter, M. S. (2009). Graduating nurses' self-evaluation of information technology competencies. *Journal of Nursing Education, 48(2),* 86–90.

Leavitt, M. O. (2005). *Statement on health information technology (IT) before The Committee on the Budget, United States Senate.* Washington, DC: U.S. Department of Health & Human Services. Retrieved from http://www.hhs.gov/asl/testify/t050720.html

National League for Nursing. (2008). *Preparing the next generation of nurses to practice in a technology-rich environment: An informatics agenda* [Position statement]. Retrieved from http://www.nln.org/aboutnln/PositionStatements/informatics_052808.pdf

Prensky, M. (2001, October). Digital natives, digital immigrants. *On the horizon.* Retrieved from http://www.marcprensky.com/writing/Prensky%20-%20Digital%20Natives,%20Digital%20Immigrants%20-%20Part1.pdf

Technology Informatics Guiding Educational Reform (TIGER). (2009a). *Tiger informatics competencies collaborative (TICC).* Retrieved from http://tigercompetencies.pbworks.com/f/TICC_Final.pdf

TIGER Initiative. (2009b). *Collaborating to integrate evidence and informatics into nursing practice and education: An executive summary.* Retrieved from http://www.tigersummit.com/uploads/TIGER_Collaborative_Exec_Summary_040509.pdf

TIGER Initiative. (2009c). *Informatics competencies for every practicing nurse: Recommendations from the TIGER collaborative.* Retrieved from http://www.tigersummit.com/uploads/3.Tiger.Report_Competencies_final.pdf

TIGER Initiative. (2009d). *Transforming education for an informatics agenda: TIGER education and faculty development collaborative.* Retrieved from http://www.tigersummit.com/uploads/Educ.Tiger.Report_final4.pdf

Weiner, E. E. (Ed.). (2008) *Technology: The interface to nursing educational informatics.* Philadelphia, PA: W. B. Saunders.

Chapter 14

Staff Development and Employee Training

Barb Schreiner, PhD, RN, CDE, BC-ADM

The vice president of nursing at Mercy Hospital was alarmed with a recent quality assurance report highlighting medication errors by nurses administering insulin. Many of the errors were related to either poor knowledge about the pharmacokinetics of insulin or to poor judgment in applying the physicians' orders about when to give the doses. The quality team initiated a performance improvement plan, which included both a training component and a nontraining intervention. The blended training plan included an online course followed by a classroom session and an online quiz. In addition, the training was supported by job aids at the medication stations. Collectively, the interventions resulted in a dramatic decrease in medication errors and increased knowledge among the staff nurses. The hospital's mission—critical goals for excellence and safe patient care were addressed.

THE PLACE FOR WORKPLACE LEARNING

Nurses and other health-care professionals are important and expensive assets for the health-care organization. As a result, workplace learning (WPL) holds an increasingly prominent place in an organization's array of performance improvement strategies. As technology simplifies tasks, nurses and other health-care providers become knowledge workers, ever more responsible for the critical thinking and interpretation of sophisticated data. For health-care enterprises, nurses are the largest source of intellectual capital that must be nurtured and supported. WPL is one of the most important performance improvement tools for building a knowledgeable, competent nursing staff.

The process of responding to a performance improvement issue is evident in the Mercy Hospital case. The flow of analyzing and responding to the problem is illustrated in Table 14.1. The vice president first identified a performance issue when the quality assurance report hit her desk. From an organizational perspective, she knew that Mercy Hospital embraced excellence in the provision of safe patient care delivered by skilled providers. A gap analysis quickly revealed the discrepancy between a desired safe environment and the current state of medication errors.

Could the cause of the errors be system-related or employee-related? Were environmental resources lacking? Were there knowledge or skill deficits among the staff? After a careful cause analysis, the quality team determined that the nurses needed additional education about insulin. The quality team initiated virtual learning approaches followed by competency assessments for the nursing staff. The team also knew that new knowledge and behaviors resulting

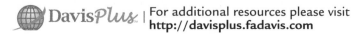

DavisPlus | For additional resources please visit
http://davisplus.fadavis.com

TABLE 14.1

Mercy Hospital's Medication Errors

Problem	Insulin dosing errors by nursing staff: • Doses delivered when patient hypoglycemic. • Doses delivered when patient had already received a dose 2 hours before.
Organizational goals	Nursing care excellence; safe delivery of patient care
Desired state	No medication errors
Current state	12 insulin errors in last quarter
Cause analysis	• Nurses lack knowledge about how insulin works. • Nurses lack critical thinking about when to deliver a sliding scale insulin dose.
Training solution	In-service education and certification
Nontraining solution	Job aids on medication carts
Implementation date	July 1, 2011
Content	Insulin pharmacokinetics and action curves Decision making and insulin dosing
Delivery method	Archived online course F-2-f session to answer questions and practice Online quiz for certification Job aid about insulin action on medication carts

Project Plan

Milestone	Completion Date	Responsible
Determine learning objectives	May 15, 2011	Quality team and training team
Determine evaluation mechanism	May 16, 2011	Quality team and training team
Build content and assessment questions	May 22, 2011	Training team
Build online lessons and quiz	June 6, 2011	Training team

TABLE 14.1—cont'd		
Mercy Hospital's Medication Errors		
Milestone	Completion Date	Responsible
Plan agenda for classroom session	June 11, 2011	Training team
Finalize job aid	June 18, 2011	Training team
Final review of materials	June 20, 2011	Quality team and training team
Begin scheduling staff	June 25, 2011	Training team and Nursing management
Deliver course	July 1, 2011	Training team
Review evaluation data	August 4, 2011	Quality team

from training needed to be supported within the work environment with nontraining materials, such as job aids.

Employee performance is the result of synergy among organizational resources, employee knowledge and motivation, and work processes all linked to the organization's mission or goals (VanTiem, Moseley, & Conway Dessinger, 2004) (see Davis Plus for a blank performance improvement template). In this example, WPL aligned directly to the hospital's mission or business goals: safe care and excellence.

THE SIX Cs OF WORKPLACE LEARNING

WPL meets six important performance needs (Table 14.2): communication, competency, compliance, certification, continuing education, and community/culture.

Communicate

Information often must be rapidly disseminated within an organization. For instance, employees must be informed of institutional changes, processes, or policies. On demand or "fingertip information" is often critical to immediately providing care. Unlike training or certification, information tends to be more informally prepared and rapidly delivered. The organization's intranet is often the vehicle for disseminating information. Bulletin boards and e-newsletters also are effective tools. Podcasts and audio conference calls are newer electronic approaches to rapid deployment of information across a health-care enterprise.

Competency

Nurses and other health-care providers rely on important technical skills and supporting knowledge. Virtual training can enhance these requirements. Consider the blended training approach used by Palomar Pomerado Health system (Spivey, 2009). Nurses are expected to

TABLE 14.2		
Performance Needs Addressed by Workplace Learning Strategies		
Types of Workplace Learning	**Examples**	**Methods**
Communicate information	Human resources (HR) information; holiday schedule	E-mail, newsletters, posters, conference calls, podcasts, Webcasts (live, archived)
Competency: skills and knowledge	New devices; new medications; onboarding	E-course, skills laboratory, Webcasts
Compliance/regulatory	HIPAA; Occupational Safety & Health Administration (OSHA)	E-course, job aids, simulations
Certification	ICU, neonatal transport team	E-course, instructor led, examinations
Continuing education	Disease state training; journal clubs	Any, case study
Community and culture	Onboarding, mentoring, employee retention programs	Social networking formats (e.g., Facebook, Myspace, Second Life, LinkedIn), Wiki, blogs, e-mentoring, FAQ, discussion groups, collaborative systems

provide point-of-care blood glucose checks in a consistent and accurate fashion. When quality measures indicated discrepancies among staff, the training team created a blended learning intervention including a training video; an interactive, virtual training session; and a final assessment. Using e-learning approaches meant that training was consistent in content and approach.

Compliance

Hospitals and other health-care agencies live in a tightly regulated environment. Employees are required to consistently follow approved procedures and processes. Many regulations require frequent review by employees, often annually. Virtual training approaches, using e-courses or archived Webcasts are effective strategies. For instance, the Children's Hospital and Clinics of Minneapolis improved the completion rate for compliance training to more than 95% using an online format (Johnson, 2004). Before the e-learning program, mandatory training consisted of a 30-page safety procedures manual. No wonder the completion rate hovered around 50% in those days. With the new technology, employees beat the hospital's metrics for compliance training within 1 month.

Certification

Compliance and regulatory training often results in certification of a skill or knowledge. Slotte and Herbert (2006) compared the effectiveness of a food industry certification offered online with the same certification provided in a traditional print format. Although both groups achieved equivalent mastery of the content, the e-learning group required less employee time to do so. Such savings in employee time translated to cost savings across the organization.

Another organization successfully using online training is the Child Health Corporation of America (CHCA). CHCA, a consortium of children's hospitals, uses an online format to deliver standardized, pediatric-specific training to more than 73,000 learners (Johnson, 2004). As a member of CHCA, Children's Hospital of Dallas enjoyed a 41% decrease in overall training costs by employing online training.

In another example, educators at MD Anderson Cancer Center effectively implemented CPR competency evaluation for 2500 hospital personnel while saving more than $160,000 (Abraham, 2007).

Continuing Education

Continuous learning is the hallmark of a learning organization and quite necessary for a competitive advantage (Senge, 1990). Continuing education has been positively linked to job satisfaction, employee retention, and quality of care (Jukkula, Henly, & Lindeke, 2008). Administrators at Miami Children's Hospital recognize the employee benefits of providing continuing education for their staff. In addition to saving costs of travel and time away from work, virtual continuing education demonstrates the hospital's commitment to its licensed employees and is viewed as a critical tool for retention (Johnson, 2004).

Across the country, Kaiser Permanente uses extensive distance learning programs to both onboard new employees and to update the skills of established staff. The system's Nursing

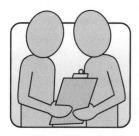

Pathways, a career developmental model, incorporates clinical e-learning, Web videos, Webinars, and home-study programs (Knapp, 2004).

Continuing education also may promote career developmental outside the organization. In another example, educators at the Texas Tech University Health Sciences Center developed a synchronous continuing education program for health-care professionals to address the burgeoning effect of diabetes in the state (Irons, Vickers, Esperat, Valdez, Dadich, Boswell, & Cannon, 2007). As a result of the program, many nurses planned to certify as diabetes educators effectively doubling the existing pool of educators in west Texas.

Community and Culture

WPL also can have an effect on employee recruitment and retention through the building of learning communities or communities of practice (Paloff & Pratt, 2007). One mechanism is that continuing education in the workplace fosters meaningful connections among nurses leading to career satisfaction (Perry, 2008). Goldsworthy, Graham, Robinson, and Campkin (2008) reported successful use of an e-learning program for critical care nurses. The blended program incorporated online sessions, simulated classes and a precepted practicum. An additional, nontraining tool included a handheld computer packed with three reference books to use at the bedside. The program encouraged staff nurses to choose critical care nursing as a career and supported existing critical care staff.

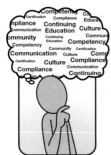

Atack (2003) studied a group of nurses enrolled in a 16-week Web-based course designed to develop case management skills. The nurses were largely novice to e-learning and inexperienced with computer use. They collectively experienced steep learning curves in the early weeks of the course as they overcame technology hurdles. What maintained their enrollment in the course, however, was the support from their online community of learners. The experience fostered an ongoing interest in continuing education.

WPL is an effective tool in addressing six key organizational needs: communication, competency, compliance, certification, continuing education, and community/culture. However, not all performance improvement issues require a training intervention.

DOES A PERFORMANCE ISSUE ALWAYS REQUIRE A TRAINING APPROACH?

The short answer to the question is: No. Not all performance issues require education. Gilbert identified two broad sources of performance problems: the organization and the employee. Gilbert's Behavioral Engineering model in Table 14.3 further delineates six influences on performance (Gilbert, 1996). Notice that most challenges to performance are not necessarily a

TABLE 14.3			
Factors Linked to Human Performance in the Workplace			
	Information	**Instrumentation**	**Motivation**
Work environment	Data • Clear expectations for performance are articulated. • Relevant feedback to employee about performance. • Functional communication channels.	Resources • Tools and materials are available. • Time and resources match the performance needs.	Incentives • Adequate financial incentives. • Opportunities for career development. • Clearly articulated consequences for nonperformance.
Employee	Knowledge • Ability to learn. • Effective training matched to performance need. • Matching employee knowledge and skill to task.	Capacity • Scheduling matches peak need. • Disability support. • Individual ability to flex.	Motives • Understanding employee's motives to work. • Matching employee interests and motivation to tasks.

deficiency in the employee. Many of the influences are system or environmental problems. Some are human resource concerns, such as a lack of adequate staff or incentives. Some performance issues result from poor communication across teams or departments.

Training strategies work best when a cause analysis points directly to a lack of knowledge or skill in the employee. Increasingly, technology-enabled learning (e-learning) strategies are used to address this gap.

Goettner (2000) characterized effective e-learning as a "learner-centered experience with rich content in a relevant context." Consider the example of virtual rounds led by an advanced intensive care nurse (Karpowicz, 2008). Bedside nurses on the night shift are supported with "on demand" information by an experienced intensive care unit (ICU) nurse. The ICU nurse in turn has access to a blog loaded with evidence-based information, decision support tools, and Web access to the hospital's library. The immediate need for relevant information is brokered through the experienced ICU nurse who provides "just-in-time" content.

If the performance issue truly dictates a learning strategy, an instructional designer or nurse educator with training in instructional design has a variety of methods from which to choose. Will the instruction be face-to-face (f-2-f), virtual, or a blend of both? What virtual learning approach will work best? This text has explored the variety and application of several e-learning approaches. Regardless of the strategy chosen, the instructional designer or nurse educator must address such learning concepts as cognitive load, knowledge transfer to action, and evaluation.

Cognitive Load

Cognitive load theory is grounded in an understanding of human learning processes and the limitations of human cognition and memory (Clark, Nguyen, & Sweller, 2006). Cognitive load is the collective effect of the complexity of the content, the mental work required by instructional activities, and any irrelevant distractions. In developing any type of learning, the instructional designer or nurse educator should consider ways to lighten the load on working memory, allowing for more efficient processing of information and improved retention of content.

Acquiring new information requires an elegant coordination between working memory and long-term storage. Working memory is very limited in capacity. An individual can only process a handful of information, shifting some to long-term memory and discarding (forgetting) others. Working memory is adversely affected by several distractions including what cognitive scientists call contiguity effect, coherence effect, modality effect, and redundancy effect (Nelson & Erlandson, 2008). These distractions contribute to the cognitive load of processing and remembering content.

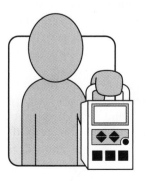

Contiguity Effect. The training department is creating a slide presentation to demonstrate a new infusion pump. Diagrams guide the learner in the process of setting up the pump. A diagram of the pump with its parts numbered is at the top of the slide. Bulleted text at the bottom of the slide lists the number of the part and its corresponding name. What is wrong with this approach?

The working memory is forced to gather information from multiple sources and mental processing slows as a result. By splitting attention between the diagram and the text, working memory experiences increased cognitive load.

To minimize split attention, the text and the diagram should be in close proximity. For instance, label the pump with the names and avoid the added step of matching a number to its name.

Coherence Effect. An educator is preparing an engaging slide deck to be used in an upcoming Webinar. Knowing it is difficult to engage and hold the learner's attention, the educator adds background music at times and interesting or inspiring quotations at other times.

In another example, imagine a typical slide-show presentation complete with bullet-pointed text, clip art, and swirling titles. The working memory is challenged by such content as the mind struggles to sift through the media for the core message—what should be remembered. Although the animation may be attention-grabbing, it becomes a distraction as the brain splits its attention between motion and static content.

Although these tactics may seem attractive or appealing, they are placing unnecessary demands on mental processing. The learner's brain is forced to sort the "nice to knows" from the "need to knows" at the expense of efficient learning. Graphics, sounds, and text should all support the core message. Extraneous background music, unrelated photographs, or nonessential stories will derail even the most focused learner.

Modality Effect. Our brains are remarkable processors of information relying on two channels to gather input. Visual and auditory channels continuously collect and process information. Effective training materials exploit the visual and auditory channels to improve cognitive processing. Materials presenting graphics and text overload the visual channel. When narration and graphics are employed, both processing conduits are activated and learning is enhanced. The takeaway is: when possible, use speech rather than on-screen text (Clark & Mayer, 2008).

Redundancy Effect. While tapping the auditory pathway is important, there is at least one situation in which narration can add to cognitive overload. When narration is repeating on-screen text, the redundancy effect takes over. The brain tries to compare and reconcile what is heard with what is seen resulting in processing, which is extraneous to the learning task. Narration works best when there are no competing graphics and plenty of time to process the content.

Knowledge Transfer. Educators should "build instruction to impact what people can do *in the real world*, not what they can do during instruction" (Shank, 2004, p.7). In 2005, more than $50 billion was budgeted for formal training with another $13.5 billion spent on products and services for training (Dolezalek, 2005). Yet, statistics regarding transfer of training are dismal with many authors claiming that only 10% to 20% of training initiatives ever result in transfer to performance on the job (Broad & Newstrom, 1992; Broad, 2000). Even when training is transferred, it may be transient. Dolezalek (2005) reported, "90% of all sales training programs do yield an increase in sales productivity," an increase that lasts only 90 to 120 days (p. 34).

Transfer theory considers all three components: the employee, the training, and the environment. Training strategies must help learners to understand the relevance of the training to the job and to build cognitive connections between old information and new knowledge. If training content is directly associated with desired outcomes, "near transfer" will occur. If, however, training focuses on building conceptual or theoretical knowledge to be applied in new contexts or situations, "far transfer" is expected.

TECHNOLOGY TIP 14.1

One way to build "far transfer" capabilities is to use job-specific cases. Check the capabilities with BioWorld, a multimedia online environment to encourage critical reasoning and thinking skills at http://www.education.mcgill.ca/cognitionlab/bioworld/

Brinkerhoff and Montesino (1995) suggested that management interventions can be effective in facilitating transfer and listed specific actions such as pre- and postcourse discussion between supervisors and employees, provision of adequate resources, and ongoing feedback. Broad (2000) found that employees were more likely to transfer behavior when managers expected accountability, provided pretraining information, required attendance at training, and were present for all or part of the training.

Chat rooms, message boards, and routinely scheduled conference calls are ways to maintain and sustain learning transfer following training. When a learner reflects on the learning session or builds an action plan, learning is more likely to be transferred to workplace behavior. For example, practical nurses used Web-based discussions to build reflection skills (Hulkari & Mahlamaki-Kultanen, 2008). Over the course of the training, the reflections matured in both content and depth indicating further learning had occurred.

Virtual WPL strategies must address the challenges of transferring learning to practice. The content must be relevant and within the context of workplace need. Will the learning activity apply to current skills or to future problem-solving needs? To promote transfer, the instructional designer or nurse educator should consider: aligning of learning with actual job performance, linking new knowledge to previous knowledge, repeating and practicing extensively and in varied contexts, and incorporating reflection and action planning (Shank, 2004).

Staff education in health-care environments provides extensive training for events the staff may be exposed to only once or twice a year. Provision of mandatory updates using case studies and implementation of required tools (e.g., skin assessment and procedure checklists) are two ways of increasing long-term retention.

EVALUATION

When developing WPL and in-service programs, start with the end in mind. Effective WPL programs link intimately to organizational goals. The programs exist because a performance gap was identified between the desired state (zero new skin breakdowns) and the existing state of behavior (15% incidence of skin breakdowns after admission). The programs exist because the key stakeholders (administrators, managers) had expectations for performance that were not being met. Surely then, a program's effectiveness must measure change in

TECHNOLOGY TIP 14.2

Build opportunities for reflection within and around training. Try online journals or learning logs to encourage reflection among learners. Use an "a-ha" blog to capture reflections following a virtual training session. Encourage participants to record their key takeways on the whiteboard before a Webcast ends.

performance. Yet so many training programs simply measure learner satisfaction or change in knowledge or skill. Long-term retention of learning and application of knowledge in the workplace are as important to evaluate as outcome measures. Knowledge of why the learning has or has not improved outcomes will assist the educator in program improvement (Evidence-Based Practice Box 14.1).

Increasingly, training departments are being asked to demonstrate performance improvement on the job to measure effectiveness and efficiency (van Adelsberg & Trolley, 1999). The Kirkpatrick model (1998) of summative evaluation uses four levels of training assessment (Table 14.4). All four levels of evaluation are needed to provide effective training programs.

- Level 1 (reaction) evaluation typically is measured using "smile sheets" or postprogram surveys designed to assess the learner's satisfaction with program content, teaching methods, or faculty educator. Most WPL programs rely on Level 1 evaluations because of the simplicity and ease of obtaining data.
- Level 2 (learning) evaluation measures knowledge acquisition and typically is achieved with quizzes or return demonstrations.
- Level 3 (behavior) evaluation measures transfer of learning to the job.
- Level 4 evaluation focuses on organizational results. Although this level is the most challenging of the four, it may be the most valuable to business planners.

It is important in the planning stage of program development for the educator to understand from key stakeholders how success should be defined. In our first example of Mercy Hospital, success was simple: decrease medication errors. A Level 3 evaluation would address this outcome. If training was successful, and the nontraining materials were

---

EVIDENCE-BASED PRACTICE BOX 14.1

Evaluation of Interactive Online Courses for Advanced Practice Nurses

Issue: How Effective Is Online Learning for Advanced Practice Nurses?

The study examined the effect of two online training modules that incorporated powerful, interactive challenges and case studies close to real-world scenarios. The scenarios attempted to foster apprenticelike learning. A pre- and post-test provided Level 2 evaluation. A descriptive survey collected Level 1 evaluation.

Study Findings

Mean knowledge scores improved significantly following the online training sessions. The 73 advanced practice nurses appreciated the interactive case study approach. They commented that their computer skills had improved over the course of the program and that they did not miss the f-2-f interaction with other learners. Learners complained about technology issues, such as broken links or navigation issues. The other problem was lack of immediate feedback to the assessment questions.

Nursing Implications

- Case studies that are rich and complex are effective teaching tools for advanced practice nurses.
- Adult learners prefer constructive feedback when interacting with training tools.
- Technology issues must be addressed for learners to have a successful experience with online learning (Huckstadt & Hayes, 2005).

TABLE 14.4			
Evaluation Levels			
Level	Measures	Question to be Answered	Source
1	Reaction; satisfaction	What did the learners like and dislike about the training?	Feedback or satisfaction score sheets
2	Learning	What did learners learn? How much was learned or remembered?	Quizzes Skill checklists
3	Behavior; transfer of learning	Is the knowledge or skill being used in the workplace?	Job performance Quality measures
4	Results	How is the training having an effect on the organization?	Business indicators Cost effect

supportive, then fewer medication errors would occur. Provision should be made for short- and long-term effectiveness in the reduction of medication errors.

Sheen, Chang, Chen, Chao, and Tseng (2008) compared the outcomes from an e-learning course with a traditional classroom course. Satisfaction scores were comparable (level one evaluation) between the two groups. Knowledge scores, however, were statistically higher for some traditional classroom content that used highly interactive strategies (Level 2 evaluation). Clearly missing in the report was the effect on performance. How well did the nurses perform back at the bedside given their new set of skills? Was the effect on nursing care still present 1 year after the WPL program?

Pullen (2006), on the other hand, reported the outcomes of a Web-based course for nurses in satisfaction and learner achievement (i.e., knowledge and behavior). The author explored three questions: (a) Do the learners like the experience? (b) Do the learners gain knowledge? and (c) Do the learners apply the knowledge in their work? Learners liked the flexibility of the course, increased their knowledge significantly, and reported a transfer of that knowledge to their jobs.

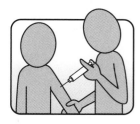

Peddocord, Holsclaw, Jacobson, Kwizera, Rose, Gersberg, and Macias-Reynolds (2007) also used three levels of evaluation in a study of public health training. Following the terrorist attacks, the Centers for Disease Control and Prevention (CDC) with others provided a nationwide satellite broadcast on mass vaccinations. More than 1600 health-care providers attended the program. Immediately following the program, learners completed opinion or satisfaction surveys and knowledge/attitude questionnaires. A unique follow-up was then conducted 6 weeks after the program. Learners completed a Web-based questionnaire that asked whether they had taken action to change their health department's emergency preparedness plan (i.e., a Level 3 evaluation). More than 80% had taken action following the training.

Effective WPL considers not only the learning objectives and strategies, but also the anticipated outcomes during the instructional design process. Effective program evaluation moves beyond "smile sheets" and quizzes to measure transfer of learning to performance and outcomes that is retained over time (Evidence-Based Practice Box 14.2).

THE CHALLENGES OF WPL

Although WPL has a prominent place in health-care organizations, it is not without challenges. How and when should training be offered? Should employees be expected to engage in virtual learning activities from their homes? Should all required training be paid training? Should professionals be expected to invest personal time in their continuing learning?

Some of these are philosophical questions while some may have legal or labor law implications. For some organizations, required training cannot incur overtime hours. In such environments, training times must be flexible and computer access readily available for the busy employee. Courses must be brief and highly focused to a particular topic. The Veterans Health Administration, for instance, has developed a Web-based campus with more than 1200 online courses designed to be taken in 15- to 30-minute intervals (Rick, Kearns, & Thompson, 2003).

In addition to the challenge of delivery time and place, technology-enabled WPL also had implications for the employee. What competencies and resources are necessary for

---

EVIDENCE-BASED PRACTICE BOX 14.2

Issue: How Effective Is a Blended Learning Program in Enhancing Collaborative Practice of Health-Care Professionals Working in Long-Term Care Facilities?

Collaborative practice across health-care disciplines is important in providing consistent patient care. The study evaluated the effect of a multimodule training course on learner knowledge, attitudes, and transfer of knowledge to practice. Nurses, family physicians, and pharmacists completed a series of online, self-paced modules and several team meetings. The program planners used online surveys to gather information before, during, and 2 months after the training. Additionally, the program planners used focus group interviews to further understand how well the program delivered on its objectives. The planners expanded on Kirkpatrick's evaluation model by also assessing the effect of the program on patient outcomes.

Study Findings

Learning objectives were achieved and participants held positive feelings about the program. Performance significantly improved across several dimensions including planning patient care together, making cooperative decisions, and respecting others' contributions. Quality-of-life changes for the patients were too early to measure by survey but the focus groups interviews suggested that change was already starting. The flexibility and convenience of online learning was most valued among the participants.

Nursing Implications

- Virtual learning programs are not only valuable in changing knowledge and attitudes, but in building teams and collaboration.
- Program evaluation is more than satisfaction questionnaires and knowledge quizzes. Evaluations of behavior change, knowledge transfer, and the affect on customers or patients validate the importance of training for stakeholders (Chambers, Conklin, Dalziel, MacDonald, & Stodel, 2008).

employees to be successful e-learners? Do they have adequate ethical and computer skills? Do they have reliable access to hardware and software? Corry and Watkins (2007) suggest that educators consider not only the technical or scientific content in training. Employees may need help with time-management skills as they take asynchronous online courses, for example. They may need better reading skills. They may need suggestions on how to organize their files and notes. Finally, employees may need to learn the fine art and etiquette of communicating online, knowing how to adjust for limited nonverbal communication cues. For WPL to be effective, virtual-training strategies must be supported by the organization in the form of time for training, consistent, easy access to the training, and technology support for the learner.

BEYOND WPL: DISTANCE MENTORING

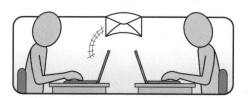

Training must translate to behavior change and action to be effective. Learners must effectively transfer learning to the work environment. One method is to provide continued support beyond the f-2-f training session through mentoring activities.

With technology, mentoring is more widely accessible. Yet, while business coaching and online mentoring have taken hold in the corporate world (Kampa-Kokesch & Anderson, 2001), the nursing literature is only beginning to report instances of cyberspace mentoring. Kasprisin, Single, Single, and Muller (2003) studied e-mentoring with nursing students, and while those students participating in online mentoring were more satisfied with and more involved in the mentoring experience, there was no data collected about behavioral outcomes. Russell and Perris (2003) explored the effect of online mentoring as an adjunct to the traditional preceptorship in a community nursing agency. Participants reported overall satisfaction with the technology and demonstrated improved clinical practice.

Bierema and Merriam (2002) echoed such a use of online mentoring, stating that e-mentoring "is a mutually beneficial relationship that is highly versatile and can be adapted to work in a variety of settings" (p. 219). O'Neill, Weiler, and Sha (2005) described a software package capable of supporting mentorship relationships, matching novices with mentors, and providing access for just-in-time learning. Still, online mentoring is not without its challenges, including the potential for miscommunication, the difficulty mentors have in modeling behaviors, the requirement for writing and computer skills, and confidentiality concerns (Ensher, Heun, & Blanchard, 2003).

Additionally, an online relationship may be slower to develop than a f-2-f one. The authors encourage mentors and mentees to use overlapping methods to communicate with each other, including phone contact.

"Developing the levels of trust and confidence to sustain the [online] relationship takes time, familiarity, and work" (Bierema & Merriam, 2002, p. 221). Because participants in a f-2-f training program have already begun a relationship with the faculty, the concern about relationship-building may be less of an issue when online mentoring is used as a follow-up tool. Further, "providing ongoing support via an online mentor after the conclusion of a training program would be an excellent way to reinforce and improve transfer of learning" (Ensher, Heun, & Blanchard, 2003, p. 284).

Molinari, Monserud, and Hudzinski (2008) described the use of e-mentoring in the Rural Nurse Internship program. Nurses from geographically disparate hospitals attend Web-based training sessions and receive ongoing support from expert rural nurse mentors. Mentors use telephone and e-mail to maintain the relationship over the course of a year. Specialist nurses also provide just-in-time support and information to the program attendees. Through these tools, the internship program successfully retained valuable human capital.

When the Missouri Department of Health noticed a progressive decline in numbers of public health nurses, a novel training program was designed that relied on e-mentors (Miller, Devaney, Kelly, & Kuehn, 2008). Population-based health-care concepts were rolled out to novice public health nurses through a Web-based platform. In addition, an e-mentoring program was designed to support the learner and to develop new leadership skills in the experienced nurse mentor. E-mail and discussion boards were used extensively. Both knowledge gain and employee retention occurred among the learners. The mentors learned new skills of coaching and guiding. The state of Missouri benefited from a strengthened public health nursing network.

CONCLUSION

Performance improvement is fundamental to an organization's ability to realize its mission and demonstrate its values. Performance improvement initiatives address gaps between the desired or expected state and the actual state. Once identified, the gaps are filled with training or nontraining interventions.

When training is the solution, e-learning options are frequently the most efficient, consistent, and economical choices. Many of the strategies explored in this text could be readily applied to the six Cs of WPL: communication, competency, compliance, certification, continuing education, and community/culture. Review Chapters 5 to 9 for discussions around online learning strategies and Chapters 15 to 16 for further exploration of technology tools for staff development.

In preparing programs for WPL, the educator must carefully consider the effect of cognitive load, the challenges of knowledge transfer, and the importance of meaningful evaluation. E-learning has taken hold in the health-care industry and is a viable tool for delivering continuous learning to a most mission-critical asset: the health-care professional.

REFERENCES

Abraham, M. J. (2007). Blended learning: Integrating an e-learning component for competency validation [Abstract]. *Advances in Teaching and Learning Day*. Houston, TX: Houston Academy of Medicine-Texas Medical Center. Retrieved at http://digitalcommons.library.tmc.edu/uthshis atldayabs/18

Atack, L. (2003). Becoming a web-based learner: Registered nurses' experiences. *Journal of Advanced Nursing, 44*(3), 289–297.

Bierema, L. L., & Merriam, S. B. (2002). E-mentoring: Using computer mediated communication to enhance the mentoring process. *Innovative Higher Education, 26*(3), 211–227.

Brinkerhoff, R. O., & Montesino, M. U. (1995). Partnerships for training transfer: Lessons from a corporate study. *Human Resource Development Quarterly, 6*(3), 263–274.

Broad, M. L. (2000). Ensuring transfer of learning to the job. In G. M. Piskurich, P. Beckschi, & B. Hall (Eds.), *The ASTD handbook of training design and delivery* (pp. 430–452). New York, NY: McGraw-Hill.

Broad, M. L., & Newstrom, J. W. (1992). *Transfer of training: Action -packed strategies to ensure high payoff from training investments*. Reading, MA: Perseus Books.

Chambers, L. W. ,Conklin, J., Dalziel, W. B., MacDonald, C. J., & Stodel, E. J. (2008). E-learning education to promote interprofessional education with physicians, pharmacists, nurses and nurse practitioners in (LTC) facilities: Promising potential solutions. *International Journal of Biomedical Engineering and Technology, 1*(3), 233–249.

Clark, R. C., & Mayer, R. E. (2008). *E-learning and the science of instruction*. San Francisco, CA: Pfeiffer.

Clark, R., Nguyen, F., & Sweller, J. (2006). *Efficiency in learning: Evidence-based guidelines to manage cognitive load*. San Francisco, CA: Pfeiffer.

Corry, M., & Watkins, R. (2007). Strategy for the learner: A student's guide to e-learning success. In Brandon, B. (Ed.), *The eLearning guild's handbook of e-learning strategy*. Santa Rosa, CA: E Learning Guild, (pp. 63–68).

Dolezalek, H. (2005). 2005 industry report. *Training, 42*(12), 14–28.

Ensher, E. A., Heun, C., & Blanchard, A. (2003). Online mentoring and computer-mediated communication: New directions in research. *Journal of Vocational Behavior, 63*(2), 264–288.

Gilbert, T. F. (1996). *Human competence: Engineering worthy performance (ISPI tribute edition)*. New York, NY: McGraw Hill.

Goettner, P. (December, 2000). Effective e-learning for health care. Health management technology. *Health Management Technologies*. Retrieved from http://archive.healthmgttech.com/cgi-bin/arttop.asp?Page=1200viewpoint.htm

Goldsworthy, S., Graham, L., Robinson, J., & Campkin, M. (2008). Learning at your fingertips: New directions for accessible critical care education—A Canadian perspective [Abstract]. *Critical Care Nurse, 28*(2), e36.

Huckstadt, A., & Hayes, K. (2005). Evaluation of interactive online courses for advanced practice nurses. *Journal of the American Academy of Nurse Practitioners, 17*(3), 85–89.

Hulkari, K., & Mahlamaki-Kultanen, S. (2008). Reflection through web discussions: Assessing nursing students' work-based learning. *Journal of Workplace Learning, 20*(3), 157–164.

Irons, B. K., Vickers, P., Esperat, C., Valdez, G. M., Dadich, K. A., Boswell, C., & Cannon, S. (2007). The need for a community diabetes education curriculum for healthcare professionals. *The Journal of Continuing Education in Nursing, 38*(5), 227–231.

Johnson, K. (2004, October 18). Increasing training compliance rates at children's hospitals with e-learning. *The e-Learning Developers' Journal*, 1–12.

Jukkula, A. M., Henly, S. J., & Lindeke, L. L. (2008). Rural perceptions of continuing professional education. *The Journal of Continuing Education in Nursing, 39*(12), 555–563.

Kampa-Kokesch, S., & Anderson, M. Z. (2001). Executive coaching: A comprehensive review of the literature. *Consulting Psychology Journal: Practice and Research, 53*(4), 205–228.

Karpowicz, M. (2008). Continuum of competence: Trials of educating in a tele-ICU [Abstract]. *Critical Care Nurse, 28*(2), e5.

Kasprisin, C. A., Single, P. B., Single, R. M., & Muller, C. B. (2003). Building a better bridge: Testing e-training to improve e-mentoring programmes in higher education. *Mentoring & Tutoring: Partnership in Learning, 11*(1), 67–78.

Kirkpatrick, D. L. (1998). *Evaluating training programs* (2nd ed.). San Francisco, CA: Berrett-Koehler Publishers, Inc.

Knapp, B. (2004). Competency: An essential component of caring in nursing. *Nursing Administration Quarterly, 28*(4), 285–287.

Miller, L. C., Devaney, S. W. , Kelly, G. L., & Kuehn, A. F. (2008). E-mentoring in public health nursing practice. *The Journal of Continuing Education in Nursing, 39*(9), 394–399.

Molinari, D. L., Monserud, M., & Hudzinski, D. (2008). A new type of rural nurse residency. *The Journal of Continuing Education in Nursing, 39*(1), 42–46.

Nelson, B. C., & Erlandson, B. E. (2008). Managing cognitive load in educational multi-user virtual environments: Reflection on design practice. *Educational Technology, Research and Development, 56,* 619–641.

O'Neill, D. K., Weiler, M., & Sha, L. (2005). Software support for online mentoring programs:

A research-inspired design. *Mentoring & Tutoring: Partnership in Learning, 13*(1), 109–131.

Paloff, R. M. & Pratt, K. (2007). *Building online learning communities: Effective strategies for the virtual classroom*. San Francisco, CA: Wiley.

Peddocord, K. M., Holsclaw, P., Jacobson, I. G., Kwizera, L., Rose, K., Gersberg, R., & Macias-Reynolds, V. (2007). Nationwide satellite training for public health professionals: Web-based follow-up. *Journal of Continuing Education in the Health Professions, 27*(2), 111–117.

Perry, B. (2008). Shine on: Achieving career satisfaction as a registered nurse. *Journal of Continuing Education in Nursing, 39*(1), 17–25.

Pullen, D. L. (2006). An evaluative case study of online learning for healthcare professionals. *The Journal of Continuing Education in Nursing, 37*(5), 225–232.

Rick, C., Kearns, M. A., & Thompson, N. A. (2003). The reality of virtual learning for nurses in the largest integrated health care system in the nation. *Nursing Administration Quarterly, 27*(1), 41–57.

Russell, A., & Perris, K. (2003). Telementoring in community nursing: A shift from dyadic to communal models of learning and professional development. *Mentoring & Tutoring: Partnership in Learning, 11*(2), 227–238.

Senge, P. (1990). *The fifth discipline: The art and practice of the learning organization*. New York, NY: Currency Doubleday.

Shank, P. (2004, September 7). Can they do it in the real world? Designing for transfer of learning. *The e-Learning Developers' Journal*, 1–7.

Sheen, S., Chang, W., Chen, H., Chao, H., & Tseng, C. (2008) E-learning education program for registered nurses: The experience of a teaching medical center. *Journal of Nursing Research, 16(3)*, 195–200.

Slotte, V., & Herbert, A. (2006). Putting professional development online: Integrating learning as productive activity. *Journal of Workplace Learning, 18*(4), 235–247.

Spivey, D. (2009). The OODA loop and learning. *Chief Learning Officer, 8*(10), 30–33.

van Adelsberg, D., & Trolley, E. A. (1999). *Running training like a business: Delivering unmistakable value*. San Francisco, CA: Berrett-Koehler.

VanTiem, D. M., Moseley, J. L., & Conway Dessinger, J. (2004). *Fundamentals of performance technology: A guide to improving people, process, and performance* (2nd ed.). Silver Spring, MD: International Society for Performance Improvement.

Chapter 15

Technology Tools

Joann M. Oliver, MNEd, BSN, RN, CNE • Marie E. Oliver, AS, AA

During clinical post conference, the nurse educator asks the fundamentals registered nurse (RN) students to share components of their nursing care plans, incorporating a component from each student into an integrated care plan for a "composite" client. Students are asked to concept map the different aspects of nursing care without faculty guidance onto an interactive whiteboard. At the end of the session, a copy of the developed concept map is printed and given to the nursing students who are asked to post their reactions to this learning activity on the course's discussion board. One student's reaction, "When I got home from clinical, I was too tired to even think! But this morning when I looked at the concept map again—I got it! I did not realize the extent of the effect of this client's mild brain injury on both the physical and psychosocial aspects of this client's care and functioning!"

One of the difficulties in writing a chapter on technology tools is that in the current competitive market technology tools often become outdated after a short life span. One of the challenges facing the nurse educator is to attempt to select technology tools that will transcend these rapid changes and remain focused on the delivery of high-quality, learner-centered content (while staying within department budgets).

While acknowledging that this work is primarily concerned with e-learning, it is nonetheless beneficial to review technology tools that facilitate classroom learning environments as online courses may have face-to-face (f-2-f) lectures, seminars, testing, or directed laboratory components. In these learning environments, using technology tools may enhance and reinforce key concepts by allowing the nurse educator the opportunity to deliver content via additional mediums (i.e., audio, video, and electronic or print versions) that support online course content.

Implementing new technology related teaching tools can range from the simple to the complex. Although many technology tools are easily adapted to nursing instruction, the nurse educator may consider partnering with a technology consultant during the initial implementation. Despite the potential pitfalls of using unfamiliar technology, many do offer worthwhile benefits to the nurse educator and students.

The nurse educator may fear that despite careful advanced planning, the actual implementation of technology-based learning strategies will result in loss of actual teaching time because of a lengthy orientation to the tool or the need to troubleshoot and/or remediate for students who fail to understand or use the tool correctly. Careful advanced planning that includes a

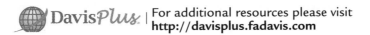 **DavisPlus** | For additional resources please visit http://davisplus.fadavis.com

thorough understanding of the tool's strengths and limitations often can be arranged with vendors to aid in managing the transition to an enhanced learning environment. Most companies are willing to provide custom training to faculty and will provide the same for nursing students who are using their products as well. Emphasis should be placed on phasing in the new tools in such a way as to not overload the faculty and students.

Finally, when implementing technology tools, the nurse educator needs to be open to the need to review learning objectives and revise outcome assessments so as to acknowledge and optimize the learning that technology tools facilitate for the nursing student.

The purpose of this chapter is to introduce nurse educators to some of the most commonly available technology tools. Through the discussion of the selected technology tool's features and applications, this chapter promotes the development of digitally savvy nurse educator.

TECHNOLOGY TOOLS FOR THE CLASSROOM ENVIRONMENT THAT ENHANCE CONTENT DELIVERY AND UTILIZATION

Interactive Whiteboards

Interactive whiteboards are touch-sensitive devices with imbedded or attached sensors that electronically convert what is "written" on the board into a digital image that can be displayed on an associated computer's monitor. They require a dedicated stylus or pen-type tool that must be used on the board's surface in order for the system to produce the computer image. The electronic content can then be saved to a file on the computer, archived, downloaded to an online teaching platform, or printed as a paper copy.

The interactive whiteboard requires little advanced preparation to use, and allows for highly interactive learning activities. It promotes active learning processes, involves social learning strategies that can be directed toward an entire class, and is a great teaching strategy to facilitate the learning of visual and kinesthetic learners.

Constructivism-based critical thinking activities such as concept mapping can be easily generated, modified, reviewed, saved, archived, and/or distributed following classroom-based interactions. Dosage calculation can be demonstrated, practiced, and saved for distribution or online "postings." Nursing process steps can be diagramed and learning outcomes can be assessed by providing nurse educators with the opportunity to observe the student's processing of required course material. Finally, the nurse educator can use this content generated on the interactive whiteboard to document the learner's progress and objective mastery for evaluative purposes.

Interactive whiteboards can greatly facilitate learning and information retention by providing the opportunity to retain copies of work, review materials presented and developed during class, document brainstorming sessions and track spontaneous outcomes of classroom learning activities. They can be used to balance the contributions of those class participants who are less verbal with their more verbal classmates by selectively assigning these learners the opportunity to represent themselves in writing or via images rather than verbally. Although some learners may express reluctance at working with whiteboard technology because they do not like to feel singled out, or be embarrassed should they may make a mistake in front of a classroom of peers, in general, whiteboards do facilitate learning when used to their fullest potential. Further, some whiteboard models provide an adaptive technology "writing tool" that can be used by the learner with physical disabilities thereby promoting a greater degree of interaction for them within the classroom setting.

TECHNOLOGY TIP 15.1

Interactive whiteboards are excellent resources on which to have nursing students develop mind maps or concept maps.

Students can work in small groups to create a concept map on the interactive whiteboard. Students could also place different steps in the nursing process on the board, and then show the relationships between the components using arrows and connecting lines. Have the students discuss and debate their choices until all of the participants are satisfied with the nursing care plan. The nursing educator can guide the learning with prompts only if the students are struggling. Information on interactive whiteboards can be found at: http://smarttech.com/ or http://www.luidia.com/products/ebeam-edge-for-education-page.html

Audience Response System Technology—Clickers

Clickers are handheld devices that allow the faculty to elicit inputs from the learners about specific questions posed during class either through PowerPoint presentations or other means. The most common use of clickers is eliciting multiple-choice responses to questions posed during classroom activities. Other types of data that can be obtained include responses to true/false, yes/no, ranking of item significance, and numeric or text entry, depending upon the response system used.

Audience response systems (ARSs) also can be used to poll learners to determine their level of critical thinking about content or to determine the level of background knowledge the learner has in a particular subject area. Clickers have been shown to motivate students, increase class attendance, and improve student course grades (Korvick, 2009). In the near future, smartphone technology will be linked to ARSs so that the learner may use the touch screen of their phones or other handheld devices to indicate their responses instead of using a separate clicker (Figs. 15.1 and 15.2).

Learners prefer this technology tool because it allows nursing faculty to analyze student understanding while retaining individual anonymity. It also allows the learner to analyze his or her own learning and comprehension before examinations or quizzes.

Smart Podiums

The smart podium provides the faculty with an efficient method of using and switching between various associated electronic or digital resources. Smart podiums usually consist of

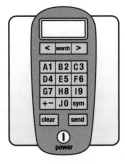

Figure 15.1 Clickers.

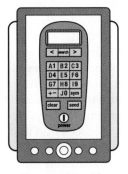

Figure 15.2 Phones as clickers.

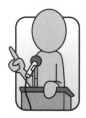

a computer, projector, monitor, digital video disc (DVD) player, document camera, and a touch-screen panel that functions as the control device for the system. The touch-screen controller allows the faculty to turn on and off projectors, select among data sources, and adjust sound settings on speakers. The document camera uses high-resolution technology to project the image of an object or document in real time. Although document cameras are normally used to project pages or information from textbooks, they can just as easily be used to project three-dimensional (3-D) items, such as anatomical models or client care-related equipment or supplies.

The advantage of teaching in a classroom with this technology tool is the ease with which the nurse educator can switch between the computer, DVD player, document camera, and any other media source without having to access that device's specific controls or controller. When coupled with screen capture video, this allows the educator to generate a student-oriented multimedia presentation that can be reproduced as needed to meet curricular and program outcomes.

DISTANCE LEARNING CLASSROOMS

Distance learning refers to educational experiences that occur when the instructor and learner are not physically located in the same setting. Strategies for electronic delivery of remote course learning content are becoming readily available with user-friendly low-tech interfaces. With affordable, high-tech options becoming increasing available many institutions of higher education and patient care facilities are opting to incorporate distance learning into their learning management system. Through careful selection of course content and instructional design, the nurse educator can optimize the learning experience (see Chapters 3 and 11).

Videoconferencing Systems

Live distance learning offers the nurse educator the opportunity to communicate content to learners in the live classroom setting while simultaneously interacting with the learners who are located at remote sites. The educator in the live distance learning classroom is referred to as the lead teacher, while the remote sites have a faculty or staff member who is responsible for assisting learners in the remote classrooms. Videoconferencing classrooms need to have controllers/computers, multiple cameras, display screens or projectors, and audio equipment for processing and sending audio, video, and electronic documents between locations. Cameras placed in the front and rear of the classroom, along with strategically placed monitors allow learners and educators to interact with each other during class. Microphones allow for communication between the faculty and learners thus promoting "regular" classroom interactions. Local and remote controls allow the lead teacher to manage the technology interface thus facilitating educational activities occurring in the classroom.

There are advantages and limitations of videoconferencing classroom systems. The greater the experience the nurse educator has with the videoconferencing classroom system, the better the transitions between media formats and the more fluid the classroom activities will be. Even the experienced lead teacher needs to practice ahead of time with the videoconferencing technology tools to ensure continuity in the teaching learning process and to maintain his or her expertise in handling the requisite technology tools. Hardware and software support needs to be readily available to the lead teacher and at the remote locations should technical difficulties arise.

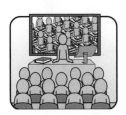

To facilitate student interactions, seat arrangement in live distance learning classrooms needs to allow optimal viewing of the students by the cameras mounted in preset positions. Likewise, monitors need to be located so that all learners are able to clearly view classroom demonstrations. Faculty need to be cognizant that because demonstrations are being broadcast in a two-dimensional (2-D) media, the remote learner may not receive the same benefit from the demonstration as the live classroom learner. Compensation for this limitation can be made during the demonstration of procedures by providing all learners with a clear field of view, performing the demonstration with a slight exaggeration of hand movements, and by repeating the procedure with the cameras set from multiple angles.

When moving between lecture content, document sharing, and interactions that are occurring in the distance learning classroom, the faculty needs to attend to monitors and respond promptly to learner cues. Microphones need to be positioned to maximize audio pickup while not impeding the communication process. Some distance learning systems have the capability of muting input from the student microphones thus minimizing extraneous noise from nonverbal paper rustling, and student movement that can result in distraction within the learning environment. When classroom noise muting is in effect a signaling system then needs to be available to the remote learners to indicate that they have a question or comment. Such a system also aids the learner in remote classrooms who are reluctant to interrupt the flow of instruction or call attention to him- or herself. The faculty or staff member who is located at the remote site also can serve this function.

Distance learning classroom environments can meet a variety of learning styles, preferences, and needs. Individuals with social or verbal learning styles enjoy the interaction within the classroom. This synchronous learning environment appeals to extrinsically motivated learners by addressing their needs for interaction and participation. Incorporating multimedia will appeal to the auditory and visual learners. When used to demonstrate procedures and nursing skills, this learning environment supports the preferences of the tactile and kinesthetic learner (Hrastinski, 2008).

In addition to regularly scheduled classes, the distance learning classroom can be used for videoconferencing. It provides an excellent medium for grand rounds, conferences, Webinars, and case studies. When using video-capture technology (i.e., recording), content presented in distance learning classroom can be archived for future distribution and review. See Table 15.1 for Live Distant Learning "Classroom Readiness" Checklist.

SUPPLEMENTS TO CLASSROOM, LABORATORY, OR CLINICAL LEARNING ACTIVITIES

Web 2.0 Tools

Web 2.0 Tools offer many opportunities to enhance learning in nursing education. These include blogs, instant messaging, podcasts, RSS feeds, and Wikis. Other Web 2.0 Tools also can be incorporated in the learning management system by the nurse educator to assist the learner organize, coordinate, and integrate content.

TABLE 15.1	
Live Distant Learning "Classroom Readiness" Checklist	
Done	**Task or Activity**
	Begin checklist 10–15 minutes before the session is scheduled to begin.
	Turn on all equipment.
	Check audio equipment: Microphones, speakers, or headphones; set volume.
	Check video equipment: Set camera locations, zooms, and monitors.
	Determine that distance learning classrooms audio and video are turned on and ready to function.
	Set the "Student wishes to speak" option to be notified when participants want to speak; set video cameras to view distance classes.
	Set audio to mute.
	Load multimedia files and other course materials.
	Close all nonessential applications.
	Check recording equipment if planning to record session; set to standby.
	Practice any skills or demonstrations ahead of time to determine best camera angles for viewing; note settings for later use.
	Begin class on time.
	Note: Always have a number of technical services on hand, just in case.

RSS Feeds

Rich site summary or really simple syndication (RSS) is a format that lets users subscribe to frequently updated online content using an RSS "reader" or "aggregator." RSS feeds allow for extensible markup language (XML) formatted content to be automatically downloaded to the user's computer or handheld device and to existing online learning platforms or course management systems. This creates a mechanism for educators to readily share information with the learners enrolled in their classes, clinical laboratories, or clinical sites. RSS downloads may consist of blogs, headlines, audio or video "feeds," or channels. RSS is an excellent vehicle for distributing frequently used content by the nurse educator. It also can serve as an online repository of course-related materials and content (EDUCAUSE Learning Initiative, 2007). RSS content includes the added benefit of frequently using metadata formats.

When using RSS as a technology tool, the educator needs to identify Web sites that contain content that is most useful, reliable, and trustworthy for inclusion in his or her course. Increasingly RSS feeds are being used in education to include college or university wide news, course content, resources, and blogs. RSS feeds can be used by educators and learners as a technology tool to provide a location where pertinent journal and online resource can be delivered and maintained. The communication of learning resources and content could be integrated into the learner's primary e-mail, as a component of a Web-based course delivery system.

To access an XML file for download to an RSS feed reader, the user has to enter the universal resource locator (URL) into the RSS "search line" on the receiving computer or handheld device, or by clicking on the universal RSS icon on the desired document.

Web 2.0 Tools as Online Personal Information Organizers

Web 2.0 Tools have the distinctive ability to allow the user to interact within the online environment to manage and organize data. Web 2.0 participants can create virtual online communities where members can engage in collective thought and shared ideas and where physical distance is no boundary (Hazari, North, & Moreland, 2009). Additional Web 2.0 Tools, such as digital "Post-it" note-card generators and discussion sites allow students to reframe didactic content, create concept maps, construct theories within single courses, and retain content over multiple courses within their nursing curriculum.

The nurse educator can promote use of Web 2.0 Tools by preselecting Web sites that articulate with learning outcome goals. Many Web 2.0 Tools promote interactive learning and resource sharing. This also gives learners the opportunity to explore the use of these tools as professionals would in the health-care industry. Because of Health Insurance Portability and Accountability (HIPAA) requirements, this is important as many learners do not understand how to apply patient privacy principles to Web 2.0 and social media.

As the learners interact and share insights, the participating community of self-selected (or assigned) learners actively pool knowledge, master skills, produce, and learn content. Alag has described this process as creating a situation where "collective" intelligence occurs (2008).

Faculty can also use Web 2.0 Tools to provide "scaffolding," or structure for a learning activity, while requiring the learner to interact in the f-2-f or online line learning environment to meet specific course learning objectives. The learner's level of engagement in the process is reinforced by the social interaction and thereby enhances learning. Multiple perspectives can be attained and critical thinking/clinical reasoning skills improved through the processes of relating, interacting, and evaluating content. Millennial learners are active participants in social networks and appreciate incorporation into their learning environments. The use of Web 2.0 Tools would have the greatest appeal to the nursing student who is a social, logical, and physical learner.

Metadata

The term *metadata* is used to describe how a specific set of data or information is managed, catalogued, or stored. Corporate and educational institutions may use metadata to manage resources, database, and organize electronically stored information. Libraries may use metadata to catalog information. Metadata may be used to denote descriptive aspects of databases and flowcharts, such as the number of characters per row or the number of fields per table. Metadata can be stored external to the data it relates to or it can be embedded in the electronic document itself.

Metadata formats also can be used to identify data associated to the primary content area of a document. Hypertext markup language (HTML) formats for metadata, as when used in RSS feeds, allow for keywords to be embedded within the text of the feed. When this is the case, these keywords often are in bold or highlighted text and can serve to clarify content or link to related information. Metadata links can be used by the learner to review vocabulary, concepts, investigate subject matter more fully, and connect to additional resources or authors on a particular subject depending upon the metadata format and links of the content.

Metadata can be used to aide in the development of a test bank for a nursing program or consortium of programs linking test question content to learning outcome objectives or specific concepts in client care.

Legal issues have arisen when documents and files with imbedded metadata content inadvertently reveal details that identify individuals or violate personal privacy. This occurs due to the distribution of data that has not been properly "wiped" of internally imbedded metadata parameters (Pelman, 2009).

PORTABLE DEVICES AND DOWNLOADABLE SOFTWARE

There are a wide variety of handheld devices on the market with increasing diversity to meet the needs of a technologically demanding consumer. Although operating systems vary according to the type of device and manufacturer, the devices often incorporate many similar or overlapping features. Handheld devices offer the nursing profession the opportunity to deliver client care more safely and efficiently. In nursing education, handheld devices can serve to aid and enhance student learning and promote the delivery of high-quality client care through the application of knowledge gained using handheld devices and downloadable software.

The process of deciding to incorporate handheld technology into a nursing curriculum can be daunting for the educator who has limited personal experience with using such devices as part of their learning management system. One of the most critical steps in this decision-making process includes articulating the role of the device as it is intended to be used to support student learning and progression within the curriculum (see *Incorporating Handheld Technology* in Davis Plus Online). Attention to the process of selecting and implementing a handheld device will aid the nurse educator in achieving his or her implementation and utilization goals. Additional steps include the determination as to whether specific software is to be used, or if the learner is to be provided with "specifications" that he or she needs to meet in his or her selection of "open-source" materials. Technical support and training on the device may be a significant consideration depending upon the device and capabilities of the users. Funding for the devices for the faculty and students also may be significant considerations. If the device and software are required for the student to purchase, the effect on the learner's financial aid should be considered. If on the other hand, the

TECHNOLOGY TIP 15.2

Do a Web search on Web 2.0 and click on the Videos tab. Watch a few videos that describe Web 2.0. Share a video with your students and ask them about the effect on health care and nursing in particular.

device is distributed to students by the nursing program, then responsibility for software, tracking of devices, and technical support needs to be considered. Some programs charge students additional fees and others seek grants to help cover the costs (see Chapter 4, The Strategic Plan).

The nursing department will want to consider how students will be perceived during clinical experiences when they are observed with handheld devices while providing patient care. Explanations and open discussions with health-care facility staff and administrators can help educate colleagues and avoid misunderstandings. Some nursing programs may even offer to provide staff in-services about the use of handheld devices as a way of partnering with clinical agencies. Faculty need to determine policies for use of PDAs, sanctions for misuse, and guidelines for the classroom (to include examinations), clinical and laboratory environments. Openly discussing these policies helps promote professionalism in the students related to technology.

Currently available Internet connectable devices with personal digital assistant (PDA) capabilities include the BlackBerry, the iPod Touch, Droid, iPad, Samsung Galaxy, and others. PDA components are being merged into sophisticated smartphones of all types. Book readers and notepads or tablets also are popular because of their portability and the ease of use for their intended function. These handheld devices need to be charged via a cable or universal serial bus (USB) connection and can be synchronized and updated as noted. Each category of device will be addressed in turn.

PERSONAL DIGITAL ASSISTANTS

The classic version of the PDA had a user interface that allowed data (i.e., calculator, calendar, tasks, notes, contact information, etc.) to be entered into the device by the user (Zurmehly, 2010). Furthermore, the "old" PDAs could be synchronized with a computer either via cable or wirelessly to download compatible software that could then be viewed at a later time. Currently the phrase PDA has come to encompass most nonphone handheld devices that have downloadable, Web-based content. These devices also can be used as MP3 players (educational podcasting or entertainment), global positioning system (GPS), calendars, handheld games, and serve many additional functions.

BlackBerry

The BlackBerry is a mobile e-device with a color screen and a QWERTY keyboard that allows for data input. A BlackBerry can be used in much the same manner as the older PDAs, but has the added feature of being able to access e-mail, send texts, and automatically download available software and software updates when an Internet connection is available. Newer versions also may have such features as a Web browser, MP3 player, video player, camera, GPS, and RSS feed support. Internet access is via cable or wireless network and smartphone capabilities.

iPod Touch

The Apple iPod Touch evolved from the iPod, which originally was an audio media player. Current iPod Touch devices have a touch-screen display for data input, play music and videos, and contain standard PDA features, such as a calendar, clock, contacts, etc.

Apple products use "apps" or applications from the Apple iTunes store as a way of adding software and functionality to the iPod Touch. Many of the Apple apps are free to the user. The iPod Touch is available with different amounts of memory. It does not have an expansion slot for a memory storage card. Synchronization of the device to a computer occurs via a cable or by connecting to a wireless network with software downloads occurring automatically when an Internet connection becomes available.

The case of use of the iPod Touch coupled with the flexibility, storage capacity, and accessibility of materials available to promote student learning has made the iPod Touch and similar devices popular as the go-to handheld device for use by faculty and learners.

With the inclusion of PDA technology and apps on handheld devices, it appears to the author that students are even more willing to be engaged with the technology. Davenport states that PDAs allow nurses to be more effective and organized by providing them with access to material and content that aides in efficiently organizing client care needs, and track treatments 265and assessments as they are done (2004). Nursing students benefit in the classroom and clinical setting by having rapid access to information about medications, laboratory data, nursing care, and client conditions thus enabling them to better formulate and review care plans while gaining insights into the complexities of client conditions (Zurmehly, 2010).

Anecdotal experience had demonstrated that, as in other areas of nursing, faculty that model and promote the use of handheld devices have students that use their handheld devices to the highest degree. When this technology tool is introduced to fundamental nursing students, along with a structured approach to its contents and applications, the learner's response to using the handheld device is consistently positive and students are observed to be actively engaged using this tool in the clinical learning environment.

SMARTPHONES

Smartphones are a hybrid mix of PDA and cellular or mobile phone technologies. Some PDAs have telephone capabilities, such as the Palm Pre or the HTC Droid. Cellular phones, such as the HTC Droid have incorporated the capabilities of a PDA into its operating systems, and have eight megapixel cameras, front videoconferencing camera, Gmail, YouTube, GPS with Google Maps plus built-in Microsoft (MS) Exchange support, Bluetooth, and Wi-Fi. Smartphones are manufactured by wide variety of companies and commonly have one of the following identifying words in their name: Symbian, Windows, Palm, BlackBerry, iPhone, or Android Google. A few smartphones offer handwriting recognition. Others have data input through a touch screen or "slide-out," thumb-sized QWERTY keyboard (see Fig. 15.3).

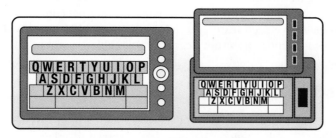

Figure 15.3 Smartphone keyboards.

Service contracts that allow smartphones to access the Internet, allow the user to download software directly or through apps that enable the process. Synchronizations of documents, calendars, and tasks with a computer is another PDA function that smartphones provide. In addition, many smartphones are video capable, MP3 compatible, and contain GPS navigation systems.

SOFTWARE AND DOWNLOADS FOR HANDHELD DEVICES AND SMARTPHONES

Many companies offer content specific to nursing for handheld devices. These downloads may consist of textbooks, standards of care, clinical calculators, or reference materials. These tools can address client conditions, treatments, or nursing care considerations. Content from some content companies is "bundled" and contains metadata tags throughout that links data to related content areas and additional resources. This feature allows the user to explore topics in greater depth and provides access to linked data about the subject without needing to actively close one program to open and access a different content source for additional information.

Companies that offer PDA-specific software include Skyscape, Epocrates, Pepid and others. One software bundle by Skyscape, *Nursing Constellation* includes drug and laboratory guides, clinically applicable nursing content, a medical calculator, guides to procedures and diseases, and tools that include a variety of other resources. Topics are searchable by index and table of contents within their respective tabs. Navigation buttons allow the user to move between pages, which are displayed in a linear manner. A process for evaluating PDAs with software can be found online in Davis Plus.

There also are many open-source downloads for the PDA and smartphone user. Using a search engine to locate "free nursing PDA smartphone downloads" results in a large variety of sites that provides free tools for handheld devices. Some of these sites offer free software and resources, while other offer free trial downloads of their products along with paid subscriptions. One such site, Epocrates, offers free downloads of drug information, which includes a drug interaction guide.

Additional software may be available from textbook publishers who offer companion software (such as skills videos) with their nursing textbooks. It is common for publishers of reference type textbooks, such as nursing dictionaries, drug guides, laboratory manuals, etc., to include a downloaded compact disk (CD) with the textbook that can be installed on the handheld device.

PDA software can be purchased by subscription lasting 1 or 2 years, allowing the user to have access to all updates and revisions that occur within the time frame of the subscription. The greater the number of features, downloaded items, and internal links within the software program, the greater the cost for the subscription. If the user opts for a onetime download without updates, the cost of the book or resource is usually similar to the cost of the paper edition.

To download the purchased software for a device that is not wireless involves several steps that begin with loading device software onto the user's computer. This software then acts as a desktop manager and conduit between the online software site and the PDA. The user will need to create an account with the company from which the software is purchased to access user or unlock codes, provide the software company with information about the serial number of the device on which to download the subscription's content, and to register products. Downloading is managed through the desktop manager associated with the PDA or directly by the handheld device itself. Moving software from one device to another usually requires a transfer of information by the technology support division of the software company and cannot be done independently by the software user.

E-READERS: E-BOOK READERS, TABLETS, KINDLES, AND NOOKS

In selecting specific technologies for nursing students, it may be extremely helpful for the learner to have a lightweight, electronic way to carry reference information with them. While handheld devices and smartphones seem to be the preferred method of accessing this information, electronic books also can be used. Kindles and other e-book readers are larger than a PDA-style handheld device and although their initial application was for personal entertainment and convenience of use, their potential for use as a handheld nursing resource could be realized in the near future. Their screens tend to have limited color availability or may be just grayscale and many allow searching a document for a specific word or phrase. The major downside of electronic books is that the desired information must already be in an electronic format, such as an e-book or in a portable document format (PDF). In addition, electronic books often have proprietary formats that can be hard to manipulate or require a computer to convert the original electronic format.

E-book readers, tablets, Amazon's Kindle, Barnes & Noble's Nook, and the Apple iPad are mobile devices that can be used to download and view e-books, including textbooks and other digital media. The batteries of these technology tools come in a variety of sizes and forms and often limit the amount of time the device can be used without an external power source. Some of these devices are the size of a PDA and others are the size of a netbook. All are considered portable; although the size of the device will dictate how portable it actually is for the user. In general, e-readers have Internet connectivity and most are powered by at least a 500-MHz RAM processor (as are PDAs, smartphones, and many calculators). This connectivity allows some e-readers a level of functionality equal to a netbook computer. This current generation of devices can have a touch screen; some have sliding keyboards as well.

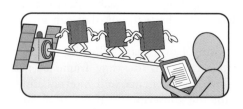

The Amazon Kindle has a keyboard input and screen that displays in 16 shades of gray. The Apple iPad and the Barnes and Noble Nook are the newest additions to this grouping of handheld devices. The Nook is an e-book reader that has a small color touch screen for data input.

The Apple iPad is a small tablet computer that runs on a modified operating system used by the iPhone and iPod touch that is intended for personal entertainment, which also can function as an e-book reader. It has a touch screen and works in all planes supporting content in portrait and landscape orientations. It is not intended to compete with laptop computers or table computers, it is intended to bridge the technology "gap" between the current PDA-style device and the fully functional computer.

Most of these devices originally had their own file formats—.AZW (Amazon.com), .TXT, and .MOBI, and separate downloadable materials, but now almost all support PDF downloads as well. For downloaded books the formats used depends on the specific devices.

Downloads are achieved over a USB connection or via wireless networks. The currently available smartbook technology, depending upon the device and platform version, allows the user to bookmark text, hyperlink to other content, and quickly search a large number of documents for key words and previous bookmarks.

The actual screen size and device capabilities are important features to consider if selecting from this category of handheld devices. Most of these portable devices have video players and can allow the user to download video content, such as lectures, client care procedures, nursing conference proceedings, Webinars, and other pertinent learning resources. The networked aspect of these devices can help support asynchronous or distance learners by engaging them in videoconferenced and other Web-based video content.

Besides downloading e-books and files, many of these technology tools have online search capability. Because of the popularity and marketability of these products, manufacturers have made available a wide variety of applications and more are soon to be released. In addition, manufacturers are seeking to produce e-readers with even more powerful processors that will allow their devices to operate full 3-D software. This software will allow the user to rotate, flip, and resize screen content to optimize viewing and allow for multiple open screens simultaneously as with the iPad. Such technology will offer the inventive educator and learner unlimited opportunity to imagine and apply content. One example of upcoming technology will be the linking of an image that has been downloaded to the device from a camera or other source with descriptive information that is available through an online search (e.g., taking a picture of a pill that results in the identification of the drug alone with pharmacological information and nursing considerations for the client taking it). Another example presented to the author that will soon be available to the learner would be to look at a wound through the camera of his or her portable device, have overlaid on this image information about assessment parameters for it, suggest appropriate wound care, project the expected rate or progress of wound healing, and recommend the appropriate document for all of these nursing care steps.

SECOND LIFE AS A LEARNING ENVIRONMENT

"Second Life is the leading virtual world development platform for the creation of virtual goods and immersive, engaging and productive 3-D spaces used by individuals, artists, corporations, governments, academic institutions and nonprofits" (Copyright, Linden Research, Inc., 2009 all rights reserved). The adoption of Second Life as a teaching tool has been widely debated and discussed by many educators. For the nongaming world, Second Life is a massively multiplayer online role-playing game (MMORPG). It has enormous potential for use as a technology tool. Synchronously and asynchronously online classes can be hosted through Second Life (see Fig. 15.4). Some nursing programs have created a virtual skills laboratory that resembles a hospital room complete with a virtual patient. The learner can then interact within the virtual environment using tools and equipment as he or she would in the actual skills laboratory, perform nursing procedures and physical assessments, or respond to prescribed or instructor guided scenarios.

To use Second Life, an "island" would have to be purchased on which to build the virtual learning environment. The development of the Second-Life teaching environment requires considerable advance planning because an enormous amount of time and effort is involved in creating the virtual world environment for learning. It has been suggested that engineering,

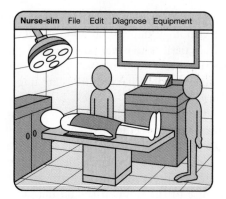

Figure 15.4   Virtual Reality Healthcare.

computer technology, or graphic arts students be engaged in the process of designing the Second-Life environment as a project for their advanced-level classes.

The individual who participates in Second Life is represented by a character called an avatar, which is accessible immediately upon logging in for the first time. The avatar is located in a place called Orientation Island. This island is where the novice avatar completes various tutorials that help familiarize them with the Second-Life program and interface. Information in the beginning tutorials includes how to customize the avatar and familiarizes the user with the various methods of moving around in the Second-Life universe. Familiarization with the environment and the Second-Life avatar can take some time and completing all the tutorials on Orientation Island takes 1 to 2 hours. See the Web bonus Chapter 18 for further discussion on virtual reality in health-care education.

SUPPLEMENTAL TEACHING CONTENT FROM TEXTBOOK PUBLISHERS

It has become increasingly common for the publishers of nursing textbooks to generate interactive learning activities that coordinate with textbook content. These supplemental activities may be made available to the learner on a companion CD or online via a dedicated site that requires a pass code or log-in to access. Traditionally included in companion resources are National Council Licensure Examination (NCLEX)-style questions, case studies, and critical thinking activities. Increasingly, publishers are expanding the focus of companion material for their textbooks to include interactive learning activities.

Teaching Tools: Client Case Scenarios

One such style of activity consists of client care scenarios with focused queries that guide the learner to develop insights into clinical conditions and to develop clinical reasoning and judgment. These scenarios can be used as classroom learning strategy or as independent learning activities. The character(s) written in the scenarios may be developed progressively over the course of time. It is the intent of many publishers for nursing students to use the text-accompanying products throughout the curriculum from the fundamental nursing courses with simple scenarios to increasing complexity nursing care as the student progresses through the nursing curriculum to the level of a graduate nurse. Nursing students are expected to respond to questions and prompts related to the scenario and manage the nursing care needed within the evolving client scenarios. Clinical reasoning is promoted through this interactive case study approach, which appeals to individual learners with virtually all learning styles.

Some publishers also have learning sites that are independent and require a separate fee to use them. The *Neighborhood* by Pearson Health Science is one such site. The *Neighborhood* contains 36 scenarios for use throughout the nursing curriculum. Elsevier also has a scenario-based learner site, called *Nurse Squared* that includes an electronic medical record. Separate electronic medical record programs also are available for purchase as stand-alone software for use in laboratory-based skill laboratories and during simulations.

INTERACTIVE CONTENT PRESENTATION

The technology tools used for nonclassroom-based distance learning may include many of the same tools used in online education. Distance learning may be synchronous, such as a Webinar or a single professional development program, or it may be asynchronous with previously presented and recorded learning content that has been archived for later broadcast. These formats allow the learner to review the content at his or her own pace and post questions to faculty through the course learning system. Delivery of such course content frequently occurs via a document or slide-show presentation, sometimes with voice-over slide features as provided by PowerPoint, Adobe Captivate, or comparable systems.

Synchronous versions of the technology tools that support the delivery of nonclassroom educational content often include audio (i.e., Skype), the ability of the learner and educator to communicate via text messages; the ability of the instructor and student to "write" on the associated whiteboard; instructor-controlled permissions that enable or disable such features as viewing the text communications of all participants, turning the microphone on for student-audio input (if audio is a component of the software); and polling features. In addition, some of these distributive technology tools, such as *Elluminate Live*, contain multiple screens that the nurse educator can use for the placement of multiple course documents and associated learning materials (see Fig. 15.5).

Audio capabilities vary from tool to tool and may use a headphone/microphone combination. Other systems use teleconferencing as the source for audio exchange during the synchronous presentation. Microphones can be muted by the presenter to prevent room noises from interfering with the audio quality.

Asynchronous learning options allow the learner time to reflect and process concepts, supporting logical and solitary learning styles. When used to model and promote psychomotor learning, online media supports the tactile and kinesthetic learner who can repeat and model behaviors again and again.

TECHNOLOGY TIP 15.3

Faculty should consider having students use the EMR for classroom and homework-based assignments. This allows them to actively synthesize the concepts being taught. When they enter data about the lecture material in an EMR, they are performing the same actions the professional does to document competent care. Students should be reminded of HIPAA requirements if actual patient scenarios are used to complete EMR activities. Overall, this realistic activity makes learning more engaging and memorable.

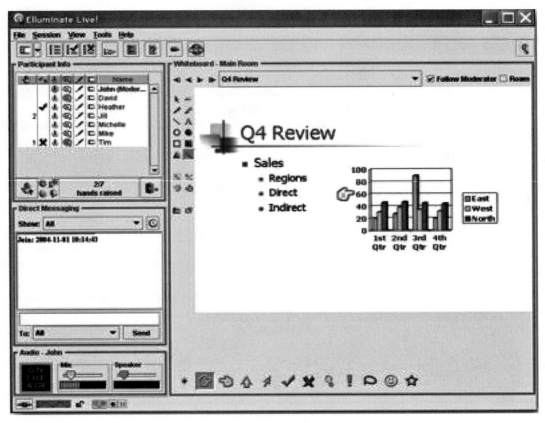

Figure 15.5 *Elluminate Live.*

AUDIO AND VIDEO CAPTURE: RECORDING OF LEARNING CONTENT

Audio recording of learning content can be readily created using widely available software ranging from MP3 recorders to elaborate software that allows for digital editing and remixing (see Table 15.2).

Screen-capture technology tools offers the nurse educator the opportunity to video record content for presentation at a later time. These technology tools afford the learner the opportunity to review content at his or her own pace and as often as he or she desires,

TECHNOLOGY TIP 15.4

Adding voice to PowerPoint slides can be learned through free tutorials on the Internet. One great site is www.office.microsoft.com. Search for "voice over" in the Help and How-to sections.

TABLE 15.2	
Keys to Creating a Podcast	
1. Content	• Chunking is best. • One concept per podcast. • 5–15 minutes.
2. Hardware	• Inexpensive microphone. • Most laptops have external microphones. • Headset for hands free.
3. Software	• Audacity-http://audacity.sourceforge.net/ • Yodio.com—http://yodio.com/ • PodBean.com—http://www.podbean.com/
4. Host	• School or University Server. • PodBean.com. • Yodio.com. • iTunes U.
5. Delivery style	• No Hollywood required/be yourself. • Turn off phone/fax; hang do not disturb sign. • Have drinking water nearby. • Track recording time.
6. Student access	• Instructions are clear. • Easy to access (keep bit rate low for MP3). • Available offline (burn CD).
7. Consider	• Talk to tech department. • Partner with students. • Test-drive your podcasts.

much as the learner who uses an audio recorder to review content at a later time. Nurse educators who frequently repeat the same lectures or content can benefit from providing recorded content to the learner, while better using the f-2-f time with their students to review concepts and emphasize key content.

TECHNOLOGY TIP 15.5

One faculty colleague has used a Webcam to record brief video clips (usually under 3 minutes in length) that describe a concept as an introduction to the current learning unit or to clarify the student's "muddiest point." Most basic Webcams work just fine for this purpose (expensive equipment is not required).

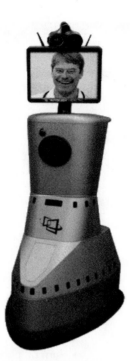

Figure 15.6   Remote faculty presence robot.

REMOTE PRESENCE ROBOTS IN NURSING EDUCATION

Remote presence robots consist of cart-mounted, mobile Webcams that link individuals for the purpose of interacting (see Fig. 15.6). Medical education has used remote presence robots to interview clients and allow participation at learning conferences and grand rounds.

The implication for use of remote presence robots in nursing education can be tremendous. Learners could access clients for interview purposes or to review care goals with them, observe procedures in real time, and actively participate in video care-planning rounds.

Distance learning centers could use this technology to "bring" remotely located learners to the clinical site to be "involved" with client care activities. Community health centers and clients could be more readily available to learners via Webcams, and teleconferencing.

The remotely activated and managed mobile technology can cost $250,000 per unit and does require a skilled operator to respond to client and equipment needs (Sloane, 2008). Less expensive tabletop units also are available as are simple Webcams with phone connectivity and/or teleconferencing for a low-tech approach to providing learners with access to opportunities to interact with clients, faculty, and health-care professionals.

CONCLUSION

Faculty need to be aware of and acknowledge that learners in their classrooms (whether online or f-2-f) are often very technologically savvy. Our learners are ready and eager for handheld technology and the use of technology tools in their classrooms.

Nursing students respond very favorably to content that is presented to them in multi-media formats, and may have had experience with interactive whiteboards, clickers, and other learning technologies from their high school or previous college classes. Most already own smartphones and MP3 players and are familiar with their use. And many of our learners are equally comfortable with reading content from a monitor or from a printed textbook. In fact, learners with diverse learning styles relate to handheld devices because the devices allow the learner to manipulate the software content in a sequence and manner that promotes a personalized approach to their accumulation of information that complements their personal learning style. These manipulations then support the learner's use of content and the subsequent critical thinking, which facilitates the transition from novice student to the nursing role. Handheld devices offer the nurse educator and the learner a wide array of options that serve to promote the development of clinical reasoning and nursing judgment. Handheld devices provide nurse educators with the need to establish departmental policies and standards for the use of devices in health-care setting that have wireless networks. Faculty need to clearly articulate expectations to learners concerning texting and use of phones during learning activities. Reinforcement of HIPAA, especially confidentiality expectations, needs to be an integral component of these discussions. In addition, the importance of behavior expected of a professional nursing student and acceptable uses of handheld devices during instruction time whether in the classroom, the skills laboratory, or the clinical site must be clearly articulated.

Many nursing faculty have highly developed skill sets related to using technology teaching tools. Some faculty, on the other hand, may be reluctant to alter their paradigms to incorporate newer learning technologies into their classrooms, laboratory sessions, or student clinical experiences. Lack of familiarity with the technical aspects of a device or technology tool is certainly a component of this reluctance, lack of faculty time to thoroughly learn the nuances of the related technology, lack of (or perceived lack of) technical support, lack of support from colleagues, lack of readily accessible funding for technology tools, and an unwillingness to be viewed as "less than" an expert at teaching are all reasons that nursing educators have given for their reluctance to step into the next generation of teaching technology.

Care and planning needs to occur to support the nursing faculty's acceptance of the implementation and comprehensive use of these technology tools. Establishing a technology implementation task group to review faculty skill sets, determine the availability of technology support, and review available hardware and software related tools is the first step toward meeting the goal of producing a technologically savvy graduate nurses who are ready to use available technology to support and enhance their professional nursing practices.

REFERENCES

Alag, S. (2008) *Collective intelligence in action*. Greenwich, CT: Manning Publications.

Hrastinski, S. (2008). Asynchronous and synchronous e-learning: A study of asynchronous and synchronous e-learning methods discovered that each supports different purpose. *Educause Quarterly*, *31*(1). Retrieved from http://www-cdn.educause.edu/EDUCAUSE+Quarterly/EDUCAUSEQuarterlyMagazineVolum/AsynchronousandSynchronousELea/163445

Interactive whiteboards and learning improving student learning outcomes and streamlining lesson planning. (2010). SMART Technologies ULC. Retrieved from http://www2.smarttech.com/

Korvick, L. (2009). *The net generation and audience response system technology* from http://www.liveclasstech.com/Pedagogy.aspx

Robson, R. Mobile learning and handheld devices in the classroom. Corvallis, OR: Eduworks Corporation. Retrieved from http://www.eduworks.com/Documents/Publications/Mobile_Learning_Handheld_Classroom.pdf

Sloane, M. M. (2008). Remote-presence robot attends patients at Ryder Trauma Center. *Nursing Spectrum–Florida News*. Retrieved from http://news.nurse.com/apps/pbcs.dll/article?AID=200880415010

Understanding Metadata. (2004) *National Information Standards Organization*. Retrieved from http://www.niso.org/publications/press/UnderstandingMetadata.pdf

Zurmehly, J. (2010). Personal digital assistants (PDAs): Review and evaluation. *Nursing Education Perspectives, 31*(3), 179–182.

Chapter 16

Simulation

Sharon Decker, PhD, MSN, RN • Teresa Gore, DNP, FNP-BC, NP-C • Cheryl Feken, RN, MS

Critical incidents during feedback sessions can initiate the faculty's own reflective thinking related to his/her personal skills. For example, during a feedback session using Socratic Questioning and posed statement (guided reflection) a student became extremely restless. She crossed and uncrossed her legs, looked up at the ceiling, and even "moaned." I became irritated and almost interrupted her. But thankfully, before I made this drastic mistake, the student yelled out, "I figured it out—if I knew my pathophysiology everything would make sense!" The student had been critiquing herself and had just developed insight into her personal learning. As I reflected on my skills, I realize how close I had come to destroying this process.

Nurse educators are faced with multiple challenges including the charge to address (1) the integration of informatics into the curricula, (2) patient safety issues, (3) the multiple comorbidities of our patients, (4) the changing demographics of society, and (5) the complex, dynamic health-care environment. At the same time, we are asked to provide evidence to validate our teaching modalities while our students continue to demonstrate difficulty identifying problems and transferring knowledge to the patient care setting (Del Bueno, 2005; Finkelman & Kenner, 2007). Nurse educators often are heard expressing concerns related to their students as "They don't know, what they don't know," or "They don't see themselves as they really are."

A proposed solution to these challenges is the integration of simulated learning experiences throughout the curricula. Research demonstrates learners express high satisfaction with teaching methods that integrate simulation (Evidence-Based Practice Box 16.1) and the use of simulation promotes the development of knowledge (Evidence-Based Practice Box 16.2) (Howard, Ross, Mitchell, & Nelson, 2010; Smith & Roehrs, 2009), skills confidence (Evidence-Based Practice Box 16.3) (Bambini, Washburn, & Perkins, 2009; Gordon & Buckley, 2009), and critical and reflective thinking (Decker, 2007; Lasater, 2007). This chapter is based on the arguments that learning is (1) associated with evidence-based teaching techniques, (2) enhanced through active involvement, and (3) dependent upon the integration of experience and reflection. We believe that simulation, when integrated appropriately, provides a technique that addresses these arguments.

DavisPlus | For additional resources please visit
http://davisplus.fadavis.com

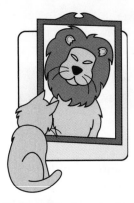

Figure 16.1 Impaired reflection.

EVIDENCE-BASED PRACTICE BOX 16.1

A quasi-experimental study used two instruments developed by the National League for Nursing (i.e., the Student Satisfaction and Self-Confidence in Learning Scale and the Simulation Design Scale) to identify student satisfaction with simulation as a teaching method. The overall mean score indicated that students were satisfied with the design characteristic of guided reflection being identified as having the highest value (Smith & Roehrs, 2009).

EVIDENCE-BASED PRACTICE BOX 16.2

A quasi-experimental, two-group, pre-/post-test design was used to compare the Health Education Systems, Inc. (HESI) scores of two educational interventions: human patient simulator (HPS) and interactive case studies. Learners who participated in the HPS intervention demonstrated a significantly higher positive perception of the learning experience and demonstrated greater understanding of concepts (Howard, Ross, Mitchell, & Nelson, 2010).

EVIDENCE-BASED PRACTICE BOX 16.3

A pairwise comparison analysis or postexperience self-efficacy scores demonstrated a significant increase in learner confidence in identified skills (i.e., performance with vital signs, breast examination, assessment of fundus, assessment of lochia, and patient teaching) after a simulated learning experience (Bambini, Washburn, & Perkins, 2009).

HISTORY

The creation of an environment or situation to practice and perfect skills has been used for centuries. Although not initially referred to as simulation, the earliest documented use of a simulated situation found was from the Roman Empire for military training. An example, of one such simulated situation consisted of a 6-foot wooden figure of an enemy solider armed with a shield and sword for jousting (Bradley, 2006). Simulation in aviation began around 1910 using the "penguin system" developed during World War I. Aviation has a long history using simulation to prepare military and commercial pilots. Nursing began using adult-sized mannequins in 1911 with the production of the first "Chase Hospital Doll" at the Hartford Hospital Training School for Nurses (Herrmann, 2000). Mrs. Chase, as she was often referred to, was used for demonstration purposes and on which student nurses could practice basic nursing skills. By 1914 a new improved adult-size Chase mannequin was developed, with an injection arm and other internal reservoirs permitting other treatments. In 1940, Chase male mannequins were developed at the request of the U.S. Army to assist in the training of medical corpsmen.

During the early 1960s, Resusci Anne was introduced. Resusci Anne was modeled after the "Girl from the River Seine" by Asmund S. Laerdal, a successful Norwegian manufacturer of plastic toys, to develop a realistic and effective training aid to teach mouth-to-mouth resuscitation (Cooper & Taqueti, 2004). Sim One, developed at the University of Southern California in the late 1960s, was the starting point for true computer-controlled simulation (Cooper & Taqueti, 2004). The simulator featured spontaneous ventilation, a heartbeat, temporal and carotid pulses, blood pressure, blinking eyes, muscle fasciculation, and a cough. When introduced in 1969, it was rejected as having no place in training, partly because computer technology was too expensive for commercialization. At the time, the prevailing belief was students had to practice on real patients; educational apprenticeship was believed to be the only model.

Dr. Michael Gordon refuted the belief of educational apprenticeship as the only model for training based on the growing use of flight simulators and Disney's then new audio animatronics. Thus, the development of Harvey was first demonstrated in 1968 at the American Heart Association Scientific Session by Dr. Gordon. Harvey was a full-sized mannequin that simulated 27 cardiac conditions. Over the next 30 years, the cost of simulators and associated technology prohibited the use of simulation in most educational programs. It was not until 1998 that simulation using advanced patient simulators appeared in the nursing literature as technology became more affordable (Cooper & Taqueti, 2004).

DEFINITIONS

To best maximize the simulation experience the creator needs a basic understanding of simulation and the components needed to create the best learning experience. These components include scenario, template, fidelity, roles, cues, and debriefing.

Simulation is an event developed to replicate some or nearly all of the essential aspects of a clinical situation so the experience may be more readily understood and managed when it occurs in the patient care setting (Morgan, 1995). Simulation has been described as a technique—not a technology. It is not designed to replace a clinical experience but to create real experiences that replicate substantial aspects of the real world (Gaba, 2004). The

National Council of State Boards of Nursing (2005) defined simulation as an educational process that imitates the working environment and requires the learner to demonstrate procedural techniques, decision making, and critical thinking. In addition, a simulated experience is composed of three parts; the prebriefing (introduction), the scenario (actual patient care activity), and the debriefing (planned feedback) session.

A scenario is described as a case study that depicts a real-life patient care situation. The scenario is the simulated event that may include but not limited to receiving of report, assessing the client, analysis of a variety of data, implementing interventions, evaluating outcomes, and collaborating with other health-care providers.

A template is a tool to assist faculty in organizing, developing, and conducting a simulation. The template includes the learning objectives and the cognitive and psychomotor skills needed for successful completion of the simulation. In addition, the template includes (1) the

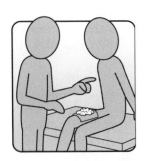

resources and equipment required to maximize the fidelity, (2) recommended mannequin responses to actions, (3) cues to assist the learner, (4) questions to be proposed during the scenario, and (5) guidelines for feedback. A variety of templates are available to assist you. For example, a scenario template is available at the National League for Nursing's Simulation Innovation Resource Center (http://www.sirc.nln.org) and on the Web sites of different companies, such as Laerdal (http://www.laerdal.com) and METI Learning (http://www.meti.com). Several regions and states have established simulation alliances and provide template examples on their Web sites. For example, the West Texas Simulation Alliance has a template available for use (requesting that the Alliance is acknowledged) at http://www.wtsaonline.org/

Fidelity refers to the extent to which a simulation mimics reality of the situation both in the environment and the mannequin. This may include the use of moulage to create wounds to provide visual cueing. Other items used to influence the fidelity include using cold packs and water sprayed onto the mannequin to represent diaphoresis. Items to maximize the reality of the environment include using appropriate medical equipment such as an IV pump. Fidelity also can refer to the type of mannequin being used and the complexity of the simulation itself.

Roles are the characters (i.e., patient, family, nurse, physician, and pharmacist) participants assume during a simulated experience. Depending on the focus of the simulation roles may be active or passive. Active roles may include nursing, physician, respiratory therapist, and family members. Participants may provide cues to guide the actions of other members in the simulation. Cues will be discussed later. Passive roles typically include some type of observation. This may include observing specific function such as communication and delegation or the sequence of interventions. A brief synopsis of the role and its responsibilities need to be included in the development of a simulation.

TECHNOLOGY TIP 16.1

For debriefing, consider having students reflect on the simulation event in an online discussion board. Have students find a professional journal article that serves as evidence for one of their nursing actions in the simulation.

Cues are assessment data, diagnostics or hints provided to direct or redirect the simulation. Cues may be used to remind participants what action needs to be taken. Such cues may be supplied by a participant in the simulation, such as a family member, a nurse supervisor, or even the simulator.

Debriefing is the planned feedback process of a simulated experience. This is a planned facilitated session where participants analyze their actions, address emotional reactions to the experience, and receive constructive input.

DEVELOPING SIMULATED LEARNING EXPERIENCES

Now that some of the basic definitions have been discussed, we will focus on developing simulated learning experiences using low, medium, and fidelity simulation. Development should be designed to meet the objectives, outcomes, and experience/educational level of the participants. The type of simulation, degree and style of prompting, and evaluation are determined by the objectives and outcomes desired from the participants and simulation experience. The objectives of the scenario should be consistent with the course objectives.

Faculty need to determine what learning experiences are appropriate for simulated activities. These might be situations the faculty identify that they want all their graduates to experience—situations that their students have minimal opportunities to experience related to the restriction placed by the agencies or the number of experience available due to the population served by agencies, or identified situations in which the patient could be placed at high risk. In addition, faculty might identify specific concepts or issues that should be integrated into all or most simulated experiences, such as patient safety, communication, resource management, prioritization, and a focused assessment.

A theoretical framework should be selected on which the simulated experience is developed, implemented, and evaluated. The authors use a modification of The Nursing Education Simulation Framework developed and tested through the National League for Nursing/Laerdal Simulation Study (Jeffries, 2007). This framework (Fig.16.2) identifies specific design characteristics to be integrated into a simulated experience: objectives, fidelity, problem-solving, student support, and debriefing.

A design template should be selected to assist in developing simulated learning experiences. Through use of a template, consistency is promoted for all participants and facilitators. Any scripting of dialogues from the simulator, family members, and health-care providers should be attached to this template. Table 16.1 lists recommended elements to be included in the template for designing a simulation.

TYPES OF SIMULATED LEARNING EXPERIENCES

Multiple simulation typologies are available to assist faculty in providing optimal learning experiences. The appropriate typology and fidelity should be selected to meet the objectives of the simulation. Table 16.2 provides a brief overview of simulation typologies. For example, a high-fidelity mannequin is not necessary for learning and validation of skills, such as Foley catheter insertion. However, if the objective of the simulated learning experience is to verify the critical thinking required during a patient situation in which a Foley catheter is inserted (to include [1] patient teaching, [2] identifying problems, [3] initiating actions,

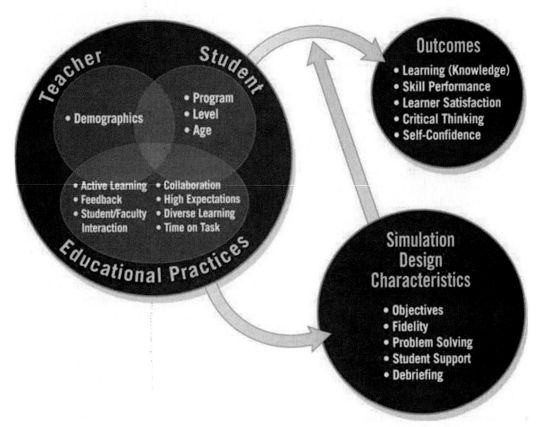

Figure 16.2 Nursing education simulation framework (Jeffries, 2007).

TABLE 16.1
Purpose of Simulation Design Template

- Recommended time for simulated learning experiences.
- Recommended participant.
- Recommended time for guided reflection/debriefing.
- Psychomotor skills and cognitive activities required.
- Learning objectives: scenario specific and program/curriculum specific objectives.
- Fidelity (level).
- Environment or setting for the simulation.
- Props required to increase the realism.
- Roles and responsibilities of participants.
- Patient overview to include health history, physical assessment, and diagnostic values.
- Reference, protocols, and evidence-based practice guidelines.

[4] communicating with other health-care providers, and [5] documenting the procedure) a high- or moderate-level fidelity simulator with use of audio-visual equipment for recording and debriefing would be appropriate.

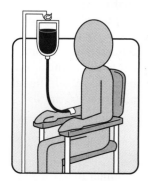

Low-fidelity mannequins are those that do not interact with the learners and are used primarily for skill acquisition. An example of this type of simulation is the insertion of an IV catheter into an IV arm and initiation of IV fluids. The next level of fidelity is medium/moderate. The realism of moderate-level fidelity is increased but still not physiologically correct. This level provides a computer based two-dimensional focus for the simulated learning experience and focuses on problem-solving and skills performance. For example, the participant is able to auscultate realistic heart and breath sounds and blood pressure, however, the chest does not rise and fall with respirations.

High-fidelity simulations are more realistic and have increased interactivity. For example, a computer-driven mannequin can depict a more physiologically correct appearance and respond in a manner that imitates real life. This provides the learner a more realistic submersion into the simulated experience. These mannequins have heart and lung sounds along with correlating pulses and chest

TABLE 16.2	
Summary of Current Simulation Typology	
Simulation Typology	**Definition**
Partial Task Simulation	A type of low-fidelity simulation that includes models or mannequins used to obtain competency in simple procedures.
Peer-to-Peer	Peer collaboration used to master specific skills.
Screen-Based Computer Simulation	A type of moderate-fidelity simulation that includes computer programs used to teach, provide feedback, and evaluate clinical knowledge, critical thinking, and clinical judgment.
Virtual Reality Simulation	A computer-generated, 3-D environment allows sensory stimuli through projection or total immersion enabling dynamic collaborative augmentation of virtual realities.
Haptic Systems	Computer generated environments that integrate tactile sensation by integrating authentic equipment into the scenario.
Standardized Patients	A type of high-fidelity simulation where volunteers or paid actors are taught to portray a patient realistically and consistently in a case scenario format.
Advanced Patient Simulators	A type of high-fidelity simulation that includes a computerized full-body mannequin programmed to provide realistic physiologic responses to a practitioner's actions.

movement and can be programmed to respond physiologically to both nursing and pharmacological interventions.

Once the level of fidelity is chosen, a decision for props is required to promote realism related to the environment, mannequin, and embedded actors. If actual equipment is not available for a scenario, notify participants of substitutions. An example of this could be a school of nursing that does not have a mechanical ventilator for the intensive care patient. To solve this dilemma, endotracheal tubes (ETT) can be purchased and hospitals can donate ventilator tubing along with in-line suction tubing that can be attached to the mannequin. This provides for some realism without the expense, storage, and maintenance of additional equipment. Remember, props are not limited to the equipment but include wigs, moulage, and clothing for the mannequins and participants.

DEVELOPING SCENARIOS

Planning and writing the scenario for a simulated learning experience is similar to writing the script for a play. Developing objectives is the most important step providing the foundation for the experience. The objectives must be congruent with module, course, and program objectives and designed to meet the experience level of the participants.

In addition, the faculty designing the experience needs to consider and document what actions the learners are expected to initiate. If the action is implement what response should occur or if the learner does not initiate the expected action what cues should be provided to assist the learner. If cues are provided, the faculty needs to include how they are presented, who or "what" will provide these cues, and at what intervals the cueing will appear.

Evidence-Based Practice and Safety Initiatives

When developing the scenario, the designer (faculty) must incorporate evidence-based practices. Multiple references are available online to assist the faculty during scenario development. For example, Quality and Safety for Nursing Education (QSEN) has followed the Institute of Medicine (IOM) safety initiatives and established teaching interventions available through its Web site (http://www.qsen.org/). The QSEN resources use Bloom's taxonomy and incorporation of knowledge, skills, and attitudes (KSAs) for different levels of learners.

Level of Experience of Participants

Simulated learning experiences should be based on the level of the participant. The difficulty of experiences should progress in complexity as learner progresses through the curriculum. We recommend developing an orientation to simulation for the students to observe before their initial experience. This orientation could be videotaped and placed on the Web for students to review before coming to the simulation center. Faculty also has used clips from movies to introduce students to simulation. Excellent examples of simulation are displayed in *Monsters, Inc.* and *Apollo 13*. Simulation should be initiated early in the curriculum with each experience building on previous experiences as content is integrated into the curriculum. As scenarios are developed, challenges (clinical problems) are strategically included to promote decision making, critical thinking, and clinical judgment.

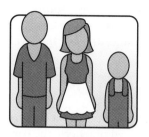

We recognize there is more than one type of learning. Ideally, a simulation should be designed to incorporate all domains of learning. Learning (behavior change) occurs when relevant objectives represent all three domains. Therefore, activities that include the three identified domains; cognitive (mental skills or knowledge), affective (feelings and attitude), and psychomotor (skills) need to be strategically integrated into the experience. We believe that for an activity to be considered a simulation, the experience should include contextually appropriate activities that require the learner to use multiple ways of knowing such as demonstrating decision making and critical thinking while performing psychomotor skills.

Role

During the development of the simulation scenario, the designer needs to identify the roles to be filled by students, faculty, and/or actors. Roles can include the primary nurse, a physician, a nurse supervisor, the patient, or a family member. The number of participants can vary from one to six and roles can be either assigned or participants may volunteer for a specific role. A problem that occurs when participants volunteer for specific roles is individuals with more dominant personalities or stronger clinically tend to assume the more active roles. Participants needing assistance with assertiveness and critical thinking, select the more passive roles. No matter how roles are assumed, learners need to understand the responsibilities associated with each role. In addition, participants should have the opportunity to experience multiple roles before program completion. A method should be employed to ensure that all participants function in a leadership or main role at least once.

We recommend when faculty participate in an experience, they avoid the role of primary nurse. In addition, the faculty member's presence or level of involvement in the scenario should depend on the level of the participants, the objectives of the simulation, and the level of facilitation required for the scenario.

Time Frames

Along with establishing objectives, time constraints should be identified when developing the case study. Research has shown that equal time for both scenario and debriefing should be allotted. Therefore, if a scenario lasts 20 minutes, then the debriefing/guided reflection should last 20 to 30 minutes. Each scenario should be timed and participants should continue until time limit reached or objectives are met.

IMPLEMENTING THE SIMULATION

Multiple factors must be considered after the simulated experience is designed. A scenario can be managed by faculty visually in the room using a handheld device, behind a partition or in another room that allows the faculty to visualize the experience through a one-way window. In addition, the scenario can be run by one or two individuals. If two individuals assist with the experience, we recommend one of them to be the faculty responsible for the students who would guide the experience. The other individual could be a staff member competent in changing the simulators parameters as instructed by the faculty or structured template for the scenario.

We also recommend a "run-through" of the scenarios before implementing the experience with learners. During this "run-through" you should identify if (1) any additional props, cues, or questions need to be integrated; (2) the instructions for the experience are appropriate; (3) the objective to be achieved in the designated time frame; and (4) the level of participant-instructor interaction appropriate for the experience.

DETERMINING THE PARTICIPANT-INSTRUCTOR INTERACTION

The role of the instructor is to guide or facilitate the learner through the experience using cueing and questioning. The level of facilitation is based on evidence-based practices, the participants, and the simulated learning experience objectives. The facilitator can function on several different levels: instructor-prompting driven, partial instructor-prompting driven, and no instructor-prompting driven. The prompting/cueing is provided through the facilitator, mannequin, or the actors' scripts embedded into the simulated learning experience. Actors may play the role of patient, family member, or other health-care workers.

Instructor-Prompting Driven

Instructor-prompting driven simulated clinical experience is used with the least experienced participants. Sometimes when participants "do not know what they do not know" maximum guidance and prompting is needed to achieve the desired outcomes. Instructor-prompting through cueing allows the instructor to guide the participants in the direction to progress in the simulated learning experience. This could be used for first semester nursing students to assess the "patient" systematically, how to detect any abnormal findings, and begin to use clinical judgment for problem-solving (Nehring & Lashley, 2010).

Partial Instructor-Prompting Driven

This type of instructor prompting requires the instructors to breakdown the scenario into parts, such as scenes in a play. Part one, the presimulation briefing, allows the participants to develop a plan of action based on the information provided. Then the participants enter the simulation area and implement the plan of care without interruptions from the 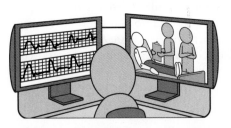 facilitator. Participants are allowed to make decisions, adjust their plan, and make corrections through group discussion. Before the simulation begins, faculty should determined what action would be initiated if the participant(s) strays from the designed pathway. Action taken by the faculty could include allowing the learner to continue with the scenario (i.e., travel down the pathway) or introduce prompting or cues by means of the "patient," actors submerged into

TECHNOLOGY TIP 16.2

Telehealth is growing rapidly in health care. One way to incorporate this into simulation is to have a computer (i.e., laptop) on a table/stand in the simulation room where the instructor (or person in the role of doctor) is being broadcast via videoconference. This can be done with a free tool, called Skype. Instead of the usual telephone call, the student communicates by speaking while looking at the image on the screen.

the scenario, or diagnostic/laboratory values results until the time limit for the activity is reached. At this point, debriefing begins and the instructor facilitates the participants into guided reflection. This will be discussed more thoroughly at the end of this chapter. The learner may then be provided the opportunity to repeat the scenario allowing the participants the ability to learn from their mistakes (Nehring & Lashley, 2010).

No Instructor Prompting

The main difference with this type of facilitation is there are no interruptions between the states for the guided reflection and changes to the plan of care. Once the plan of care is implemented or time limit has been reached, the participants leave the scenario to a faculty-led feedback session using questioning strategy (Nehring & Lashley, 2010).

QUESTIONING

Questioning can be integrated strategically throughout a simulated experience to guide the novice learners' thinking. When guiding the thinking of novice learners, faculty may be present in the room and use questioning to assist the learners in obtaining cues. For example, the faulty might ask, "After noting the abnormal respirations of 36 and shallow, what other assessment data would you gather?" For the more advanced learner, questioning may be posed by the patient, family member, or other health-care providers to identify the learner's ability to reflect-in-action. For example, requiring the learner to have a telephone conversation with a physician provides multiple opportunities for questioning or a patient might ask "How is this medication going to solve the problems I'm having?"

AUDIO-VISUAL RECORDING OF SIMULATIONS

If experiences are to be recorded, you must obtain the learners' consent. If the audio-visual recording is integrated into the planned feedback session, the faculty must be proficient with the equipment, show only critical segments (both exemplary and sessions need critical critique) of the simulated activity. Each segment of the session should be introduced with "Discuss what you were thinking..." to allow the participants the opportunity to analyze their performance and discuss activities they perceive as needing improvement.

FORMATIVE VERSUS SUMMATIVE ASSESSMENT

Simulated experiences can be used for formative and summative assessments. The type of assessment, formative versus summative, needs to be determined and communicated to the participants. Faculty should strive to provide a safe learning environment for all activity, both formative and summative. For example, trust in the facilitator and attitudes toward simulation could be impaired if participants prepare for a formative experience only to discover the experience was changed to a summative evaluation. If a simulated activity is being used as a summative assessment, faculty are challenged to develop or select valid and reliable evaluation tools. In addition, no matter if the simulated experiences are being conducted for formative or summative assessments, the learner needs to sign a confidentiality statement. This statement should include a requirement of the learner to respect the confidentiality of the experience to include both the scenario and the actions of the participants.

PLANNED FEEDBACK

All simulated experiences should include a planned feedback session using principles of debriefing, guided reflection, or a combination of the two strategies. The goal of planned feedback is to assist the participant in becoming a reflective practitioner. A reflective practitioner demonstrates reflection-on-action, reflection-in-action, and knowing-in-action while providing patient care (Benner, Sutphen, Leonard, & Day, 2009; Schön, 1987). Table 16.3 provides the definitions to the different types of reflection. In addition, a reflective practitioner consciously considers the meaning and implication of an action in an effort to assimilate KSAs into his or her pre-existing knowledge. Johns (1995) describes reflection as a process of self-discovery that serves as the window through which practitioners view themselves to confront, understand, and resolve contradictions between desired and actual practice.

Reflective thinking skills can be taught, but require the learner to be actively involved in realistic experiences facilitated by a guide (Henderson & Johnson, 2002; Johns, 2004). Recognizing reflective thinking skills does not occur automatically and barriers exist. The faculty need to address and overcome these barriers if the desired outcomes of the experience are to be achieved. Table 16.4 provides a summary of the barriers to reflective thinking and the potential outcomes once these barriers are addressed. We believe simulation provides a technique in which realistic learning experiences that require both an active engagement (i.e., the experience) and a planned feedback session will assist in promoting the development of reflective thinking skills required to improve patient care.

Planned feedback sessions (debriefing) uses multiple techniques to lead the learner is through a purposeful discussion related to a simulated experience. The feedback session is planned allowing the learner to uncover and discuss his or her thoughts, feelings, behaviors, and actions in an effort to promote insightfulness. The planned feedback session has been described as the "heart and soul" of a simulated experience (Rall, Manser, & Howard, 2000), and identified by learners as the most important component of the simulated experience (Evidence-Based Practice Box 16.4) (Gordon & Buckley, 2009; Smith & Roehrs, 2009). Jeffries (2005) cautioned knowing how to debrief is as important as

TABLE 16.3	
Definitions of the Types of Reflection	
Type	**Definition**
Reflection-on-action	The conscious review of an interaction once the action is completed.
Reflection-in-action	The self-monitoring that occurs as an individual is engaged in an experience or thinking about what is being done while the action is being performed.
Knowing-in-action	The unconscious, intuitive knowing that occurs when an individual is engaged in action or the ability to "think on your feet."

TABLE 16.4	
Barriers and Outcomes Related to Reflective Thinking	
Barriers	**Outcomes**
Perceived stress	Heightened self-confidence
Previous learning	Enhanced knowledge
Acquired fixations	Improved understanding
Resistance to change	Increased empathy
Poor communication skills	Improved patient care
Organizational culture	

knowing how to create and initiate a simulated experience. Therefore, you are challenged to develop the skills required to effectively facilitate feedback sessions. These skills include the appropriate use of the different techniques (e.g., Socratic questioning, Plus-Delta, advocacy-inquiry, and guided reflection) while addressing the learner's emotions. To achieve this, faculty need to use therapeutic communication skills, especially the tactical use of silence and active listening. Remember, if an experience caused emotional distress the feedback session must provide the support, environment, and time to discuss and defuse the situation.

Feedback (debriefing) can be integrated during or at the conclusion of a simulation experience. Frozen debriefing is when a scenario is stopped or "frozen" and immediate feedback is provided at the bedside. This technique is used to emphasize a teaching point, defuse a deteriorating situation, or limit potential embarrassment. Postscenario debriefing occurs after the experience and uses the techniques of Socratic questioning, Plus-Delta, advocacy-inquiry, or guided reflection. Postscenario debriefing can be conducted at the bedside or in a separate room, but no matter which setting all participates should either stand or sit in a circle (faculty need to avoid the appearance of being controlling or authoritative).

Postscenario debriefing should be initiated by faculty reviewing the objectives of the experience and providing ground rules for the session (Table 16.5 provides an example of ground rules for a feedback session). As a facilitator, faculty is responsible for guiding the session, allowing the learners to critique their performances, and identify the positive and negative actions implemented during the scenario (Table 16.6 provides an overview of faculty responsibilities during the feedback session). The feedback session should not be structured as a teaching conference but, if mistakes are not identified by the participants these deficiencies need to be discussed at the conclusion of the feedback session.

EVIDENCE-BASED PRACTICE BOX 16.4

Use of a questionnaire response, descriptive statistics, and a paired t-test identified formal debriefing as the most useful aspect of a simulated experience (Gordon & Buckley, 2009).

TABLE 16.5
Ground Rules for Feedback Session
• Conversations must be kept confidential, "What is said in the session—stays in the session."   • Respect each other and extend profession courtesy.   • Does not talk about anyone who is not in the room.   • Be supportive, not judgmental.   • Listen to your peers.

TABLE 16.6
Facilitator Responsibilities
• Set the expectations.   • Facilitate the session according to the needed level of engagement.   • Engage the quiet learner.   • Identify any unrecognized deficiencies.   • Provide reinforcement.

To optimize the experience, feedback sessions should be facilitated by faculty who observed the simulated experience. If appropriate feedback is not provided the learner could develop a distorted view of the experience leading to the repetition of mistakes and fixations. Fixations are beliefs acquired when an individual relates the outcome of an event to all situations similar to the witnessed situation. For example, the belief that any one experiencing a hypertensive event needs to be treated with a beta blocker no matter the underlying cause.

The outcome of the simulated experience is influenced by past relationships between the facilitator and the learners and the facilitator's debriefing skill (Evidence-Based Practice Box 16.5). For example, if teachers interject their feedback prematurely, learners stop reflecting, lose confidence, and become dependent on faculty.

As the facilitator, you need to implement the degree of facilitation based on the objectives of the experience and the participants. The degree of facilitation varies from high to intermediate to low. High facilitation is used when the participants are critical reflectors who demonstrate the ability to debrief themselves. When facilitating feedback sessions for these learners, you may only need to interject periodic comments to stimulate the discussion. For example, "Talk to me about how this experience made you feel." Low facilitation is used for learners who function at the novice or advanced beginner stage and demonstrate minimal reflective abilities (nonreflectors); whereas, intermediate facilitation requires the facilitator to tactfully assist the participants (reflectors) in analyzing the experience (Decker, 2007; Fanning & Gaba, 2007; Mezirow, 1981). Table 16.7 provides definitions for the different levels of reflective abilities.

TABLE 16.7	
Degrees of Reflecting Abilities	
Reflecting Abilities	**Characteristics**
Nonreflectors	Straightforward thinking Lower self-confidence Limited ability of self-analysis
Reflectors	Identify relationships Improved levels of self-confidence Beginning abilities related to self-analysis Perceived feelings of competence with clinical skills Identification of experiential knowledge
Critical Reflectors	Engage in self-analysis Identify relationships Ability to transfer experiential knowledge to new situations Validate outcomes of nursing actions High level of perceived self-confidence

EVIDENCE-BASED PRACTICE BOX 16.5

Learning through participating in a simulated experience is influenced by the learner's preparation, the faculty's demeanor and attitude, and the debriefing session (Cantrell, 2008).

Techniques for Providing Feedback

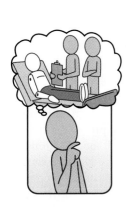

Socratic questioning can be used during the feedback session to assist the learner in identifying problems and making connections thereby facilitating critical and reflective thinking. If you use Socratic questioning, develop some questions before the activity gauging the questioning to the learner's level of competence. For example, questions used to assist the novice learning are more directed; "Discuss the cues that guided the care you initiated related to the patient's respiratory status." Whereas, a competent learner could be asked to, "Discuss the cues that guided the action you initiated during the simulated experience." In addition, faculty might include "what if" questions in the feedback session for competent and above learners, such as, "What if the patient's assessment revealed a history of smoking, how would this have affected the actions that were initiated?"

Guided reflection integrates the use of Socratic questioning and posed statements to encourage reflection-on-action. Numerous models are available to assist faculty developing these sessions. For example, Johns (2004) provides questions based on Carper's four ways of knowing. A modification of Johns' questions is provided (see Facilitator's Tool for Guided Reflection Session in the Practical Tool Kit on Davis Plus).

The Plus-Delta technique can be used for all levels of learners. This technique requires the learner to actively engage in the critique of the experience by identifying actions initiated appropriately, indicating actions requiring change, and discussing how the change would occur (see Plus-Delta Tool for Feedback in the Practical Tools Kit on Davis Plus). Although the Plus-Delta technique can be used for individual or team debriefing. When using this technique for team debriefing it requires participants to complete the assessment as a group and not identify or isolate specific members of the team (Decker, Moore, Thal, Opton, Caballero, & Beasley, 2010; Fanning & Gaba, 2007).

"Debriefing with good judgment" approach was developed by the Center for Medical Simulation at Harvard Medical School (see its Web site at http://www.harvardmedsim.org/). This rigorous technique, based on cognitive science, endeavors to identify the "frames of reference" used by individuals when making decisions. Faculty explores these frames with the participant, link them to actions, and through feedback facilitates the learner in developing other frames and actions for future situations (Rudolph, Simon, Rivard, Dufresne, & Raemer, 2007).

Faculty have modified the structured feedback session to include the use of the Outcome Present State-Test Model of clinical reasoning developed by Pesut and Herman (1999) (see the discussion in the article by Kuiper, Heinrich, Matthias, Graham, & Bell-Kotwall available at http://www.bepress.com/ijnes/vol5/iss1/art17). Other faculty has integrated the use of concept mapping and cause and effect diagramming. Discussion related to these strategies are included in an article by Decker, Moore, Thal, Opton, Caballero, and Beasley (2010). Other strategies implemented by faculty to promote reflective thinking after simulated learning experiences include written journals and Web-based discussions.

Recognizing faculty's need to obtain the KSA required to becoming competent in teaching with simulation, multiple simulation centers provide extensive workshops. Networking and resources are available through professional organizations related to simulation, for example; International Nursing Association for Clinical Simulation and Learning (INACSL) at http://www.inacsl.org, the Society for Simulation in Healthcare (SSH) at http://www.ssih.org, and the Association of Standardized Patient Educators (ASPE) at http://www.aspeducators.org. In addition, the National League for Nursing has online e-learning courses available through the Simulation Innovation Resource Center at http://www.nln.org.

SUCCESSFUL INTEGRATION

Successful integration of simulation throughout the curriculum or program, educational or orientation, is dependent on administrative support and buy-in by both the faculty and the learner. Commitment from the administration is required for financial support to design, build and maintain simulation centers, purchase equipment and simulators, and hire and educate support personnel and faculty. Faculty buy-in can be achieved by providing faculty development related to scenario construction and implementation along with modifications in tenure and promotion guidelines that recognize simulation as an education pedagogy. Learner buy-in is achieved by orientating the student to simulation, including the desired outcomes, the integration of feedback, and providing repeated experiences that are integrated throughout the curriculum. Curriculum integration requires faculty involvement and needs to be strategic. Faculty need to (1) identify and map key concepts and learning outcomes that can be facilitated by simulation; (2) determine the placement of specific learning activities within the curriculum; (3) determine the appropriate simulation typology for each of the activities; (4) use evidence-based findings to design the experience; (5) conduct the experience; (6) review the outcomes of the experience; and (7) modify the learning experience.

CONCLUSION

Simulation as a tool offers educators a unique learning strategy for individuals and groups, and to assess both discipline-specific and interprofessional teamwork skills. Simulation has specific advantages to assist learners in developing the KSAs required for interprofessional teamwork. These advantages include scenarios designed to present specific challenging situations, opportunities for cross-training, and shared debriefing (Gaba, Howard, Smith, & Sowb, 2001). As reflected in the literature, opportunities to practice and develop competence in a simulated "consequence-free" environment where the learners is provided constructive feedback is essential to the mastery of team-related skills (Shapiro, Gardner, Godwin, & Jay, 2008). In addition, study participants from various disciplines indicated the interprofessional simulated learning experience promoted an understanding of the roles and responsibilities of other health-care providers and fostered mutual trust.

Educators are challenged to provide empirical data to validate the use of simulation as a learning and an evaluation tool. We believe simulation has a potential to assist in assessing clinical competencies but, educators need to acquire the knowledge and skills needed to use this educational strategy. We challenge educators to continue their endeavors toward validating the use of simulation as an evaluation tool.

The future of simulation is only limited by our imaginations. The future will provide us advances in technology that will improve realism and through enhanced technologies, such as the use of gaming platforms, will allow individuals from different locations to participate in activities together. We can use our imagination to visualize the potential opportunities of virtual reality (VR) and how it will affect our future when it is available. The unique VR will allow environments for real-time exploration, manipulation of 3-D objects, and learning in situations impossible to achieve in the real world due to patient safety issues. Yet, we must continue to provide the evidence to assist us in determine the best way in which to use our current and future tools to support our learners.

REFERENCES

Bambini, D., Washburn, J., & Perkins, R. (2009). Outcomes of clinical simulation for novice nursing students: Communication, confidence, clinical judgment. *Nursing Education Perspectives, 30*(2), 79–82.

Benner, P., Sutphen, M., Leonard, V., & Day, L. (2009). *Educating nurses: A call for radical transformation.* The Carnegie Foundation for the Advancement of Teaching. San Francisco, CA: Jossey-Bass.

Bradley, P. (2006). The history of simulation in medical education and possible future directions. *Medical Education History, 40,* 245–262.

Cantrell, M. A. (2008). The importance of debriefing in clinical simulation. *Clinical Simulation in Nursing, 4,* e19–e23.

Cooper, J. B., & Taqueti, V. R. (2004). A brief history of development mannequin simulators for clinical education and training. *Quality Safe Health Care 13*(Supp 1), i11–i18.

Decker, S. I. (2007). *Simulation as an educational strategy in the development of critical and reflective thinking: A qualitative exploration* (Unpublished doctoral dissertation). Denton, TX: Texas Woman's University.

Decker, S., Moore, A., Thal, W., Opton, L., Caballero, S., & Beasley, M. (2010). Synergistic integration of concept mapping and cause and effect diagramming into simulated experiences (Manuscript submitted for publication). *Clinical Simulation in Nursing*.

Del Bueno, D. (2005). A crisis in critical thinking [Electronic version]. *Nursing Education Perspectives, 26*(5), 278–282.

Fanning, R. M., & Gaba, D. M. (2007). The role of debriefing in simulation-based learning. *Simulation in Healthcare: The Journal of the Society for Simulation in Healthcare, 2*(2), 115–125.

Finkelman, A., & Kenner, C. (2007). *Teaching IOM: Implications of the IOM report for nursing education*. Silver Spring, MD: American Nurses Association.

Gaba, D. (2004). The future vision of simulation in health care. *Quality and Safety in Healthcare, 13*(Suppl 1), i2–i10.

Gaba, D. M., Howard, S. K., Smith, B. E., & Sowb, Y. A. (2001). Simulation-based training in anesthesia crisis resource management (ACRM): A decade of experiences. *Simulation and Gaming, 69*, 387–394.

Gordon, C. J., & Buckley, T. (2009). The effects of high-fidelity simulation training on medical-surgical graduate nurses' perceived ability to respond to patient clinical emergencies. *The Journal of Continuing Education in Nursing, 40*(11), 491–498.

Henderson, P., & Johnson, M. H. (2002). An innovative approach to developing the reflective skills of medical students [Electronic version]. *BioMed Central BMC Medical Education, 2*(4), 1–4.

Herrmann, E. K. (2000, March–May). Connecticut nursing history vignettes. *Connecticut Nursing News*. Retrieved from http://homepage.ntlworld.com/bleep/SimHist1.html

Howard, V. M., Ross, C., Mitchell, A. M., & Nelson, G. M. (2010). Human patient simulators and interactive case studies a comparative analysis of learning outcomes and student perceptions. *Computers, Informatics, Nursing, 28*(1), 42–48.

Jeffries, P. R. (Ed.). (2007). *Simulation in nursing education for conceptualization to evaluation*. New York, NY: National League for Nursing.

Jeffries, P. R. (2005). A framework for designing, implementing and evaluating simulations used as teaching strategies in nursing. *Nursing Education Perspectives, 26*(2), 96–103.

Johns, C. (1995). Framing learning through reflection within Carper's fundamental ways of knowing in nursing. *Journal of Advanced Nursing, 22*(2), 226–234.

Johns, C. (2004). *Becoming a reflective practitioner* (2nd ed.). Malden, MA: Blackwell Publishing Inc.

Lasater, K. (2007). High-fidelity simulation and the development of clinical judgment: Students' experiences. *Journal of Nursing Education, 46*(6), 269–275.

Mezirow, J. (1981). *Transformative dimensions of adult learning*. San Francisco, CA: Jossey-Bass.

Morgan, P. G. (1995) Creating a laboratory that simulates the critical care environment. *Critical Care Nurse, 16*(6), 76–81.

National Council of State Boards of Nursing (NCSBN). (2005). *Clinical instruction in prelicensure nursing programs*. Retrieved from http:/www.ncsbn.org/pdfs/Final_Clinical_Instruction_Prelicensure_Nursing_Programs.pdf

Nehring, W. N., & Lashley, F. R. (2010). *High-fidelity patient simulation*. Boston, MA: Jones and Bartlett Publishers.

Pesut, D. J., & Herman, J. (1999). *Clinical reasoning: The art and science of critical and creative thinking*. Albany, NY: Delmar Publishers.

Rall, M., Manser, T., & Howard, S. K. (2000). Key elements of debriefing for simulator training. *European Journal of Anaesthesiology, 17*(8), 516–517.

Rudolph. J. W., Simon, R., Rivard, P., Dufresne, R. L., & Raemer, D. B. (2007). Debriefing with good judgment: Combining rigorous feedback with genuine inquiry. *Anesthesiology Clinics, 25*, 361–376.

Schön, D. A. (1987). *Educating the reflective practitioner*. Hoboken, NJ: Jossey-Bass Printing.

Shapiro, M. J., Gardner, R., Godwin, S., & Jay, G. (2008). Defining team performance for simulation-based training: Methodology, metrics, and opportunities for emergency medicine. *Academic Emergency Medicine, 15*(11), 1088–1097.

Smith, S. J., & Roehrs, C. J. (2009). High-fidelity simulation: Factors correlated with nursing students satisfaction and self-confidence. *Nursing Education Perspectives, 30*(2), 74–78.

Chapter 17

Program Approval and Accreditation

Linda Caputi, EdD, MSN, RN, ANEF, CNE

The faculty of a small community college in a mountainous area of Colorado are preparing for their initial National League for Nursing Accrediting Commission, Inc. (NLNAC) accreditation visit. The main campus is in one location and three offsite campuses, each approximately 100 miles from the main campus offering the program to a small cadre of students through Web-based and interactive conferencing delivery systems. The faculty member leading the effort read Standard 4.9, which states: For programs with distance education: Learning activities, instructional materials, and evaluation methods are appropriate for the delivery format and consistent with student learning outcomes. The faculty engage in discussion about what that means and how to address that criterion.

Although approval and accreditation vary in nature and purpose, their approach to distance education and other technologies reflect the same underlying belief. That belief is that no matter which alternative methods are used to deliver the instruction, the program must meet the same standards as the face-to-face (f-2-f) or traditional format. This means, among other things, the online version is congruent with the stated mission, goals, and objectives of the program and the student outcomes are met. Ensuring that this consistency is maintained is the challenge educators engaged in distance education must meet. This chapter addresses some of the specific aspects that must be considered when addressing both approval and accreditation of nursing programs using these technologies.

APPROVAL AND ACCREDITATION

Approval

Nursing education is a regulated practice. That is, there is a regulatory body that holds legislative power to ensure that nursing schools provide the education necessary for the safe care of the citizens of the jurisdiction in which the nursing program resides. Regulation, as it relates to the nurse, refers to individuals being granted legal authority to engage in professional practice after meeting specific qualifications and demonstrating minimal entry-level competencies. Nursing is regulated because of the potential for a nurse who is unprepared or unqualified to cause harm to a patient (Spector, 2010). Preparing a nurse to provide safe, effective care is a primary goal of nursing programs. Regulation is necessary to

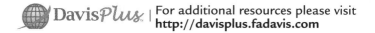

For additional resources please visit
http://davisplus.fadavis.com

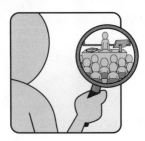

ensure nursing programs do just that, and regulation is the work of the individual boards of nursing. Currently, there is a board of nursing for each of the 50 states, the District of Columbia, and four United States territories—Guam, Virgin Islands, American Samoa, and the Northern Mariana. Programs are designated to be an approved program through one of these boards of nursing. The National Council of State Boards of Nursing (NCSBN) was established in 1977. One purpose of the NCSBN is to provide an organization through which the individual boards of nursing can counsel together on matters of common interest (https://www.ncsbn.org/about.htm).

Of interest to the approving board of nursing is the manner in which nurses are prepared for practice. Nurses must graduate from an approved program of study as a requirement to write the national licensing examination to practice. Because distance education and technologies, such as simulations currently are used to deliver instruction in schools of nursing and those technologies bear on learner outcomes, the boards of nursing and the NCSBN look at these pedagogies with interest.

Evidence-Based Practice

The NCSBN's work is firmly supported by evidence. Therefore, they are a leader in evidence-based practice. The NCSBN conducts its own research on a variety of topics including distance education and innovative practice, in addition to providing links to other credible sites that provide evidence for best practices. Visit https://www.ncsbn.org/373.htm for information on distance education and https://www.ncsbn.org/1927.htm for information on innovations in nursing education.

Accreditation

Accreditation, unlike approval, is not required, but voluntary. Accreditation bodies that focus specifically on nursing programs are the NLNAC and the Commission on Collegiate Nursing Education (CCNE). NLNAC accredits all levels of nursing programs including practical, associate, baccalaureate, master's, and doctoral programs. The CCNE accredits only baccalaureate and higher-level programs.

Accreditation provides an additional level of quality and rigor. Voluntary accreditation ensures excellence in both process and outcomes. The program is developed using established standards and the outcomes are evaluated to provide evidence the program is achieving its mission and stated outcomes (Newsome & Tanner, 2010). Nursing has a long history of accreditation in the United States beginning in 1893 with the American Society of Superintendents of Training Schools for Nursing and continuing today through the work of the nursing accrediting bodies (NLN, 2008, www.nln.org/aboutnln/info-history.htm).

These accreditation bodies also are extremely interested in distance education and technology, such as simulations. Their purpose is to ensure the program curriculum is implemented to achieve the program outcomes, regardless of the media used in the teaching/learning process. However, they also encourage innovation in implementing a nursing program, support the application of evidence-based teaching.

DISTANCE EDUCATION

Regulatory Agencies

There are many definitions in the nursing literature for the various technologies used in nursing education. Regulatory agencies have adopted definitions for their specific use when evaluating nursing programs. On its Web site, the NCSBN offers definitions for dozens of terms that apply to using technology in teaching. Each definition is referenced, demonstrating their definitions are derived from the literature. Faculty engaging in distance education should be familiar with these definitions. The NCSBN offers definitions for the following terms on its Web site at https://www.ncsbn.org/836.htm:

- Distance Education.
- Distance Education Technologies.
- Distance Medium.
- Distributed Learning.

In fulfilling its mission to provide an avenue for counsel to its member boards of nursing, the NCSBN has established recommendations for those member boards for use when approving nursing programs that use distance learning to deliver courses. They state that distance education methods must be congruent with the program's curriculum plan and serve the same purpose as all other methods of delivery; that is, to meet the goals and competencies of the educational program and to be in compliance with the standards of the board by which the program is regulated. The NCSBN's recommendations for distance education as presented on their Web site at https://www.ncsbn.org/373.htm

Individual Boards of Nursing

It is important to keep in mind the purpose of the NCSBN. As previously stated, the NCSBN provides an avenue for boards to act together and counsel; it does not dictate what the individual boards of nursing must do. Each board provides legislative action that it deems best serves its constituents (i.e., citizens) in its region. All faculty in each state and territory should be familiar with the rules and regulations of the board of nursing that governs their practice. These rules and regulations can vary greatly from state to state. Following are some examples.

Illinois Nurse Practice Act

The Illinois Nurse Practice Act does not provide a definition of distance education. Section 1300 on the approval of nursing programs, offers a brief paragraph on distance learning. This section states:

> *If portions of the required clinical or theoretical curriculum are offered at different geographical sites or by distance learning, the curriculum must be planned, supervised, administered, and evaluated in concert with appropriate faculty committees, department chairmen and administrative officers of the parent school (http://www.ilga.gov/commission/jcar/admincode/068/068013000000400R.html).*

The Illinois Nurse Practice Act does not specifically state the distance education program needs to be congruent with the f-2-f version, but rather takes the approach that it does not differentiate distance learning from f-2-f, handling all delivery methods as one program. It does address requirements regarding the curriculum, ensuring the curriculum is "in concert with" personnel of the parent school, which in turn provides congruency.

North Dakota Nurse Practice Act

As with the Illinois Practice Act, the North Dakota Board of Nursing does not offer a definition of distance education. It does reference distance education in Article 54-03.2 of its Rules which states:

> Delivery of instruction by distance education methods must meet the standards for nursing education according to article 54-03.2 (Author's note: Article 54-03.2 is this state's article describing expectations for curriculum), be congruent with the nursing program curriculum plan, and enable students to meet the goals, competencies, and objectives of the education program and standards of the board (http://www.legis.nd.gov/information/acdata/pdf/54-03.2-06.pdf).

North Dakota's statement is very similar to the NCSBN's recommendations.

Louisiana Nurse Practice Act

The Louisiana Nurse Practice Act provides definitions in Section 3501 of its Rules and Regulations that are somewhat abbreviated from those offered by the NCSBN. These are:

Distance Education—teaching learning strategies to meet the needs of students who are physically separated from the faculty.

Distance Education Technology—the methods and technical support used to teach students who may be physically distant from the faculty. The methods may include audio conference, compressed video, electronic mail, and the World Wide Web. Distance education programming is consistent with the mission and goals of the nursing unit and the governing organization.

Section 3511 of the Louisiana Nurse Practice Act Rules and Regulations states a program offered by distance education must be consistent with the mission and goals of the nursing unit and the governing organization (http://www.lsbn.state.la.us/documents/rules/fullrules.pdf). This is consistent with the recommendations of the NCSBN.

Summary of Regulation

All nursing programs must meet their board of nursing requirements to be granted approval, including any sections that relate to distance education. Nursing faculty and program administrators must be aware of all board of nursing requirements as they are planning distance education courses. They must demonstrate the delivery method does not compromise the quality of the program.

ACCREDITATION

The Council for Higher Education Accreditation (CHEA) is an association comprised of accrediting agencies (http://www.chea.org). CHEA published a document in 2002 reporting that 1979 institutions offered distance education at that time (CHEA Institute for Research and Study of Accreditation and Quality Assurance, 2002). CHEA's 2002 report stated that many specialized accreditors treat distance learning as an alternative delivery system which would not require developing separate standards, policies, and procedures.

The eight regional accreditation agencies of the Higher Learning Commission issued a document agreeing to adopt a common platform for review of distance learning (Anonymous 1, n.d.). The platform, based on the *Best Practices for Electronically Offered Degree and Certificate Programs* (Anonymous 2, n.d.) lists five components:

1. Institutional context and commitment
2. Curriculum and instruction
3. Faculty support
4. Student support
5. Evaluation

The importance of a specific focus in the accreditation process on distance education to ensure the same quality as f-2-f instruction had been established with these efforts.

Accreditation in Nursing Education

In 2005, the *Alliance for Nursing Accreditation Statement on Distance Education Policies*, published a policy statement that includes the following (http://www.aacn.nche.edu/education/disstate.htm):

> All nursing education programs delivered solely or in part through distance learning technologies must meet the same academic program and learning support standards and accreditation criteria as programs provided in f-2-f formats, including the following:
> • Student outcomes are consistent with the stated mission, goals, and objectives of the program; and
> • The institution assumes the responsibility for establishing a means to assess student outcomes. This assessment includes overall program outcomes, in addition to specific course outcomes, and a process for using the results for continuous program improvement.

This policy continues on to include that distance education programs must also address other components of a quality program, such as faculty development, technical support, clinical competence, professional role socialization, and availability of resources (AACN, 2005).

Both CCNE (2008) and NLNAC (2008), in their most recent standards for accreditation for nursing programs, include distance education. A brief review of these standards follows.

TECHNOLOGY TIP 17.1

Writing a self-study can be a daunting task. Most faculty form groups with a number of faculty working together on a standard. Technology can assist with this process. For example, all files can reside on a common place on the college's server. All faculty would access the files residing on that server as they work through revisions. With this approach all faculty can access the latest versions without uploading, sending, and downloading files and the subsequent task of keeping track of the latest version.

CCNE

Page 6 of the *CCNE Accreditation Manual* that took effect January, 2009, states: "All programs seeking CCNE accreditation, including those offered via distance or 'distributed' learning, are expected to meet the standards presented in this document." The CCNE defined both distance education and distance education program on page 18 of its manual as follows:

Distance Education: Teaching-learning activities characterized by the separation, in time or place, between instructor and student. Courses may be offered through the use of print, electronic, or other media.

Distance Education Program: A program in which 50% or more of the required academic credit hours in nursing, excluding practicum, are accrued through distance education activities.

CCNE integrated distance education into the four overall standards of the new guidelines, which are:

- Standard I: Program Quality: Mission and Governance.
- Standard II: Program Quality: Institutional Commitment and Resources.
- Standard II: Program Quality: Curriculum, Teaching-Learning Practices, and Individual Student Learning Outcomes.
- Standard IV: Program Effectiveness: Aggregate Student Performance and Faculty Accomplishments.

Distance education is mentioned under three of these four standards as follows:

- Under Standard I: Roles of the faculty and students in the governance of the program, including those involved in distance education are clearly defined and enable meaningful participation (CCNE, 2008, p. 7).
- Under Standard II: Academic support services (e.g., library, technology, distance education support, research support, admission, and advising services) are adequate (CCNE, 2008, p. 9).
- Under Standard III: Teaching-learning practices and environments (classroom, clinical, laboratory, simulation, distance education) support achievement of expected individual student learning outcomes (CCNE, 2008, p. 14).

NLNAC

The 2008 *Accreditation Manual* includes a policy specifically addressing distance education, Policy 15: Distance Education (NLNAC, 2008). The policy begins with a definition of distance education:

Distance Education—An educational process in which the majority of the instruction occurs when a student and instructor are not in the same place. Instruction may be

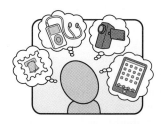

synchronous or asynchronous. Distance education may employ correspondence study, audio, video, and/or computer technologies (NLNAC, 2008, p. 49).

The policy then goes on to list critical elements of distance education to include:

- Congruence with governing organization mission.
- Instructional design and delivery method of the course(s).
- Preparation and competence of the faculty.
- Quality and accessibility of the support services.
- Accessibility, currency, and relevancy of learning resources.
- Currency and appropriateness of the offerings relative to the method of delivery.
- Provision for faculty/student and student/student interaction.
- Ongoing evaluation of student learning (NLNAC, 2008, p. 49).

For all levels of programs (i.e., practical, associate, diploma, baccalaureate, master's, and clinical doctorate), the NLNAC integrates distance learning into each of the standards:

- Standard 1: Mission and Administrative Capacity.
- Standard 2: Faculty and Staff.
- Standard 3: Students.
- Standard 4: Curriculum.
- Standard 5: Resources.
- Standard 6: Outcomes.

Some Recommendations

When addressing accreditation standards, faculty must demonstrate certain elements of development and management of distance education. Here are some recommendations to help manage issues in this process.

Mission and outcome congruence. Suggestions offered to address this area include: The nursing program must present its definition of distance education and explain how it fits into the overall structure of both the nursing unit and that of the governing organization. It must provide a mechanism for distance education students to file a complaint and demonstrate ways students are able to contribute to the governance of the nursing program. Describe how student can contribute to a student association. Address policies related to distance education courses that may be somewhat different. For example, most schools have a time frame in which students may drop a course during the first week of class. Discuss the considerations that are made for an online student who has technical problems and is not able to access the course until after that time period (Nelson, 2010).

Faculty development and support. Suggestions offered to address this area include: The nursing program might demonstrate the availability of technology support, how faculty are taught to use the technology, and how faculty demonstrate their competency in using the technology. Ensure faculty support is available and discuss faculty development related to distance education. Also important is how faculty learn about the types of instructional methods and evaluation methods that are best practices for distance education. Teaching online may use different instructional methods than teaching f-2-f; the important factor is to demonstrate that the distance education methods result in the same learning outcomes.

Technology requirements and policies. Suggestions offered to address this area include: Faculty might explain how the online students receive information about the technology requirements and related policies. Some schools require completion of an assessment to determine the student's readiness for an online course and a tutorial that teaches them about the course management system. Faculty also may address how they determine students have the necessary technology and what technological assistance is available to students. Provide information about how students receive faculty advising for services, such as setting academic and professional goals and developing a plan of study. It might be important to inform students where they can access information about the nursing education program, the parent institution, policies, and all other important information, especially if students are never physically present on campus.

Appropriate instructional design. Suggestions offered to address this include: The curriculum for a distance education program must ensure both the rigor and quality of instruction of a f-2-f program. Students should interact with both the faculty and other online students. The materials used in online instruction should be current and appropriate for delivery through distance education.

Sufficient resources. Suggestions offered to address this area include: Schools must provide evidence they have the required equipment and technical expertise to deliver distance education and the budget provides for ongoing support. Also important to address are the learning resources. If students are not physically on campus, is there an online library available and other online resources? Do the online resources include an adequate collection of journals, texts, and references? Is there an online librarian available? Do students receive an orientation to the online library? Do the students use these online resources? Other services to include are an online bookstore for purchasing texts and online registration.

Evaluation and outcomes. Suggestions offered to address this area include: If the nursing program offers two formats, a totally online program and a f-2-f program, how do student and program outcomes compare? Compare the attrition rate, National Council Licensure Examination (NCLEX) pass rates, student satisfaction, and employer satisfaction of the two groups of students. The programs should be comparable. Both groups are evaluated based on established benchmarks. If only specific courses are offered online rather than an entire program, compare the outcomes for courses offered online with those offered f-2-f. This information would be used to make decisions regarding the admission of students, policies related to the distance education program, and revisions to the distance education offerings.

TECHNOLOGY TIP 17.2

Both state boards of nursing and national accrediting agencies require collection of data from students and stakeholders. Data is used to make informed decisions. Data, however, has been difficult to collect using paper-pencil surveys delivered via the traditional mail. Some faculty have had success using online questionnaires delivered via Internet survey (Baker & Perkins, 2008). Using free Internet survey software the cost of the sending surveys is substantially reduced. Because the use of computers is commonplace, recipients of the surveys are accustomed to, and appreciate, using the computer as a tool for effective and efficient work patterns. A survey conducted online takes less time than filling out a paper-pencil survey and returning it via the U.S. mail. In addition, the data collected in the survey is stored in a database and readily analyzed and downloaded to a spreadsheet or statistical program.

SIMULATIONS

The use of simulations as a teaching strategy has become commonplace in many schools of nursing. The use of simulations to teach students how to deal with real situations they may never encounter in school is for the purpose of the graduate being prepared to deal with like situations in the real world. Dr. Elaine Tagliareni, in her *President's Message* column of the March/April issue of *Nursing Education Perspectives*, provided an excellent and compelling rationale for using simulations (Tagliareni, 2009). Dr. Tagliareni summarized how pilot, Chesley Sullenberger, safely landed a disabled airplane in the Hudson River in January, 2009. This pilot had no experience piloting a wounded plane; however, he had prepared for years for this occasion through the use of simulations. What an amazing feat!

Nursing students may never experience an emergency situation in the real world of their clinical courses that requires quick thinking and life-or-death decisions. But, they can now be educated in handling such situations through the use of simulations. What a comforting thought. This comparison presents a compelling argument for the use of simulations in nursing education with teach nursing professionals how to respond to situations that they may never encounter in school, but may encounter after entering the workforce.

The notion that simulations are an effective means of preparing students for actual patient care also is evident in more subtle ways. For example, the word "authentic" is being used to describe simulation experiences. Smith (2009) published a brief article titled, *Creative Clinical Solutions: Aligning Simulation with Authentic Clinical Experiences*. This implies that a simulated clinical experience using a high-fidelity simulation mannequin can substitute as an "authentic" direct patient care experience. With the number of clinical sites shrinking, the simulated laboratory offers a viable alternative experience; even perhaps a better experience than may be afforded in the clinical.

NCSBN and Simulations

The NSCBN defines simulation in its position paper titled, *Clinical Instruction in Prelicensure Nursing Programs*. The NSCBN's definition is as follows:

> *Simulation—Simulations are activities that mimic the reality of a clinical environment and are designed to demonstrate procedures, decision making and critical thinking through techniques, such as role-playing and the use of devices, such as interactive videos or mannequins. A simulation may be very detailed and closely simulate reality, or it can be a grouping of components that are combined to provide some semblance of reality (Jeffries, 2005). However, simulation shall not take the place of clinical experiences with actual patients (p. 2).*

Simulations cannot be used in place of clinical experiences with actual patients; however, that same document states that "prelicensure nursing education programs shall include clinical experiences with actual patients; they might also include innovative teaching strategies that complement clinical experiences for entry into practice competency (NCSBN, 2005, p. 1)." The NCSBN's definition of hands-on clinical instruction states:

> *Hands-on clinical instruction—Hands-on learning situations are those where students directly care for patients within the relevant setting. "Sufficient" hands-on*

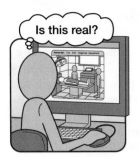

clinical instruction means adequate time spent directly with patients under the supervision of a qualified faculty member, so that program outcomes are met (p. 2).

There is no set number of clinical hours the NCSBN requires.

Individual Boards of Nursing and Simulations

The NCSBN provides advice and information for state boards of nursing, but each board makes its own decisions. Some state boards of nursing are beginning to look at the issue of using experiences in the simulation laboratory in place of clinical hours. Some states present their expectations very clearly in their rules. For example, the following is from the Colorado Board of Nursing (http://www.dora.state.co.us/NURSING/education/PhaseIIApplication.pdf):

> *Rule II Section 3.13 C 4. a., b. & 5. a., b.:*
> *Professional nursing programs consist of a minimum of 450 clock hours in theory instruction in nursing and 750 clock hours in clinical practice. Practical nursing programs include a minimum of 300 clock hours in theory instruction and 400 clock hours in clinical practice.*
> *Rule II Section 3.13 C. 4 c.—Clinical delivery using simulation does not exceed standard set in Section 3.13 C. 4c:*
> - *List the courses with simulation.*
> - *List the number of hours these courses have allotted to simulation in place of clinical hours. What percent of the total clinical hours in each course are simulation hours?*
> - *What percent of the total clinical hours in the whole curriculum are simulation hours?*
> - *Provide evidence of equivalence between the simulation experience planned for the student and what a student would experience in a clinical situation with patients.*
> *NOTE: Nursing education programs can allocate no more than 15% of clinical hours to simulation for any one clinical course and no more than 15% of the total clinical hours in the total curriculum.*
> *Rule II Section 3.15 D.—The program plan for utilizing the clinical laboratory and/or clinical simulation laboratory, if these experiences will deliver part of the minimum clinical hours.*
> - *Document equivalency of the simulation experience with the live patient. Include the following in the equivalency information: (a) diagnostic symptoms/nursing diagnosis, (b) focused assessment demands, (c) expected care needs, (d) decisions that have to be made in delivering the care, (e) the interventions that are expected to be used, (e) the reassessment expected, (f) the planned patient outcome if all of the expected care is delivered.*

Other states are not as prescriptive but offer more general guidelines. For example, the Iowa Board of Nursing provides the following (http://www.legis.state.ia.us/aspx/ACODocs/DOCS/3-25-2009.655.2.pdf):

> *"Lab/simulation" means activities that mimic the reality of a clinical environment and that are designed to demonstrate procedures, decision making and critical thinking*

through techniques, such as role-playing and through the use of devices, such as interactive videos or mannequins. "Lab/simulation" shall not take the place of clinical experiences with actual patients.

Because there are no specific hours for clinical required by the Iowa Board of Nursing, a course could be readjusted to provide less clinical time and more lab/simulation time. The amount of clinical time would need to be sufficient for students to meet the learning outcomes of the course.

Accrediting Bodies and Simulations

Neither the NLNAC nor the CCNE specifically address the use of simulations other than in a general sense to ensure use of this teaching strategy meets the learning outcomes. For example, CCNE states in Standard IIID:

> Elaboration: *Teaching-learning practices and environments (classroom, clinical, laboratory, simulation, distance education) support achievement of expected individual student learning outcomes identified in course, unit, and/or level objectives.*

NLNAC's Standard 4.3 states:

> *The student learning outcomes are used to organize the curriculum, guide the delivery of instruction, direct learning activities, and evaluate student progress.*

Both accrediting bodies expect faculty who use simulations to explain how that teaching pedagogy is used to support learning outcomes. This means the use of simulations should be based on evidence and used when it is the best means for teaching to the student outcomes. This is, of course, good instructional design and should be the guiding principles for the selection of all teaching strategies, not just those that use technology.

Summary

Widespread use of high-fidelity simulators is relatively new in nursing education. There is a growing number of researchers looking at the use of simulations and how this technology can replace clinical time. Jeffries (2009) reports a few states are now allowing the use of simulation to account for up to 25% of real clinical time. Jeffries predicts that, "Based on evidence and quality outcomes from the use of this pedagogy, simulation could eventually be used for the majority of clinical time in nursing education (p. 71)." Regulatory agencies and accrediting bodies will be watching as the future of simulations unfolds.

CONCLUSION

Both the regulatory approval process and the voluntary accreditation process are important to nursing education. Both processes have different purposes, but both ensure quality programs. Because nursing programs are using technology in greater numbers and in increasingly creative ways, it is important these agencies consider these pedagogies during the evaluation process. It would be helpful for faculty to be cognizant of their state regulations and accreditation standards when planning the use of technology in their programs.

REFERENCES

American Association of Colleges of Nursing. (2005). *Alliance for nursing accreditation statement on distance education policies*. Retrieved from http://www.aacn.nche.edu/education/disstate.htm

Anonymous (1). (n.d.). *Statement of commitment by the regional accrediting commissions for the evaluation of electronically offered degree and certificate programs*. Retrieved from https://content.springcm.com/content/DownloadDocuments.ashx?Selection=Document%2C594864b3-4e91-df11-9372-001cc448da6a%3B&accountId=5968

Anonymous (2). (n.d.). *Best practices for electronically offered degree and certificate programs*. Retrieved from www.ncahlc.org/download/Best_Pract_DEd.pdf

Baker, B. H., & Perkins, G. B. (2008). Internet surveys: Obtaining feedback from clinical site coordinators. *Nurse Educator, 13*(3), 128–130.

Commission on Collegiate Nursing Education. (2008). *Standards for accreditation of baccalaureate and graduate degree nursing programs*. Retrieved from http://www.aacn.nche.edu/Accreditation/index.htm

Council for Higher Education [CHEA] Institute for Research and Study of Accreditation and Quality Assurance. (2002). *Accreditation and assuring quality in distance education* [CHEA Monograph Series 2002, No. 1]. Retrieved from http://www.chea.org/pdf/mono_2_spec-accred_02.pdf

Jeffries, P. (2005). A framework for designing, implementing and evaluating simulations used as teaching strategies in nursing. *Nursing Education Perspectives, 26*, 96–103.

Jeffries, P. (2009). Dreams for the future for clinical simulation. *Nursing Education Perspectives, 30*(2), 71.

National Council of State Boards of Nursing. (2005). *Clinical instruction in prelicensure nursing programs*. Retrieved from https://www.ncsbn.org/Final_Clinical_Instr_Pre_Nsg_programs.pdf

National League for Nursing. (2008). About the NLN: History. Retrieved from http://www.nln.org/aboutnln/info-history.htm

National League for Nursing Accreditation Commission [NLNAC]. (2008). *NLNAC accreditation manual*. New York, NY: NLNAC. Retrieved from http://www.nlnac.org/manuals/Manual2008.htm

Nelson, R. (2010, in press). Distance education technology: Implications for nursing education. In L. Caputi, *Teaching nursing: The art and science, Vol 2.* (2nd ed.). Glen Ellyn, IL: College of DuPage Press.

Newsome, G., & Tanner, S. (2010, in press). Nursing accreditation: Context and evolution. In L. Caputi, *Teaching nursing: The art and science, Vol 3.* (2nd ed.). Glen Ellyn, IL: College of DuPage Press.

Smith, M. M. (2009). Creative clinical solutions: Aligning simulation with authentic clinical experiences. *Nursing Education Perspectives, 30*(2), 126–128.

Spector, N. (2010, in press). Approval: National council of state boards of nursing. In L. Caputi, *Teaching nursing: The art and science, Vol 3.* (2nd ed.). Glen Ellyn, IL: College of DuPage Press.

Tagliareni, M. E. (2009). Beyond the realities of current practice: Preparing students to provide safe and effective care. *Nursing Education Perspectives, 30*(2), 69.

Appendix A

HIPAA Tips for Educators

For information on the Health Insurance Portability and Accountability Act of 1996 visit http://www.hhs.gov/ocr/privacy/

1. Review HIPAA often. Professionals in health care encounter HIPAA constantly. To create a habit of being HIPAA conscious, have your students encounter client privacy in multiple learning activities.
2. Students create policy. Have students create HIPAA-friendly policy for learning activities. This can be done for laboratory practice experiences, online discussions, text-messaging activities, and community health fairs, etc.
3. Involve professionals from practice. Discuss learning activities with professionals knowledgeable about HIPAA. Ask them to identify the potential problems.
4. Share bad examples. Talk frequently about potential and actual breeches.
   - The nurse did not log off and a family member browsed the record of another client.
   - The nurse text messaged (from his personal phone) laboratory values to the physician.
   - The physician took a picture of a wound for the chart with her PDA.
   - The respiratory therapist shares her frustrations with a noncompliant patient on Facebook.
   - The student mentioned the patient's first name in the online clinical video journal.
   - The clinical instructor looked up laboratory values for his neighbor.
5. Students create case studies. Review the HIPAA policy from a local facility with your students. Then have students work in groups of three to four to develop case studies about HIPAA violations.
6. Examinations. HIPAA standards and violations should be a part of examinations and other assessments. Like patient safety, privacy is important in all aspects of health care. Subsequently, examinations in all areas should reflect this importance.

Copyright, 2010, NurseTim, Inc. All rights reserved.

307

Internet Safety and Professionalism for Nurses, Faculty, and Students

Safety

- Avoid linking to family members (especially your children as this gives others personal information).
- Avoid sharing professional affiliations (unless that is the specific purpose of that Web site/space and you were referred).
- Change passwords every 3 months.
- Never share a password with anyone/anywhere (e.g., online, on the phone, in-person, e-mail, etc.).
- Avoid clicking links in unfamiliar e-mails/posts (even if you know the sender). Wait 2 to 3 days for an alert that the e-mail may be malicious.
- Never reply to a forwarded e-mail.
- Never forward an e-mail that has been forwarded to you.

Professionalism

- Avoid jokes and sharing jokes with professional colleagues.
- Use care when "friending" professional colleagues as they may see all personal information, photos, etc. It is hard to predict who will forward your message to others.
- Remember that any information, comments, and thoughts you share digitally is stored on a server somewhere and may return to visit you.
- Address your reader and sign your communication.
- Avoid slang and sarcasm.
- After creating an audio/video recording watch/listen for embarrassing/inappropriate content.
- After creating an audio/video recording, ask a trusted colleague to proof for embarrassing/inappropriate content.
- Check all posts/comments/e-mails for correct grammar, spelling, and attachments.
- Double-check recipients of all communications before you click send/post.

School of Nursing (SON) Faculty Mentoring/ Monitoring Tool

SON Faculty Mentoring/Monitoring Tool

Faculty: _____ **Course #:** _____ **Section:** _____ **Term:** _____

Audit Date: _____ **Auditor:** _____ **Course Enrollment #:** _____

Directions: Enter assessment in appropriate column using key: M=met, NI=needs improvement (see notes).

Fac Eval	Self Eval	Element	#	Criteria	Comments
		Course Home	1.	Completes course setup 5 days before start date.	
			2.	Posts instructor bio and contact info with phone number and office hours.	
			3.	Provides weekly announcements.	
		Student Lounge	4.	Posts instructor introduction in the student lounge and greets students individually within the first week of class.	
		Q & A	5.	Responds to questions within 48 hours.	
		Interaction	6.	Is present in discussion a minimum of 4 days a week or secures coverage when illness/vacation necessitates absence.	
		Discussion:	7.	Week 1 - Responds to 2/3 of students.	
		(a) Presence	8.	Week 2 - Responds to 2/3 of students.	
			9.	Week 3 - Responds to 2/3 of students.	
			10.	Week 4 - Responds to 2/3 of students.	
			11.	Week 5 - Responds to 2/3 of students.	
			12.	Week 6 - Responds to 2/3 of students.	
			13.	Week 7 - Responds to 2/3 of students.	
			14.	Week 8 - Responds to 2/3 of students.	
		(b) Content	15.	Facilitates mutual respect and scholarly dialogue among students.	
			16.	Responses are learner-centered and individualized.	
			17.	Writing is essentially error-free.	
			18.	Tone is positive, respectful, and helpful.	
		(c) Feedback	19.	Encourages independent thinking.	
			20.	Gradebook feedback is individualized.	
		Evaluation of Assignments	21.	Provides assignment feedback within 7 working (business) days.	
			22.	Offers constructive and individualized feedback.	
			23.	Tone is positive, respectful, and helpful.	
			24.	Follows established grading policies/ guidelines; Submits final Banner grades within 5 days from the last day of class.	
			25.	Addresses elements such as requirements, content, quality of writing, and/or ways of improving work.	

Additional Comments and/or Recommendations:

Faculty Mentor Monitor/Self-Monitoring Form. Reprinted with permission by Walden University School of Nursing.

Agents: The term used by learning management system software (e.g., ANGEL, Blackboard, eCollege) to describe actions that the system can complete upon the completion of another action, such as an e-mail generated to confirm submission of a quiz after the quiz has been completed by a student.

Andragogy: The art and science of teaching adults, which focuses on the unique needs of adult learners and the need to be learner-centered when teaching adults. Sometimes referred to as adult learning and is based on works by Malcolm Knowles.

Asynchronous: Activities that are conducted at times of the individual's choice; participants do not have to be online at the same time to complete these activities together.

Authentic Learning: Learning by doing using real-world problems that allow the students to experience and discuss the learning that has occurred.

Avatar: A character created online to represent the user in an online environment. Usually these characters are fully configurable in which the user can select gender, height, weight, build, clothing, shoes, skin color, and many other attributes.

Blackboard: A popular learning management system and virtual classroom; one of the largest in the country.

Blog (Web log): An online journal usually written by one individual located at a specific Web address. Users follow a person's journal, which may be updated hourly, daily, weekly, or monthly.

Browser: A program that connects a user to the Internet. This is the software interface that translates the information sent from the Internet into a readable form for the user.

Bulletin-Board System (BBS): A message board that people use to dial directly into their own computers to send and receive messages about various subjects.

Clinical Decision Support (CDS): Technology that offers appropriate information (i.e., patient data, clinical information, etc.) and alerts at the appropriate time; includes e-books on a PDA and other types of just-in-time tools.

Cloud: Referring to the Internet, often used to describe storing or backing up data to the Internet.

Cognitive Load: The amount and intensity of material that can be put into short-term memory before the working memory can no longer use or process it.

Cognitive Load Theory: A theory based in recent study of information processing by the human brain. Because the brain has limited-working memory, extraneous demands can impede efficient processing and information storage and retention.

Coherence Effect: A type of distraction contributing to cognitive load in which the brain must sift through information to find the core message.

Community: A group of individuals with common goals working together to meet those goals. Building community with and between online learners helps improve retention.

Compliance Training: Education that addresses processes and procedures required to meet specific requirements defined by a regulatory organization or government.

Computer-Assisted Instruction (CAI): Using technology to provide learning activities. The CAI can happen online or on the computer. The learning can be in a fully online course or face-to-face course. It also could come from the disc in the back of the textbook.

Computer-Supported Collaborative Learning: Collaborative learning strategies are used via computer and/or the Internet to encourage and enhance peer interaction and group work among students.

Constructivism: Learning as the result of activities and schedules planned and controlled by the learner.

Contiguity Effect: A type of distraction contributing to cognitive load in which the brain must split its attention to gather information from dissimilar sources.

Course Management System (CMS): A collection of applications used to create a learning environment and manage educational activities (e.g.. Angel, eCollege, Blackboard, Moodle, etc.). A CMS sometimes is considered a learning management system.

Diffusion of Innovation: Reflecting the work of Rodgers, the theory of diffusion of innovation describes the process by which an innovation is communicated through certain channels over time among members of a social system.

Distributed Learning: A learning model in which the student, content, and instructors are all located in different geographic areas.

Early Adopter: An individual who readily accepts and tries new ideas and technologies when he or she is introduced without waiting for improvements and enhancements from large-scale testing.

E-Book Reader: A device that can store many books purchased from the Internet to read on the device wherever the user is. A popular book reader is the Kindle.

Electronic Health Record System (EHRS): A database-management system that holds all information about a patient including financial information, scheduling information, and clinical information.

Electronic Medical Record (EMR): A database that holds only the clinical information about a patient. This is one part of the electronic health record system.

E-mentoring: Coaching and supporting a protégé (or mentee) using virtual/electronic methods or systems.

E-portfolio: An online collection of job experience and educational accomplishments presented in a pleasant format and used to highlight a user's experience and skill sets.

Emoticons: Graphical pictures used to represent an emotion ☺ or activity ;-).

f-2-f (face to face): The process of meeting someone in person (e.g., education, employment, socializing, etc.).

Facebook: A large, social networking site used to connect people in which each individual can have his or her own online page and share this page with whomever he or she selects to be an online Facebook friend.

Far Transfer: Application of conceptual or theoretical knowledge to new contexts or situations.

Flash: An application that plays a specific encoded-compressed video format for universal viewing on many different platforms. It can be animation, video, or presentation.

Friending: The process of adding someone to the private area of your social network page. Often we say that you will friend someone.

Handhelds: Devices that are easily transported. Usually refers to a PDA or a smartphone. See personal digital assistant.

High Fidelity: A simulation event or tool with a high level of realism.

Homophily: The tendency of individuals to associate and bond with similar others.

HTML (Hypertext Markup Language): A universally accepted format language used to deliver documents over the Internet to a wide variety of devices. This is the main format most Internet browsers use in displaying information from Web pages.

Hybrid: Educational courses that meet face-to-face at specific times, but also have a significant amount of coursework done between class sessions in an online environment.

Hyperlink: An area on a Web page that the user can select to jump to a different page or location; usually underlined blue text. Words that are hyperlinks are considered HOT or Hot Links.

Informatics Nurse (IN): Registered nurse who has experience with electronic health record systems; may have an informatics certification or degree specialty.

Informatics Nurse Specialist (INS): Registered nurse who has studied informatics or a related field at the graduate level.

Instant Messaging (IM): A form of synchronous online communication in which an online user can converse with another user. Both have to be present in front of their computers at the same time. Information entered on one user's computer automatically shows on the computer of another user.

Instructivism: An approach to learning in which the expert determines what is needed by passive learners and delivers content.

IPod: A device made famous by Apple for storing and playing portable digital audio, video, and data.

ITouch: A form of iPod that has increased functionality to include data management, Wi-Fi, Internet, telephone, e-mail, Web searching, touch screen, etc. When an iTouch has cellular phone capability, it is called an iPhone.

Job Aid: A tool to assist employees in the conduct of their jobs. Job aids are best used when information is needed on demand and when time allows the interruption to use the tool.

Learning Community: A group of people who share common values and beliefs and are actively engaged in learning together from each other.

Learning Management System (LMS): A large network in which information pertaining to a degree program, school, or university is available to anyone who has access. This is a collection of applications and databases for administrators, staff, instructors, students, and even alumni.

Learning Object: An application or file that helps the user to develop understanding about concepts.

Listserv: An online mailing list that uses electronic mail to send and receive messages to and from groups of people.

Local Area Network (LAN): A group of computers in one geographic area connected together to share information and complete tasks.

Mashup: Two or more applications on the Internet are combined to make a new service. Conduct a Web search on "cloud computing" for more information.

Metadata: A description of how certain data is managed, catalogued, and stored.

Modality Effect: Information processing is enhanced when the content is delivered through both the visual and auditory channels of the brain.

Moodle: A popular "open-source" learning management system, which is configurable.

MP3 (MPEG Layer 3): A popular digital audio-encoding format used for audio files. The advantage of saving audio in this format is its ability to compress the information to reduce the transfer time online and required need for storage.

Multiuser Virtual Environment (MUVE): An online simulated graphical piece of software that allows users to create characters of themselves (called avatars) and explore a three-dimensional online environment.

Near Transfer: Application of training content directly associated with desired performance outcomes.

Netbook: A small laptop computer (screen is about 10.1" diagonal); usually does not include a DVD/CD drive/burner but has similar functionality to a laptop computer.

Netiquette: Socially accepted communication strategies for digital/virtual communication. For example, ALL CAPS is considered screaming.

Nursing Informatics: A specialty that integrates nursing science, computer science, and information science to manage and communicate data, information, knowledge, and wisdom in nursing practice.

Online: As it pertains to learning, refers to the use of Internet technologies to provide course activities.

Online Community of (Professional) Practice: A group of people from different departments or organizations who meet on the Internet to work toward a common goal. For example, nurses and nursing students taking the same course together online.

Pedagogy: The art and science of being a teacher. Pedagogy is sometimes referred to as the study of being a teacher of children whereas andragogy is the study of teaching adults.

Personal Digital Assistant (PDA): A portable device used to store personal information, manage data, manage media, and communicate (if the device has access to technology such as Wi-Fi) for immediate retrieval. Information can include but is not limited to contact information, calendars, pictures, videos, and more.

Personal Health Record (PHR): Health data that patients collect and maintain.

Podcast: An audio recording saved in a digital format with the ability to download to a portable audio player (popularly known as an MP3 player).

Portable Document Format (PDF): A file format that allows viewing and printing of a file using free, readily available software that is available for many different computer systems and mobile devices.

Problem-Based Learning: An instructional method in which students work cooperatively to seek solutions to real-world problems.

Pushed: The act of a network sending information to your e-mail, cell phone, pager, or other electronic devices. This allows the information to come to the user so the user does not have to go to a specific Web site on the Internet.

Redundancy Effect: Information process is impaired when narration is repeating visual text.

RSS (Really Simple Syndication or Rich Site Summary): Software used to send continuously updated information directly to the user in a browser (see pushed).

Scaffolding: In education, a support or basis of education and experience that helps the learner build and develop more skills and concepts for enhanced learning.

Screencast: Digital recording of a computer screen used to instruct users in how to perform certain computer-software functions. Also known as a video capture of a computer screen.

Screenshot: A still picture of a computer screen usually used for sample or instructional purposes.

Search Engine: An Internet software tool used to search the entire Internet for specific content. Popular search engines include Google, Bing, and Yahoo.

Short Message Service (SMS): See texting.

Smartphone: A cell phone combined with a PDA (see personal digital assistant). This phone also does a variety of things including the ability to browse the Internet, keep information on contacts, schedules, take pictures, and even use as a global positioning service (GPS) device.

Social Bookmark: A list of Web-site addresses accessible to a group of users for the purpose of sharing popular resources.

Social Learning: A theory that focuses on the learning that occurs within a social context, reflecting learning from one another, imitation, modeling, and observation.

Social Networks: An online network used as a meeting place for anyone who has access to the Internet for purposes of social interaction, sharing of personal experiences, and other artifacts including pictures, videos, and favorite places, etc.

Spam: Advertising sent by e-mail; commonly known as the junk mail of the Internet.

Streaming: The process of sending audio and video directly to the computer for immediate playback and can be done instead of downloading audio or video for play at a later time.

Student-Centered Learning: An approach to education focusing on the needs of the students more than the needs of the faculty or the system.

Syllabism: Reliance upon the course syllabus without concern for individuals, current practice, or flexibility.

Synchronize: The act of sharing information between one database and another so that changes can be made to both separately, and updated on both when synchronized. It is common to synchronize a smartphone with a computer. "Sync your contacts with Google."

Synchronous: Activities that are completed in real time, such as online chats, where all participants are involved in the same activity at the same time.

Tablet: A computer either without a physical keyboard or with a keyboard that is hidden by the screen. Everything is entered by pressing or writing on the screen itself. The Apple iPad is considered a tablet computer.

Techno-Learning: Use of technology to assist with the learning process.

Technology Informatics Guiding Educational Reform (TIGER) Initiative: Grassroots collaborative of clinical leaders formed to create a vision for the future of nursing, which bridges the quality chasm with information technology, enabling nurses to use informatics in practice and education to provide safer, higher-quality patient care.

Texting: Sending a written message over a network from one person to another. Short message service (SMS) is the most common technology used. Typically reserved to cell phones, the act of texting online is more accurately described as instant messaging. Text messages can however be sent from a computer to a cell phone and vice versa using an online service, such as Twitter.

Tweet: A message containing 140 characters with the online service, Twitter. The message is typed by a user and sent to anyone following that person's Twitter account.

Twitter: A service that allows anyone to send limited messages (called tweets) to other people who wish to "follow" this person. Also considered a social network or microblogging site.

Uniform Resource Locator (URL): An address location on the Internet where a specific resource or device can be found.

Virtual Classrooms: Electronic learning management platforms that create the learning space used to store course content, complete collaborative learning activities, network with peers, and submit student work—an online classroom.

Virtual Conference: A meeting of people held in a multiuser virtual environment (MUVE) using avatars for the participants. This term also may be used for a Webinar.

Virtual Reality: A simulated environment found in a computer- or Internet-based system. Users can interact with objects and others in this simulated environment as a way of gaining and disseminating information. Second Life is a popular online software tool that allows for virtual reality interactions.

Vodcast: A digital video recording that is transferable to a portable media device, such as a smartphone or other media player. Also referred to as a video podcast.

Webademia Instruction: Use of the Internet or Web-based content in an academic setting.

Web 2.0: Web applications that facilitate interactivity on a Web site allowing viewers to contribute beyond the passive readership of the "old" Internet.

Web-Based Content Management Systems: See learning management system.

Webcasting: A video capture tool that provides integration of multiple types of input (audio, video, PowerPoint, whiteboard, etc.) into one presentation. It can be viewed via a Web page live or recorded for future viewing.

WebCT: A popular online classroom and learning management system that recently has been acquired by the parent company of Blackboard.

Webinar: Meeting on the Internet through the use of special software; can include video, texting, document sharing, and activities, such as voting.

Web-Supported Learning: Course content is taught in a traditional face-to-face method (i.e., lecture, laboratory, etc.) with specifically developed content and activities offered online to supplement learning.

Wide Area Network (WAN): A group of computers connected together regardless of geographic distance from each other.

Wi-Fi: Technology that allows computers and other devices to communicate without wires. Usually found in a local area (such as business, home, or campground). Not to be confused with the wireless connectivity that comes through mobile phone providers and 3G/4G Internet service. Mobile phone providers and 3G/4G Internet services provide wireless service over a large geographical area.

Wiki: Web site used for the simple creation and editing of interlinking Web pages to create a database of interlinked topics. Most wikis can be developed by a group of people and each person's contribution/edit is tracked in a log. The most famous is Wikipedia, an online encyclopedia that allows additions and editing of information by any member.

XML (Extensible Markup Language): A set of rules used to make a document universally available across a variety of browser formats for compatibility on the Internet. Similar to HTML but more advanced.

YouTube: An online service offering video (see streaming) submitted by anyone who has membership to share with anyone who has access.

Chapter 1

Allen, I. E., & Seaman, J. (2008). *Staying the course: Online education in the United States, 2008.* Retrieved from http://www.sloan-c.org/sites/default/files/staying_the_course-2.pdf

Baker's Guide to Christian Distance Education. (2010). *Distance education timeline.* Retrieved from http://www.bakersguide.com/Distance_Education_Timeline/

Billings, D. M. (2003). Online communities of professional practice. *Journal of Nursing Education, 42*(8), 335.

Diigo. (2010). *Diigo. Research, share, collaborate.* Retrieved from http://www.diigo.com/

Georgiev, T., Georgieva, E., & Smrikarov, A. (2004). *M-learning: A new stage of E-learning.* Paper presented at the International Conference on Computer Systems and Technologies. Retrieved from http://ecet.ecs.ru.acad.bg/cst04/Docs/sIV/428.pdf

Hinkle, L. (2009a). *Distance education history: The early years of distance learning.* Retrieved from http://www.brighthub.com/education/online-learning/articles/24404.aspx

Hinkle, L. (2009b). *The future of distance learning.* Retrieved from http://www.brighthub.com/education/online-learning/articles/27955.aspx#ixzz0eJQq36x3

Kala, S., Isaramalai, S., & Pohthong, A. (2010). Electronic learning and constructivism: A model for nursing education. *Nurse Education Today, 30,* 61–66. doi:10.1016/j.nedt.2009.06.002

McArthur, D. (2002). Investing in digital resources. *New Directions for Higher Education, 119,* 77–84.

Seaman, J. (2009). *Online learning as a strategic asset. Volume II: The paradox of faculty voices: Views and experiences with online learning.* Retrieved from http://www.sloan-c.org/sites/default/files/APLU_online_strategic_asset_vol2-1.pdf

Struk, C., & Moss, J. (2009). Focus on technology: What can you do to move the vision forward? *Computers Informatics Nursing, 27*(3), 92–194. doi: 10.1097/NCN.0b013e3181a5568e

Time. (1983, January 3). Cover image: The computer moves in. *Time.* Retrieved from http://www.time.com/time/covers/0,16641,19830103,00.html

Chapter 2

Bandura, A. (2001). Social cognitive theory: An agentic perspective. *Annual Review of Psychology, 52,* 1–26.

Beaudoin, M. (1990). The instructor's changing role in distance education. *American Journal of Distance Education, 4,* 2.

Bertrand, Y. (2003). *Contemporary theories and practice in education.* Madison, WI: Atwood.

Cook-Sather, A. (2002). Authorizing students' perspectives: Toward trust, dialogue, and change in education. *Educational researcher, 31*(4), 3–14.

Dewey, J. (1933). *How we think.* Boston: Heath.

Dewey, J. (1964). My pedagogic creed. In R. D. Archambault (Ed.), *Dewey on education.* Chicago: University of Chicago Press.

Forehand, M. (2005). Bloom's taxonomy: Original and revised. In M. Orey (Ed.), *Emerging perspectives on learning, teaching, and technology.* Retrieved March 12, 2010, from http://projects.coe.uga.edu/epltt/

Gardner, H. (1991). *The unschooled mind: How children think and how schools should teach.* New York: Basic Books.

Hanna, D. E., Conceicao-Runlee, S., & Glowacki-Dudka, M. (2000). *147 practical tips for teaching online groups: Essentials of Web-based education.* Madison, WI: Atwood.

Hannafin, M. J., & Land, S. M. (1997). The foundations and assumptions of technology-enhanced student-centered learning environments. *Instructional Science, 25,* 167–202.

Knowles, M. S. (1989). *The making of an adult educator.* San Francisco: Jossey-Bass.

Knowles, M. S., Holton, E. F., & Swanson, R. A. (Eds.). (2005). *The adult learner: The definitive classic in adult education and human resource development* (6th ed.). Woburn, MA: Butterworth-Heinemann.

Merriam, S. (2001). Andragogy and self-directed learning: Pillars of adult learning theory. *New Directions for Adult and Continuing Education, 89*, 3–13.

Panitz, T. (1997). *Ted's cooperative e-book*. Retrieved from http://home.capecod.net/~tpanitz/

Piaget, J. (1952). *The origins of intelligence in children*. New York: International University Press.

Rogers, E. (2003). *Diffusion of innovations* (3rd ed.). New York: Free Press.

Thorpe, M., Edwards, R., & Hanson, A. (1993). *Culture and processes of adult learning*. New York: Routledge.

Chapter 3

Ali, S., & Salter, G. (2004). The use of templates to manage on-line discussion forums. *Electronic Journal on e-Learning, 2*(1), 11–18.

Anderson, L. W., & Krathwohl, D. R. (Eds.). (2001). *A taxonomy for learning, teaching and assessing: A revision of Bloom's taxonomy of educational objectives*. Boston: Allyn & Bacon.

Angelo, T. A., & Cross, K. P. (1993). *Classroom assessment techniques: A handbook for college teachers* (2nd ed.). San Francisco: Jossey-Bass.

Bender, T. (2003). *Discussion based online teaching to enhance student learning*. Sterling, VA: Stylus.

Brookfield, S. D. (1995). *Becoming a reflective teacher*. San Francisco: Jossey-Bass

Businessballs. (n.d.). *Blooms taxonomy of learning domains: Bloom's learning model for teaching and lesson planning*. Retrieved from http://wwwbusienssballs.com/bloomstaxonomyoflearningdomains.htm

Cagiltay, K. (2006) Scaffolding strategies in electronic performance support systems: Types and challenges. *Innovations in Education and Teaching International, 43*(1), 93–103. doi: 10.1080/14703290500467673

Center for Applied Special Technology. (2009). *UDL guidelines – version 1.0: Introduction*. Retrieved from http://www.cast.org/research/udl/index.html

Coyne, P., Ganley, P., Hall, T., Meo, G., Murray, E., & Gordon, D. (2008). Applying universal design for learning in the classroom. In D. H. Rose & A. Meyers (Eds.), *A practical reader in universal design for learning*. Cambridge, MA: Harvard Education Press.

Dick, W. (1996). The Dick and Carey model: Will it survive the decade? *Educational Technology Research and Development, 44*(3), 55–63. doi: 10.1007/BF02300425

Dick, W., Carey, L., & Carey, J.O. (2006). *The systematic design of instruction* (6th ed.). San Francisco: Berett-Koehler.

Diekelmann, N. (2002). "Too much content . . .": Epistemologies' grasp and nursing education. *Journal of Nursing Education, 41*, 469–470.

Freire, P. (1993). *Pedagogy of the oppressed* (30th ed.). New York: Continuum Press.

Gagné, R. M., Briggs, L. J., & Wager, W. W. (1992). *Principles of Instructional Design* (4th ed.). Fort Worth, TX: Harcourt Brace Jovanovich College Publishers.

Graessner, A. C., McNanara, D. S., & VanLehn, K. (2005). Scaffolding deep comprehension strategies through Point&Query, Auto Tutor, and iStart. *Educational Psychologist, 40*(4), 225–234.

Gregoire, M. (2003). Is it a challenge of a threat? A dual-process model of teachers' cognition and appraisal processing during conceptual change. *Educational Psychology Review, 15*(2), 147–179.

Gronlund, N. E., & Waugh, C. K. (2009). *Assessment of learner achievement*. New York: Allyn & Bacon.

Gustafson, K. L., & Branch, R. M. (2002). What is Instructional Design? In R. A. Reiser & J. V. Dempsey (Eds.). *Trends and issues in Instructional Design and technology*. Columbus: OH, Merrill Prentice Hall.

Molenda, M., Pershing, J. A., & Reigeluth, C. M. (1996). Designing instructional systems. In R. L. Craig (Ed.). *The ASTD training and development handbook* (4th ed., pp. 266–293). New York: McGraw-Hill.

Meyers, A., & Rose, D. H. (2005). The future is in the margins: The role of technology and disability in educational reform. In D. H. Rose, A. Meyers, & C. Hitchcock (Eds.), *The universally designed classroom: Accessible curriculum and digital technologies* (pp. 13–16). Cambridge, MA: Harvard Education Press.

National Center for Universal Design (D. H. Rose & J. Wasson, compilers). (2009). *Introduction: UDL guidelines – Version 1.0*. Retrieved from http://www.udlcenter.org/aboutudl/udlguidelines/

National League for Nursing. (2005). *Position statement: Transforming nursing education*. New York: National League for Nursing. Retrieved from: http://www.nln.org/aboutnln/positionstatements/transforming052005.pdf

Notar, C. E., Zuelke, D. C., Wilson, J. D., & Yunker, B. D. (2004). The table of specifications: Insuring accountability in teacher made tests. *Journal of Instructional Psychology*. Retrieved from http://findarticles.com/p/articles/mi_m0FCG/is_2_31/ai_n6130123/pg_4/?tag=content;col1

Reiser, R. (2001). A history of instructional design and technology: Part II: A history of instructional design. *ETR&D, 49*(2), 57–67.

Rideout, E. (2001). *Transforming nursing education through problem-based learning.* Sudbury, MA: Jones & Bartlett.

Rideout, E., England-Oxford, V., Brown, B., Fothergill-Borunnais, F., Ingram, C., Benson, G., Ross, M., & Coates, A.. (2002). A comparison of problem-based and conventional curricula in nursing education. *Advances in Health Science Education, 7,* 3–17.

Strampel, K., & Oliver, R. (2007). *Using technology to foster reflection in higher education.* Proceedings of Ascilite Singapore. Retrieved from http://www.ascilite.org.au/conferences/singapore07/procs/strampel.pdf

University of Illinois. (2010). *Instructional strategies for online courses.* Retrieved from http://www.uillinois.edu/resources/tutorials/pedagogy/instructionalstrategies.asp

Uribe, D., & Klein, J.D. (2003). The effect of case-based versus systematic problem solving in a computer–mediated collaborative environment. *Quarterly Review of Distance Education, 4*(4), 417–436.

Van den Hurk, M. M. (2006). The relation between self-regulated strategies and individual study time, prepared participation and achievement in a problem-based curriculum. *Active Learning in Higher Education, 7,* 155–169. Doi: 10.1177/469787406064752

vanMerrienboer, J. J. G., & Sluijsmams, D. M. A. (2009). Toward a synthesis of cognitive load theory, four-component instructional design, and self-directed learning. *Education Psychology Review, 21,* 55–66. Doi: 10.1007/s10648-008-9092-5

Chapter 4

American Association of Colleges of Nursing. (2008). *The essentials of baccalaureate education for professional nursing practice.* Washington, DC: Author.

Bailey, C. J., & Card, K. A. (2009). Effective pedagogical practices for online teaching: Perception of experienced instructors. *Internet and Higher Education, 12*(3), 152–155. doi:110.1016/j.iheduc.2009.1008.1002

Benner, P., Sutphen, M., Leonard, V., & Day, L. (2010). Educating nurses: A call for radical transformation. San Francisco: Jossey-Bass.

Bristol, T. (2005). *Perceptions of e-learning in Iowa nursing faculty.* Minneapolis, MN: Capella University.

Fisher, C. A., Newbold, S., & O'Neil, C. A. (2008). *Developing online learning environments in nursing education* (2nd ed.). New York: Springer.

Halstead, J. A., & Billings, D. M. (2009). Teaching and learning in online learning communities. In D. M. Billings & J. A. Halstead (Eds.), *Teaching in nursing: A guide for faculty* (3rd ed., pp. 369–389). St. Louis, MO: Elsevier.

Jeffries, P. (2007). *Simulation in nursing education: From conceptualization to evaluation.* New York: National League for Nursing.

Lake, D. (2001). Student performance and perceptions of a lecture-based course compared with the same course utilizing group discussion. *Physical Therapy, 81*(3), 896–902.

National League for Nursing Accrediting Commission. (2008). *2008 edition: NLNAC accreditation manual.* New York: Author.

Palloff, R. M., & Pratt, K. (2007). *Building online learning communities: Effective strategies for the virtual classroom.* San Francisco: John Wiley & Sons.

Rogers, E. M. (2003). Diffusion of innovations (5th ed.). New York: The Free Press.

Sitzman, K. (2010). Student-preferred caring behaviors for online nursing education. *Nursing Education Perspectives, 31*(3), 171–176.

Chapter 5

Allen, D. B., & Allen, D. W. (1996). *2+2 equals better performance: Alternative performance appraisal with feedback and encouragement.* Beijing, China: Author.

Horton, W. (2008). Knowledge management: From the graveyard to good ideas. In S. Carliner & P. Shank (Eds.), *The e-learning handbook: Past promises, present challenges* (pp. 77–107). San Francisco: Pfeiffer.

Ignatavicius, D. (2005). An introduction to developing critical thinking in nursing students. In L. Caputi & L. Engelmann (Eds.), *Teaching nursing: The art and science* (Vol. 2, pp. 622–633). Glen Ellyn, IL: College of Dupage Press.

Jonassen, D. H., & Land, S. M. (2000). *Theoretical foundations of learning environments*. Mahwah, NJ: Lawrence Erlbaum Associates.

Lake, D. (2001). Student performance and perceptions of a lecture-based course compared with the same course utilizing group discussion. *Physical Therapy, 81*(3), 896–902.

National League for Nursing. (2006). *Nurse educators 2006: A report of the faculty census survey of RN and graduate programs*. New York: Author.

Nelson, L. M. (1999). Collaborative problem-solving. In C. M. Reigeluth (Ed.), *Instructional Design theories and models* (Vol. 2, pp. 241–268). Mahwah, NJ: Lawrence Erlbaum Associates.

Palloff, R. M., & Pratt, K. (2007). *Building online learning communities: Effective strategies for the virtual classroom*. San Francisco: John Wiley & Sons.

Preece, J. (2000). *Online communities: Designing usability, supporting sociability*. New York: John Wiley & Sons.

Reigeluth, C. M. (1999). *Instructional-Design theories and models*. Mahwah, NJ: Lawrence Erlbaum Associates.

Royse, M. A., & Newton, S. E. (2007). How gaming is used as an innovative strategy for nursing education. *Nursing Education Perspectives, 28*(3), 263–267.

Shea, V. (2005). *The core rules of netiquette*. Retrieved from http://www.albion.com/netiquette/corerules.html

Sitzman, K. (2010). Student-preferred caring behaviors for online nursing education. *Nursing Education Perspectives, 31*(3), 171–176.

Yukselturk, E., & Top, E. (2005/2006). Reconsidering online course discussions: A case study. *Journal of Educational Technology Systems, 34*(3), 341–367.

Chapter 6

Abrami, P. C., & Barrett, H. (2005). Directions for research and development on electronic portfolios. *Canadian Journal of Learning and Technology, 31*(3).

Allen, E. B., Walls, R. T., & Reilly, F. D. (2008). Effects of interactive instructional techniques in a Web-based peripheral nervous system component for human anatomy. *Medical Teacher, 30*, 40–47. doi : 10.1080/01421590701753518

Angelo, T., & Cross, P. (1993). *Classroom assessment techniques*. San Francisco: Jossey-Bass.

Bartini, M. (2008). An empirical comparison of traditional and Web-enhanced classrooms. *Journal of Instructional Psychology, 35*(1), 3–11.

Billings, D. M., & Halstead, J. A. (2009). *Teaching in nursing: A guide for faculty* (3rd ed.). St. Louis, MO: Saunders.

Bouzidi, L., & Jaillet, A. (2009). Can online peer assessment be trusted? *Educational Technology & Society, 12*(4), 257–268.

Bowen, J. A. (2006). Teaching naked: Why removing technology from your classroom will improve student learning. *National Teaching and Learning Forum, 16*(1). Retrieved from http://www.ntlf.com/html/ti/naked.htm

Creative Commons. (2009, October 11). *Frequently asked questions*. Retrieved from http://wiki.creativecommons.org/Frequently_Asked_Questions

Forbes, M. O., & Hickey, M. T. (2008). Podcasting: Implementation and evaluation in an undergraduate nursing program. *Nurse Educator, 33*(5), 224–227.

Garrison, R., & Anderson, T. (2003). *E-learning in the 21st century. A framework for research and practice*. London and New York: Routledge Falmer.

Juwah, C. (2003), *Using peer assessment to develop skills and capabilities. United States Distance Learning Association Journal, 17*(1), retrieved from http://www.usdla.org/html/journal/JAN03_Issue/article04.html

Kim, B., & Reeves, T. C. (2007). Reframing research on learning with technology: In search of the meaning of cognitive tools. *Instructional Science, 35*(3), 207–256.

Knowledge Loom. (n.d.). *Good models of teaching with technology*. Retrieved from http://knowledgeloom.org

Krathwohl, D. R. (2002). A revision of Bloom's taxonomy: An overview. *Theory into Practice, 41*(4), 212–218.

Lashley, M. (2005). Teaching health assessment in the virtual classroom. *Journal of Nursing Education, 44*(8), 348–350.

Lim, J., Kim, M., Chen, S.S., & Ryder, C. E. (2008). An empirical investigation of student achievement and satisfaction in different learning environments. *Journal of Instructional Psychology, 35*(2), 113–119.

Lombardi, M. (2007, May). *Authentic learning for the 21st century: An overview* (Educause Learning Initiatives white paper). Retrieved from http://net.educause.edu/ir/library/pdf/ELI3009.pdf

Madden, M. (2009, July). *The audience for online video-sharing sites shoots up.* Retrieved from Pew Internet & American Life Project Web site: http://pewinternet.org

McBride, D., & Cohen, E. (2009). Misuse of social networking may have ethical implications for nurses. *ONS Connect, 24*(7), 17.

Nursing Education and Technology. (2006). *Learning object repository.* Retrieved from http://webcls.utmb.edu/neat/

Pozzi, F., Manca, S., Persico, D., & Sarti, L. (2007). A general framework for tracking and analyzing learning processes in computer-supported collaborative learning environments. *Innovations in Education and Teaching International, 44*(2), 169–179.

Rhoads, J., & White, C. (2008). Copyright law and distance nursing education. *Nurse Educator, 33*(1), 39–44.

Salyers, V. L. (2005). Web-enhanced and face-to-face classroom instructional methods: Effects on course outcomes and student satisfaction. *International Journal of Nursing Education Scholarship, 2*(1), 1–13.

Schmidt, B., & Stewart, S. (2009). Implementing the virtual reality learning environment: Second Life. *Nurse Educator, 34*(4), 152–155.

Simonson, M., Smaldino, S, Albright, M. & Zvacek, S. (2006) *Teaching and learning at a distance: Foundations of distance education* (3rd ed.) Upper Saddle River, NJ: Merrill Prentice Hall.

Wink, E. (2009). Sources of fully developed course materials on the Web. *Nurse Educator, 34*(4), 143–145.

Whitsed, N. (2004). Learning and teaching: An introduction to re-using learning materials in learning and teaching. *Health Information and Libraries Journal, 21*, 201–205.

Young, J. R. (2008, January 25). YouTube professors: Scholars as online video stars. *Chronicle of Higher Education, 54*, 14–16. Retrieved from http://chronicle.com

Chapter 7

Brookfield, S. D., & Preskill, S. (2005). *Discussion as a way of teaching. Tools and techniques for democratic classrooms* (2nd ed). San Francisco: Jossey-Bass.

Chickering, A., & Ehrmann, S. C. (1996). Implementing the seven principles: Technology as lever. *AAHE Bulletin, 48*, 3–6. Reprinted by the TLT Group. Retrieved from http://www.tltgroup.org/programs/seven.html

Chickering, A., & Gamson, Z. (1987). Seven principles of good practice in undergraduate education. *AAHE Bulletin, 39*, 3–7. Retrieved from http://www.aahea.org/bulletins/articles/sevenprinciples1987.htm

Churches, A. (2008). Bloom's digital taxonomy. Retrieved from http://media.ccconline.cccs.edu/ccco/FacWiki/Blooms_Taxonomy_Tutorials/Churches_2008_DigitalBloomsTaxonomyGuide.pdf

Ehrmann, S. C. (2008). New ideas and additional reading. Retrieved from the TLT Group Web site: http://www.tltgroup.org/programs/seven.html

Eskow, S. (2009, April 2). All learning is hybrid learning: The idea of the organizing technology. *Educational Technology & Change Blog Journal.* Retrieved from http://etcjournal.wordpress.com/2009/04/02/all-learning-is-hybrid-learning-the-idea-of-the-organizing-technology/

Fay, V. P., Selz, N., & Johnson, J. (2005). *Active learning in nursing education.* Houston: Center for Education and Information Resources Publications; Houston Academy of Medicine–Texas Medical Center. Retrieved from http://digitalcommons.library.tmc.edu/cgi/viewcontent.cgi?article=1000&context=uthson_ceirpubs

Ireland, J., Martindale, S., Johnson, N., Adams, D., Eboh, W., & Mowatt, E. (2009). Blended learning in education: Effects on knowledge and attitude. *British Journal of Nursing, 18*(2), 124–130.

Mueller, J. (2008). *Authentic assessment toolbox. North Central College.* Retrieved from: http://jonathan.mueller.faculty.noctrl.edu/toolbox/index.htm

Muilenburg, L., & Berge, Z. (2006). *A framework for designing questions for online learning.* Retrieved from http://www.emoderators.com/moderators/muilenburg.html

Reynard, R. (2007, May 23). Hybrid learning: Maximizing student engagement. *Campus Technology.* Retrieved from http://campustechnology.com/articles/2007/05/hybrid-learning-maximizing-student-engagement.aspx

Russell, T. L. (1999*). The no significant difference phenomenon as reported in 355 research reports, summaries and papers.* Raleigh: North Carolina State University Press.

Zimmerman, L. (2009, February 6). Hybrid, online, or F2F—It depends. *Educational Technology & Change Blog Journal.* Retrieved from http://etcjournal.wordpress.com/2009/02/06/hybird-online-f2f-it-all-depends/

Chapter 8

Abdel-Salam, T., Kauffman, P. J., & Crossman, G. (2006). Does the lack of hands-on experience in a remotely delivered laboratory course affect student learning? *European Journal of Engineering Education, 31*(6), 747–756.

CHEA Institute for Research and Study of Accreditation. (2002). *Accreditation and assuring quality in distance learning.* Washington, DC: Council for Higher Education Accreditation.

Commission on Collegiate Nursing Education. (2009). *Standards of accreditation of baccalaureate and graduate degree nursing programs.* Washington, DC: Commission on Collegiate Nursing Education.

Dougiamas, M. (1999). Developing tools to foster online educational dialogue. In K. Martin, N. Stanley, & N. Davison (Eds.), *Proceedings of the 8th annual Teaching Learning Forum* (pp. 119–123). Perth, UWA: University of Western Austrailia.

Elliott, S. J., & Kukula, E. (2007, November 1). The challenges associated with laboratory-based distance education. *Educause Quarterly, 30*(1), 37–42. Retrieved from http://www.educause.edu/EDUCAUSE+Quarterly/EDUCAUSEQuarterlyMagazineVolum/TheChallengesAssociatedwithLab/157441

Gellman-Danley, B., & Fetzner, M. J. (1998, Spring). *Asking the really tough questions: Policy issues for distance learning.* Retrieved from Penn State University Web site http://citeseerx.ist.psu.edu/viewdoc/download?doi=10.1.1.123.2784&rep=rep1&type=pdf

Google Wave. (2009, December 23). Wikipedia. Retrieved from http://en.wikipedia.org/w/index.php?title=Google_Wave&oldid=333570186

Hilbelink, J. (2009). A measure of the effectiveness of incorporating 3D human anatomy into an online undergraduate laboratory. *British Journal of Educational Technology, 40*(4), 664–672.

Lynch, M. (2002). *The online educator: Guide to creating the virtual classroom.* New York: Rutledge Falmer.

Morabito, M. G. (2009). *CALCampus: Origins.* Retrieved from http://www.calcampus.com/calc.htm

Morgan, G. (2003, May 20). *Course management systems in the history and the future of higher education.* Retrieved from Educause Center for Applied Research Web site http://net.educause.edu/ir/library/pdf/pub7101.pdf

Morris, T., & Hancock, D. (2008). Program exit examinations in nursing education: Using a value-added assessment as a measure of the impact of a new curriculum. *Educational Research Quarterly, 32*(2), 19–29.

National League for Nursing Accrediting Commission. (2008). *Accreditation manual, 2008 edition.* New York: Author.

Ogot, M., Elliott, G., & Glumac, N. (2003). An assessment of in-person and remotely operated laboratories. *Journal of Engineering Education, 92,* 57–63.

Omale, N., Hung, W.-C., Luetkehans, L., & Cooke-Plagwitz, J. (2009). Learning in 3-D multiuser virtual environments: Exploring the use of unique 3-D attributes for online problem-based learning. *British Journal of Educational Technology, 40*(3), 480–495.

O'Neil, C. A., Fisher, C. A., & Newbold, S. K. (2009). *Developing online nursing environments in nursing education.* New York: Springer.

Palloff, R. M., & Pratt, K. (2001). *Lessons from the cyberspace classroom.* San Francisco: Josey-Bass.

Palloff, R. M., & Pratt, K. (2003). *The virtual student.* San Francisco: Josey-Bass.

Rounds, L. R., & Rappaport, B. A. (2008, January/February). The successful use of problem-based learning in an online nurse practitioner course. *Nursing Education Perspectives, 29*(1), 12–16.

Saeed, N., Yang, Y., & Sinnappan, S. (2009). Emerging Web technologies in higher education: A case of incorporating blogs, podcasts and social bookmarks in a Web programming course based on students' learning styles and technology preferences. *Educational Technology & Society, 12*(4), 98–109.

Sancho, P., Moreno-Ger, P., Fuentes-Fernandez, R., & Fernandez-Manjon, B. (2009). Adaptive role-playing games: An immersive approach for problem-based learning. *Educational Technology & Society, 12*(4), 110–124.

Schmidt, B., & Stewart, S. (2009). Implementing the virtual reality learning environment: Second Life. *Nurse Educator, 34*(4), 152–155.

Spurlock, D. R., & Hunt, L. A. (2008). A study of the usefulness of the HESI Exit Exam in predicting NCLEX-RN failure. *Journal of Nursing Education, 47*(4), 157–166.

United States Securities and Exchange Commission. (2008). *Form 10-K: Blackboard, Inc. annual filing.* Washington, DC.

Vergara, V., Caudell, T., Goldsmith, T., & Alverson, D. (2008). *Knowledge-driven design of virtual patient simulations.* Retrieved from Innovate Online Web site http://www.innovateonline.info/index.php?view=article&id=579

Wang, Y., Peng, H., Huang, R., Hou, Y., & Wang, J. (2008). Characteristics of distance learning: Research on relationships of learning motivation, learning strategy, self-efficacy, attribution and learning results. *Open Learning, 23*(1), 17–28.

Wijekumar, K. (2002). *Creating effective Web-based learning environments: Relevant research and practice.* Retrieved from Innovate Online Web site www.innovateonline.info/index.php?view=article&id=26

Woo, Y., Herrington, J., Agostinho, S., & Reeves, T. C. (2007, November 3). *Implementing authentic tasks in Web-based learning environments.* Retrieved from www.educase.edu/161831

Woodill, G. (2007, April 23). *The evolution of learning management systems.* Retrieved December 26, 2009, from *HR Reporter* Web site: www.hrreporter.com

Yang, S.-H. (2009). Using blogs to enhance critical reflection and community of practice. *Educational Technology & Society, 12*(2), 11–21.

Chapter 9

Anderson, L. W., Krathwohl, D. R., Airasian, P. W., Cruikshank, K. A., Mayer, R. E., Pintrich, P. R., et al. (Eds.). (2001). *A taxonomy for learning, teaching, and assessing: A revision of Bloom's taxonomy of educational objectives.* New York: Addison Wesley Longman.

Buzzetto-More, N. A., & Alade, A. J. (2006). Best practices in e-assessment. *Journal of Information Technology Education, 5,* 251–268.

Draper, S. W. (2009). What are learners actually regulating when given feedback? *British Journal of Educational Technology, 40*(2), 306–315.

Hazari, S. (2004, Winter). Strategy for assessment of online course discussions. *Journal of Information Systems Education, 15*(4), 349–355.

Krathwohl, D. R. (2002). A revision of Bloom's taxonomy: An overview. *Theory into Practice, 41*(4), 212–218.

Milne, J. Heinrich, E., & Morrison, D. (2008). Technological support for assignment assessment: A New Zealand higher education survey. *Australasian Journal of Educational Technology, 24*(5), 487–504.

Nicol, D. J., & MacFarlane-Dick, D. (2006). Formative assessment and self-regulated learning: A model and seven principles of good feedback practice. *Studies in Higher Education, 31*(2), 199–218.

Nitko, A. J. (2004). *Educational assessment outcomes.* Columbus, OH: Pearson Merrill Prentice Hall.

Orsmond, P., Merry, S., & Reiling, K. (2005). Biology student's utilization of tutor's formative feedback: A qualitative interview study. *Assessment & Evaluation in Higher Education, 30*(4), 369–386.

Scalise, K., & Gifford, B. (2006, June). Computer-based assessment in e-learning: A framework for constructing "intermediate constraint" questions and tasks for technology platforms. *Journal of Technology, Learning, and Assessment, 4*(6). Retrieved from http://www.jtla.org

Seok, S. (2008). Teaching aspects of e-learning. *International Journal on E-Learning, 7*(4), Retrieved from http://findarticles.com/p/articles/mi_hb1408/is_200810/ai_n32297646/

Van der Linden, W.J. (2002). On complexity in CBT. In C. Mills, M. Potenza, J. Fremer, & W. Ward (Eds.), *Computer-based testing* (pp. 89–102). Mahwah, NJ: Lawrence Erlbaum Associates.

Chapter 10

Ambrose, L. (2001). *Learning online facilitation online.* Paper presented at the Moving Online Conference II, 2–4 September, Gold Coast, Australia. Retrieved from http://flexiblelearning.net.au/leaders/fl_leaders/fll00/lyn_ambrose.htm

Armstrong, T. (1994, November). Multiple intelligences: Seven Ways to approach curriculum. *Educational Leadership, 52*(3), 26–28.

Berge, Z. L. (1995). The role of the online instructor/facilitator, in facilitating computer conferencing: Recommendations from the field. *Educational Technology, 35*(1), 22–30. Retrieved from http://www.emoderators.com/moderators/teach_online.html

Boettcher, J. V. (2006). *Ten core principles for designing learning: The jungle brain meets the tundra brain.* Expanded version of Boettcher, J. V. (2003). Course management systems and learning principles: Getting to know each other. *Syllabus, 16,* 33–36. Retrieved from campustechnology.com/articles/39412/

Coates, K. (2002). *Up to the challenge. Nurses with disabilities overcome legal, social and mental hurdles to flourish in their careers.* Retrieved from http://www.nurseweek.com/news/features/02-03/disabilities.asp

De Cicco, E. (2002). *The role of the facilitator within online discussion groups: A case study.* Paper presented at the Global Summit Conference, Adelaide, Australia. Retrieved from http://www.educationau.edu.au/globalsummit/papers/ecicco.htm

Finke, L. M. (2005). Teaching in nursing: The faculty role. In D. M. Billings & J.A. Halstead (Eds.), *Teaching in nursing: A guide for faculty* (2nd ed., pp. 3–20). St. Louis, MO: Elsevier-Saunders.

Fleming, S., & Maheady, D. (2005, Spring). Homework for future nursing students with disabilities. *Minority Nurse.* Retrieved from http://www.minoritynurse.com/features/nurse_emp/01-27-02h.html

Gardner, H. (2003). Can technology exploit our many ways of knowing? Retrieved from http://www.howardgardner.com/Papers/papers.html

Gardner, H. (2005). Multiple lenses on the mind. Retrieved from http://www.howardgardner.com/Papers/papers.html

Keefe, D., & Dickinson, D. (1998). *Technology enhances Howard Gardner's eight intelligences.* Retrieved from http://www.newhorizons.org/

Kaminski, J. (2006) *P.A.T.C.H. assessment scale pretest for attitudes toward computers in healthcare.* Retrieved from http://www.nursing-informatics.com/kwantlen/patch.html

Lauer, M., & Wombwell, M. (2007). *Speaking engagement: Technology on a budget: Utilizing companion Websites to enhance the learning experience.* Paper presented at the Drexel E-Learning 2.0 Conference, Philadelphia.

Maheady, D. (2003). *Nursing students with disabilities change the course.* River Edge, NJ: Exceptional Parent Press.

Ramsey, G. (2007). *Education and accommodation are the keys to incorporating RNs with disabilities.* Retrieved from http://www.usuhs.mil/chd/Outreach/Publications/Publ-NursSptrm-Disabled-Nurses-Education-and-Accommodation-are-the-Keys-to-Incorporating-RNs-with-Disabilities.pdf The Center for Universal Design. (1997). *The principles of Universal Design, version 2.0.* Raleigh: North Carolina State University. Bettye Rose Connell, Mike Jones, Ron Mace, Jim Mueller, Abir Mullick, Elaine Ostroff, Jon Sanford, Ed Steinfeld, Molly Story, and Gregg Vanderheiden. Retrieved from http://www.design.ncsu.edu/cud/about_ud/udprinciplestext.htm

Wheeler, L., Reynolds, T., & Russell, J. (2000). *Teaching online: A guide for teachers, facilitators and mentors, RMIT.* Retrieved from http://www.learnlinks.com.au/docs/downloads/online.pdf

Chapter 11

Allen, I. E., & Seaman, J. (2003). *Seizing the opportunity: The quality and extent of online education in the United States, 2002 and 2003.* Needham, MA: The Sloan Consortium. Report. Retrieved from http://www.aln.org/resources/sizing_opportunity.pdf

American Association of Colleges of Nursing. (2009). *Nursing shortage fact sheet.* Retrieved from http://www.aacn.nche.edu/Media/pdf/NrsgShortageFS.pdf

American Association of Colleges of Nursing. (2009). *AACN applauds the Carnegie Report calling for a more highly educated nursing workforce.* Retrieved February from https://www.aacn.nche.edu/Media/NewsReleases/2010/carnegie.html

Bitler, D. (2001). Managing technological changes: Strategies for college and university leaders. *Journal of College Student Development, 42,* 80–82.

California Labor & Workforce Development Agency. (2009). $11 million Public-Private Partnership with the Governor's Nurse Education Initiative receives approval for first-in-the-nation, on-line Pre-licensure nursing education program [News release]. Retrieved from http://www.labor.ca.gov/pdf/nwsrel09-08.pdf

Dick, W., & Carey L. (1990). *The systematic design of instruction.* Glenview, IL: Scott, Foresman.

Donofrio, N. (2006). An engine of innovation. *Diverse Issues in Higher Education, 23,* 45.

Hartman, J., Dziuban, C., & Moskal, P. (2000). Faculty satisfaction in ALNs: A dependent independent variable? *Journal of Asynchronous Learning Networks, 4*(3), 155–179.

Hazari, S. I., & Borkowski, E. Y (2001). Looking beyond course development tools: Faculty training issues. *Proceedings of Educause 2001 Conference.* Retrieved from http://www.sunilhazari.com/education/documents/educause2001.htm

Hawkins, B. (2003). Making a commitment. *Educause Review, 38,* 68.

Hundert, E. M., Wakefield, M., Bootman, J. L., Cassel, C. K., Ching, W., Chow, M. P., et al. (2003). *Institute of Medicine report—Health professions education: A bridge to quality.* Washington, DC: National Academies Press.

Keegan, D. (1995). *Distance education technology for the new millennium: Compressed video teaching.* ZIFF Papiere. Hagen, Germany: Institute for Research into Distance Education.

LaRocco, S. (2006). Who will teach the nurses? *Academe, 92*(3), 38–40.

Lazarus, B. D. (2003). Teaching courses online: How much time does it take? *Journal of Asynchronous Learning Networks, 7*(3), 47–53.

Levy, S. (2003). Six factors to consider when planning online distance learning programs in higher education. *Online Journal of Distance Learning Administration, 6*(1), 1–2.

Nevada Nurses Association. (2004). Nursing faculty shortage facts and factors. *RNformation, 13*(2), 16.

Neal, E. (1999). Distance education: Prospects and problems. *Phi Kappa Phi Journal, 79*(1), 40–43.

Reigle, R. (2008). Teacher autonomy defined in online education Retrieved from http://www.eric.ed.gov/PDFS/ED503316.pdf

Sloan Consortium. (2006). *Making the grade: Online education the United States, 2006.* Retrieved from http://www.sloanconsortium.org/sites/default/files/Making_the_Grade.pdf

Schraeder, M., Swamidass, P., & Morrison, R. (2006). Employee involvement, attitudes, and reactions to technology changes. *Journal of Leadership & Organizational Studies, 12,* 85–101.

Talbert, J. (2009). Distance education: One solution to the nursing shortage? *Clinical Journal of Oncology Nursing, 13*(3), 269–270.

Chapter 12

American Nurses Association. (2008). *Nursing informatics: Scope and standards of practice.* Silver Springs, MD: Nursesbooks.org.

American Nurses Association. (2009). *Education.* Retrieved from http://nursingworld.org/MainMenuCategories/CertificationandAccreditation/AboutNursing/NumbersandDemographics/Education.aspx

Association of College and Research Libraries. (2010). *Introduction to information literacy.* Retrieved from http://www.ala.org/ala/mgrps/divs/acrl/issues/infolit/overview/intro/index.cfm

Bickford, C. J. (2007). The specialty practice of nursing informatics. *CIN: Computers, Informatics, Nursing, 25*(6), 364–366.

Courtney, K. L., Alexander, G. L., & Demiris, G. (2008). Information technology from novice to expert: Implementation implications. *Journal of Nursing Management, 16*(6), 692–699.

Elder, B. L., & Koehn, M. L. (2009). Assessment tool for nursing student computer competencies. *Nursing Education Perspectives, 30*(3), 148–152.

Enhanced Online News. (2009). Study shows 96 percent of doctors concerned about losing the unique patient story with transition to electronic health records. Retrieved from http://eon.businesswire.com/news/eon/20091221005228/en/EHR/EMR/Hitech-act

Garets, D., & Davis, M. (2006). *Electronic medical records vs. electronic health records: Yes, there is a difference—An HIMSS Analytics white paper.* Retrieved from http://www.himssanalytics.org/docs/WP_EMR_EHR.pdf

Gugerty, B., & Delaney, C. (2009). TIGER informatics competencies collaborative (TICC) final report. Retrieved from http://tigercompetencies.pbworks.com/f/TICC_Final.pdf

Hart, M. D. (2008). Informatics competency and development within the U.S. nursing population workforce: A systematic literature review. *CIN: Computers, Informatics, Nursing, 26*(6), 32031–32031.

Health Resources and Services Administration. (2004). The registered nurse population: Findings from the 2004 National Sample Survey of Registered Nurses. Washington, DC. Author. Retrieved from http://bhpr.hrsa.gov/healthworkforce/rnsurvey04/

Healthcare Information and Management Systems Society. (2009). *Clinical decision support.* Retrieved from http://www.himss.org/ASP/topics_clinicalDecision.asp

Healthcare Information and Management Systems Society. (2009a). *EMR adoption model.* Retrieved from http://www.himssanalytics.org/hc_providers/emr_adoption.asp

Healthcare Information and Management Systems Society. (2009b). *HIMSS 2009 informatics nurse impact survey: Final report.* Retrieved from http://www.himss.org/content/files/HIMSS2009 NursingInformaticsImpactSurveyFullResults.pdf

Hebda, T., & Czar, P. (2009). *Handbook of informatics for nurses & healthcare professionals* (4th ed.). Upper Saddle River, NJ: Pearson Prentice Hall.

Nelson, R. (2002). Major theories supporting health care informatics. In S. P. Englebardt & R. Nelson (Eds.), *Health care informatics: An interdisciplinary approach* (pp. 3–27). St. Louis, MO: Mosby.

OpenClinical. (2005). *Electronic medical records, electronic health records.* Retrieved from http://www.openclinical.org/emr.html

Ornes, L. L., & Gassert, C. (2007). Computer competencies in a BSN program. *Journal of Nursing Education, 46*(2), 75–78.

Parker, C. D. (2009). *Crossroads of caring and technology.* Retrieved from http://www.healthcaregoes-mobile.com/content/crossroads-caring-and-technology

Prensky, M. (2001). Digital natives, digital immigrants. *MCB Press, 9*(5), 1–6. Retrieved from http://www.marcprensky.com/writing/Prensky%20-%20Digital%20Natives,%20Digital%20Immigrants%20-%20Part1.pdf

Provost, C., & Gray, M. (2007). Plugged in. Perinatal clinical decision support system: A documentation tool for patient safety. *Nursing for Women's Health, 11*(4), 407–410.

Rutherford, M. A. (2008). Standardized nursing language: What does it mean for nursing practice? *Online Journal of Issues in Nursing, 13*(1). Retrieved from www.nursingworld.org/MainMenu Categories/ANAMarketplace/ANAPeriodicals/OJIN/TableofContents/vol132008/No1Jan08/Article PreviousTopic/StandardizedNursingLanguage.aspx

Saba, V. K., & Riley, J. B. (1997). Nursing informatics in nursing education. *Student Health & Technology Information, 46,* 185–190.

Saletnik, L. A., Niedlinger, M. K., & Wilson, M. (2008). Nursing resource considerations for implementing an electronic documentation system. *AORN Journal, 87*(3), 585.

Tang, P. (2003). *Key capabilities of an electronic health record system: Letter report.* Institute of Medicine Committee on Data Standards for Patient Safety. Retrieved from http://books.nap.edu/openbook. php?isbn=NI000427

TIGER Initiative. (2007). *Evidence and informatics transforming nursing: 3-year action steps toward a 10-year vision.* Retrieved from http://www.aacn.nche.edu/Education/pdf/TIGER.pdf

Wyatt, J., & Spiegelhalter, D. (1990). Evaluating medical expert systems: What to test and how? *Medical Informatics, 15,* 205–217.

Chapter 13

American Association of Colleges of Nursing. (2008). *The essentials of baccalaureate education for professional nursing practice.* Washington, DC: Author.

American Nurses Association. (2008). *Nursing informatics: Scope and standards of practice.* Silver Spring, MD: Author.

Benner, P., Sutphen, M., Leonard, V., & Day, L. (2010). *Educating nurses: A call for radical transformation.* San Francisco: Jossey-Bass.

Berner, E. S. (2009, June). *Clinical decision support systems: State of the art.* Rockville, MD: Agency for Healthcare Research and Quality. (AHRQ Publication No. 09-0069)

Cronenwett, L., Sherwood, G., Barnsteiner, J., Disch, J., Johnson, J., Mitchell, P., et al. (2007). Quality and safety education for nurses. *Nursing Outlook, 55*(3), 122–131.

Curran, C. R. (2008). Faculty development initiatives for integration of informatics competencies and point-of-care technologies in undergraduate nursing education. *The Nursing Clinics of North America, 43*(4), 523–533.

Fetter, M. S. (2007). Curriculum strategies to improve baccalaureate nursing information technology outcomes. *Journal of Nursing Education, 48*(2), 78–85.

Fetter, M. S. (2009). Graduating nurses' self-evaluation of information technology competencies. *Journal of Nursing Education, 48*(2), 86–90.

Ironside, P.M. (n.d.). *Exploring the complexity of advocacy: Balancing patient-centered care and safety.* Retrieved from http://www.qsen.org/teachingstrategy.php?id=58

Leavitt, M. O. (2005). *Statement on health information technology (IT) before the Committee on the Budget, United States Senate*. Retrieved from http://www.hhs.gov/asl/testify/t050720.html

National League for Nursing. (2008). *Preparing the next generation of nurses to practice in a technology-rich environment: An informatics agenda* [Position statement]. Retrieved from http://www.nln.org/aboutnln/PositionStatements/informatics_052808.pdf

Prensky, M. (2001). Digital natives, digital immigrants. *MCB Press, 9*(5), 1–6. Retrieved from http://www.marcprensky.com/writing/Prensky%20-%20Digital%20Natives,%20Digital%20Immigrants%20-%20Part1.pdf

Technology Informatics Guiding Educational Reform. (2009a). *TIGER informatics competencies collaborative (TICC)*. Retrieved from http://tigercompetencies.pbworks.com/f/TICC_Final.pdf

TIGER Initiative. (2009b). *Collaborating to integrate evidence and informatics into nursing practice and education: An executive summary*. Retrieved from http://www.tigersummit.com/uploads/TIGER_Collaborative_Exec_Summary_040509.pdf

TIGER Initiative. (2009c). *Informatics competencies for every practicing nurse: Recommendations from the TIGER collaborative*. Retrieved from http://www.tigersummit.com/uploads/3.Tiger.Report_Competencies_final.pdf

TIGER Initiative. (2009d). *Transforming education for an informatics agenda: TIGER education and faculty development collaborative*. Retrieved from http://www.tigersummit.com/uploads/Educ.Tiger.Report_final4.pdf

Weiner, E. E. (Ed.). (2008) *Technology: The interface to nursing educational informatics*. Philadelphia: W. B. Saunders.

Chapter 14

Abraham, M. J. (2007). Blended learning: Integrating an e-learning component for competency validation [Abstract]. *Advances in Teaching and Learning Day Abstracts, 18*. Houston Academy of Medicine-Texas Medical Center. Retrieved from http://digitalcommons.library.tmc.edu/uthshis_atldayabs/18/

Atack, L. (2003). Becoming a Web-based learner: Registered nurses' experiences. *Journal of Advanced Nursing, 44*(3), 289–297.

Bierema, L. L., & Merriam, S. B. (2002). E-mentoring: Using computer mediated communication to enhance the mentoring process. *Innovative Higher Education, 26*(3), 211–227.

Brinkerhoff, R. O., & Montesino, M. U. (1995). Partnerships for training transfer: Lessons from a corporate study. *Human Resource Development Quarterly, 6*(3), 263–274.

Broad, M. L. (2000). Ensuring transfer of learning to the job. In G. M. Piskurich, P. Beckschi, & B. Hall (Eds.), *The ASTD handbook of training design and delivery* (pp. 430–452). New York: McGraw-Hill.

Broad, M. L., & Newstrom, J. W. (1992). *Transfer of training: Action-packed strategies to ensure high payoff from training investments*. Reading, MA: Perseus.

Chambers, L. W.,Conklin, J., Dalziel, W. B., MacDonald, C. J., & Stodel, E. J. (2008). E-learning education to promote interprofessional education with physicians, pharmacists, nurses and nurse practitioners in long-term care facilities: Promising potential solutions. *International Journal of Biomedical Engineering and Technology, 1*(3), 233–249.

Clark, R. C. & Mayer, R. E. (2008). *E-learning and the science of instruction*. San Francisco: Pfeiffer.

Clark, R., Nguyen, F., & Sweller, J. (2006). *Efficiency in learning: Evidence-based guidelines to manage cognitive load*. San Francisco: Pfeiffer.

Corry, M., & Watkins, R. (2007). Strategy for the learner: A student's guide to e-learning success. In B. Brandon (Ed.), *The e-learning guild's handbook of e-learning strategy* (ch. 6), pp. 63–68.

Dolezalek, H. (2005). 2005 industry report. *Training, 42*(12), 14–28.

Ensher, E. A., Heun, C., & Blanchard, A. (2003). Online mentoring and computer-mediated communication: New directions in research. *Journal of Vocational Behavior, 63*(2), 264–288.

Gilbert, T. F. (1996). *Human competence: Engineering worthy performance*. New York: McGraw Hill.

Goettner, P. (2000, December). Effective e-learning for health care. *Health Management Technology, 21*(12), 64.

Goldsworthy, S., Graham, L., Robinson, J. & Campkin, M. (2008). Learning at your fingertips: New directions for accessible critical care education—A Canadian perspective [Abstract]. *Critical Care Nurse, 28*(2), e36.

Huckstadt, A., & Hayes, K. (2005). Evaluation of interactive online courses for advanced practice nurses. *Journal of the American Academy of Nurse Practitioners, 17*(3), 85–89.

Hulkari, K., & Mahlamaki-Kultanen, S. (2008). Reflection through Web discussions: Assessing nursing students' work-based learning. *Journal of Workplace Learning, 20*(3), 157–164.

Irons, B. K., Vickers, P., Esperat, C., Valdez, G. M., Dadich, K. A., Boswell, C., & Cannon, S. (2007). The need for a community diabetes education curriculum for healthcare professionals. *Journal of Continuing Education in Nursing, 38*(5), 227–231.

Johnson, K. (2004, October 18). Increasing training compliance rates at children's hospitals with e-learning. *E-Learning Developers' Journal,* 1–12.

Jukkula, A. M., Henly, S. J., & Lindeke, L.L. (2008). Rural perceptions of continuing professional education. *Journal of Continuing Education in Nursing, 39*(12), 555–563.

Kampa-Kokesch, S., & Anderson, M. Z. (2001). Executive coaching: A comprehensive review of the literature. *Consulting Psychology Journal: Practice and Research, 53*(4), 205–228.

Karpowicz, M. (2008). Continuum of competence: Trials of educating in a tele-ICU [Abstract]. *Critical Care Nurse, 28*(2), e5.

Kasprisin, C. A., Single, P. B., Single, R. M., & Muller, C. B. (2003). Building a better bridge: Testing e-training to improve e-mentoring programmes in higher education. *Mentoring & Tutoring: Partnership in Learning, 11*(1), 67–78.

Kirkpatrick, D. L. (1998). *Evaluating training programs* (2nd ed.). San Francisco: Berrett-Koehler.

Knapp, B. (2004). Competency: An essential component of caring in nursing. *Nursing Administration Quarterly, 28*(4), 285–287.

Miller, L. C., Devaney, S. W. , Kelly, G. L., & Kuehn, A. F. (2008). E-mentoring in public health nursing practice. *Journal of Continuing Education in Nursing, 39*(9), 394–399.

Molinari, D. L., Monserud, M., & Hudzinski, D. (2008). A new type of rural nurse residency. *Journal of Continuing Education in Nursing, 39*(1), 42–46.

Nelson, B. C., & Erlandson, B. E. (2008). Managing cognitive load in educational multi-user virtual environments: reflection on design practice. *Educational Technology, Research and Development, 56,* 619–641.

O'Neill, D. K., Weiler, M., & Sha, L. (2005). Software support for online mentoring programs: A research-inspired design. *Mentoring & Tutoring: Partnership in Learning, 13*(1), 109–131.

Paloff, R. M., & Pratt, K. (2007). *Building online learning communities: Effective strategies for the virtual classroom.* San Francisco: Wiley.

Peddocord, K. M., Holsclaw, P., Jacobson, I. G., Kwizera, L., Rose, K., Gersberg, R., & Macias-Reynolds, V. (2007). Nationwide satellite training for public health professionals: Web-based follow-up. *Journal of Continuing Education in the Health Professions, 27*(2), 111–117.

Perry, B. (2008). Shine on: Achieving career satisfaction as a registered nurse. *Journal of Continuing Education in Nursing, 39*(1), 17–25.

Pullen, D. L. (2006). An evaluative case study of online learning for healthcare professionals. *Journal of Continuing Education in Nursing, 37*(5), 225–232.

Rick, C., Kearns, M. A., & Thompson, N. A. (2003). The reality of virtual learning for nurses in the largest integrated health care system in the nation. *Nursing Administration Quarterly, 27*(1), 41–57.

Russell, A., & Perris, K. (2003). Telementoring in community nursing: A shift from dyadic to communal models of learning and professional development. *Mentoring & Tutoring: Partnership in Learning, 11*(2), 227–238.

Senge, P. (1990). *The fifth discipline: The art and practice of the learning organization.* New York: Currency Doubleday.

Shank, P. (2004, September 7). Can they do it in the real world? Designing for transfer of learning. *E-Learning Developers' Journal,* 1–7.

Sheen, S., Chang, W., Chen, H., Chao, H., & Tseng, C. (2008) E-learning education program for registered nurses: The experience of a teaching medical center. *Journal of Nursing Research, 16*(3), 195–200.

Slotte, V., & Herbert, A. (2006). Putting professional development online: Integrating learning as productive activity. *Journal of Workplace Learning, 18*(4), 235–247.

Spivey, D. (2009). The OODA loop and learning. *Chief Learning Officer, 8*(10), 30–33.

Van Adelsberg, D., & Trolley, E. A. (1999). *Running training like a business: Delivering unmistakable value.* San Francisco: Berrett-Koehler.

VanTiem, D. M., Moseley, J. L., & Conway Dessinger, J. (2004). *Fundamentals of performance technology: A guide to improving people, process, and performance* (2nd ed.). Silver Spring, MD: International Society for Performance Improvement.

Chapter 15

Alag, S. (2008) *Collective intelligence in action*. Greenwich, CT: Manning.

Davenport, C. B. (2004, October). What nurses need to know about personal digital assistants (PDAs). *Online Journal of Nursing Informatics, 8*(3). Retrieved from http://ojni.org/8_3/davenport.htm

Geroge, L. E., & Davidson, L. J. (2005). PDA use in nursing education: Prepared for today, posed for tomorrow. *Online Journal of Nursing Informatics, 9*(2). Retrieved from http://ojni.org/9_2/george.htm

Hrastinski, S. (2008). *Asynchronous and synchronous e-learning: A study of asynchronous and synchronous e-learning methods discovered that each supports different purpose. Educause Quarterly, 31*(1). Retrieved from http://www.cdn.educause.edu/EDUCAUSE+Quarterly/EDUCAUSEQuarterlyMagazineVolum/AsynchronousandSynchronousELea/163445

Korvick, L. (2009) *The net generation and audience response system technology.* Retrieved from wwwhttp://.liveclasstech.com/LinkClick.aspx?fileticket=nA1OL46f%2fyY%3d&tabid=91

Mason, S., & Davis, M. (2000) *A teacher's guide to videoconferencing: How to plan, produce, present, manage, and assess a distance learning class*. Retrieved from Northwest Regional Educational Laboratory Web site http://www.netc.org/digitalbridges/teachersguide/toc.html

Pelman, A. M. (2009, September). The legal ethics of metadata mining. *Akron Law Review* (forthcoming), *9*(40). Retrieved from Suffolk University Law School Web Site: http://ssrn.com/abstract=1472712

Sloane, M. M. (2008). Remote-presence robot attends patients at Ryder Trauma Center. *Nursing Spectrum–Florida News*. Retrieved from http://news.nurse.com/apps/pbcs.dll/article?AID=200880415010

Agnihotri, R. (2009). The effective use of technology in personal knowledge management: A framework of skills, tools, and user content. *Online Information Review, 33*(2), 329–342.

Bracey, G. (2009). *Robots in education*. Retrieved from http://www.huffingtonpost.com/gerald-bracey/robots-in-education_b_215883.html

Chambers, P. D. (2010). Tap the unique strengths of the millennial generation. *Nursing 2010, 2*, 48–51.

Day, C. W. (2008). Up close. *American School & University, 81*(1).

Demiray, U., & Sharma, R. C. (Eds.). (2009) Ethical practices and implications in distance learning. Hershey, PA: Information Science Reference.

Kuiper, R. A. (2010) Metacognitive factors that impact student nurse use of point of care technology in clinical settings. *International Journal of Nursing Education Scholarship, 7*(1), Article 5. Retrieved from http://www.bepress.com/ijnes/vol7/iss1/art5

LaPrad, J., & Mink, A. (2009). *The ECHO model of experiential learning*. Retrieved from http://www.facultyfocus.com/author/jim-la-prad-and-andy-mink/

Manzo, K. K. (2009, August). NAEP draft on technological literacy unveiled: Test to gauge knowledge of tools and their use and impact on society. *Education Week, 29*(1), 9.

Meedzan, N., & Fisher, K. (2009, June). Clickers in nursing education: An active learning tool in the classroom. *Online Journal of Nursing Informatics, 13*(2), 1–19. Retrieved from http://ojni.org/13_2/Meedzan_Fisher.pdf

National Information Standards Organization. (2004). *Understanding metadata*. Retrieved March 6, 2010, from http://www.niso.org/publications/press/UnderstandingMetadata.pdf

Prensky, M. (2001). *Digital natives, digital immigrants*. Retrieved from www.marcprensky.com/writing/Prensky%20%20Digital%20Natives,%20Digital%20Immigrants%20-%20Part1.pdf

Robinson, E. *Mobile learning and handheld devices in the classroom*. Corvallis, OR: Robby Robson, Eduworks Corporation. Retrieved from http://www.eduworks.com/Documents/Publications/Mobile_Learning_Handheld_Classroom.pdf

Rosenfeld, B. (2008). The challenges of teaching with technology: From computer idiocy to computer competence. *International Journal of Instructional Media, 35*(2), 157–166.

SMART Technologies ULC. (2010). *Interactive whiteboards and learning improving student learning outcomes and streamlining lesson planning*. Retrieved from http://www2.smarttech.com/

SMART Technologies ULC. (2010). *Creating classrooms for everyone: How interactive whiteboards support Universal Design for Learning* [White paper]. Retrieved from http://www2.smarttech.com/NR/rdonlyres/BAEE09C6-0871-46BE-AE23-70A787F184E0/0/Interactivewhiteboardsanduniversaldesign-forlearningJan20.pdf

Weiss, M. (2008). Reach beyond use and usability and focus on impact by combining marketing and interaction design to improve academic Website development. *Educause Quarterly, 31*(4). Retrieved from http://www.cdn.educause.edu/EDUCAUSE%2BQuarterly/EDUCAUSEQuarterlyMagazineVolum/ResultsBasedInteractionDesign/163444

Zurmehly, J. (2010). Personal digital assistants (PDAs): Review and evaluation. *Nursing Education Perspectives, 31*(3), 179–182.

Chapter 16

Bambini, D., Washburn, J., & Perkins, R. (2009). Outcomes of clinical simulation for novice nursing students: Communication, confidence, clinical judgment. *Nursing Education Perspectives, 30*(2), 79–82.

Benner, P., Sutphen, M., Leonard, V., & Day, L. (2009). *Educating nurses: A call for radical transformation.* Jossey-Bass: San Francisco.

Bradley, P. (2006). The history of simulation in medical education and possible future directions. *Medical Education History, 40,* 245–262.

Cantrell, M. A., (2008). The importance of debriefing in clinical simulation. *Clinical Simulation in Nursing, 4,* e19–e23.

Cooper, J. B., & Taqueti, V. R. (2004). A brief history of development mannequin simulators for clinical education and training. *Quality Safe Health Care, 13*(Suppl. 1), i11–i18.

Decker, S. I. (2007). *Simulation as an educational strategy in the development of critical and reflective thinking: A qualitative exploration* (Unpublished doctoral dissertation). Denton: Texas Woman's University.

Decker, S., Moore, A., Thal, W., Opton, L., Caballero, S., & Beasley. (2010). Synergistic integration of concept mapping and cause and effect diagramming into simulated experiences [Manuscript submitted for publication]. *Clinical Simulation in Nursing.*

Del Bueno, D. (2005). A crisis in critical thinking [Electronic version]. *Nursing Education Perspectives, 26*(5), 278–282.

Fanning, R. M., & Gaba, D. M. (2007). The role of debriefing in simulation-based learning. *Simulation in Healthcare: The Journal of the Society for Simulation in Healthcare, 2*(2), 115–125.

Finkelman, A., & Kenner, C. (2007). *Teaching IOM: Implications of the IOM report for nursing education.* Silver Spring, MD: American Nurses Association.

Gaba, D. (2004). The future vision of simulation in health care. *Quality and Safety in Healthcare, 13*(Suppl. 1), i2–i10.

Gaba, D. M., Howard, S. K., Smith, B. E., & Sowb, Y. A. (2001). Simulation-based training in anesthesia crisis resource management (ACRM): A decade of experiences. *Simulation and Gaming, 69,* 387–394.

Gordon, C. J., & Buckely, T. (2009). The effects of high-fidelity simulation training on medical–surgical graduate nurses' perceived ability to respond to patient clinical emergencies. *Journal of Continuing Education in Nursing, 40*(11), 491–498.

Henderson, P., & Johnson, M. H. (2002). An innovative approach to developing the reflective skills of medical students [Electronic version]. *BioMed Central BMC Medical Education, 2*(4), 1–4.

Herrmann, E. K. (2000, March–May). Connecticut nursing history vignettes. *Connecticut Nursing News,* Retrieved from http://homepage.ntlworld.com/bleep/SimHist1.html

Howard, V. M., Ross, C., Mitchell, A. M., & Nelson, G. M. (2010). Human patient simulators and interactive case studies a comparative analysis of learning outcomes and student perceptions. *Computers, Informatics, Nursing, 28*(1), 42–48.

Jeffries, P. R. (2005). A framework for designing, implementing and evaluating simulations used as teaching strategies in nursing. *Nursing Education Perspectives, 26*(2), 96–103.

Jeffries, P. R. (Ed.). (2007). *Simulation in nursing education for conceptualization to evaluation.* New York: National League for Nursing.

Johns, C. (1995). Framing learning through reflection within Carper's fundamental ways of knowing in nursing. *Journal of Advanced Nursing, 22*(2), 226–234.

Johns, C. (2004). *Becoming a reflective practitioner* (2nd ed.). Malden, MA: Blackwell.

Lasater, K. (2007). High-fidelity simulation and the development of clinical judgment: Students' Experiences. *Journal of Nursing Education, 46*(6), 269–275.

Mezirow, J. (1981). *Transformative dimensions of adult learning.* San Francisco: Jossey-Bass.

Morgan, P. G. (1995) Creating a laboratory that simulates the critical care environment. *Critical Care Nurse. 16*(6), 76–81.

National Council of State Boards of Nursing. (2005). *Clinical instruction in prelicensure nursing programs.* Retrieved August 22, 2006, from http:/www.ncsbn.org/pdfs/Final_Clinical_Instruction_Prelicensure_Nursing_Programs.pdf

Nehring, W. N., & Lashley, F. R. (2010). *High-fidelity patient simulation.* Boston: Jones & Bartlett.

Pesut, D. J., & Herman, J. (1999). *Clinical reasoning: The art and science of critical and creative thinking.* Albany, NY: Delmar.

Rall, M., Manser, T., & Howard, S. K. (2000). Key elements of debriefing for simulator training. *European Journal of Anaesthesiology, 17*(8), 516–517.

Rudolph. J. W., Simon, R., Rivard, P., Dufresne, R. L., & Raemer, D. B. (2007). Debriefing with good judgment: Combining rigorous feedback with genuine inquiry. *Anesthesiology Clinics, 25*(2), 361–376.

Schön, D. A. (1987). *Educating the reflective practitioner.* San Francisco: Jossey-Bass.

Shapiro, M. J., Gardner, R., Godwin, S.A., Jay, G., Lindquist, D., Salisbury, M. & Salas, E. (2008). Defining team performance for simulation-based training: Methodology, metrics, and opportunities for emergency medicine. *Academic Emergency Medicine, 15*(11), 1088–1097.

Smith, S. J., & Roehrs, C. J. (2009). High-fidelity simulation: Factors correlated with nursing students satisfaction and self-confidence. *Nursing Education Perspectives, 30*(2), 74–78.

Chapter 17

American Association of Colleges of Nursing. (2005). *Alliance for nursing accreditation statement on distance education policies.* Retrieved April 19, 2009, from http://www.aacn.nche.edu/education/disstate.htm

Baker, B. H., & Perkins, G. B. (2008). Internet surveys: Obtaining feedback from clinical site coordinators. *Nurse Educator, 13*(3), 128–130.

Commission on Collegiate Nursing Education. (2008). *Standards for accreditation of baccalaureate and graduate degree nursing programs.* Retrieved from http://www.aacn.nche.edu/Accreditation/index.htm

Council for Higher Education Institute for Research and Study of Accreditation and Quality Assurance. (2002). *Accreditation and assuring quality in distance education* [CHEA Monograph Series 2002, No. 1]. Retrieved from http://www.chea.org/pdf/mono_2_spec-accred_02.pdf

Higher Learning Commission. (n.d.-a). *Statement of commitment by the regional accrediting commissions for the evaluation of electronically offered degree and certificate programs.* Retrieved from www.hlcommission.org/index.php?option=com_docman&task=doc_download&gid=394&Itemid=236

Higher Learning Commission. (n.d.-b). *Best practices for electronically offered degree and certificate programs.* Retrieved from www.ncahlc.org/download/Best_Pract_DEd.pdf

Jeffries, P. (2005). A framework for designing, implementing and evaluating simulations used as teaching strategies in nursing. *Nursing Education Perspectives, 26,* 96–103.

Jeffries, P. (2009). Dreams for the future for clinical simulation. *Nursing Education Perspectives, 30*(2), 71.

National Council of State Boards of Nursing. (2005). *Clinical instruction in prelicensure nursing programs.* Retrieved April 19, 2009, from https://www.ncsbn.org/Final_Clinical_Instr_Pre_Nsg_programs.pdf

National League for Nursing. (2008). *About the NLN: History.* Retrieved at http://www.nln.org/aboutnln/info-history.htm

National League for Nursing Accreditation Commission. (2008) *NLNAC accreditation manual.* New York: NLNAC. Retrieved from http://www.nlnac.org/manuals/Manual2008.htm

Nelson, R. (2010). Distance education technology: Implications for nursing education. In L. Caputi (Ed.), *Teaching nursing: The art and science, vol. 2* (2nd ed.). Glen Ellyn, IL: College of DuPage Press.

Newsome, G., & Tanner, S. (2010). Nursing accreditation: Context and evolution. In L. Caputi (Ed.), *Teaching nursing: The art and science, vol. 3* (2nd ed.). Glen Ellyn, IL: College of DuPage Press.

Smith, M. M. (2009). Creative clinical solutions: Aligning simulation with authentic clinical experiences. *Nursing Education Perspectives, 30*(2), 126–128.

Spector, N. (2010). Approval: National council of state boards of nursing. In L. Caputi (Ed.), *Teaching nursing: The art and science, vol. 3* (2nd ed.). Glen Ellyn, IL: College of DuPage Press.

Tagliarenia, M. E. (2009). Beyond the realities of current practice: Preparing students to provide safe and effective care. *Nursing Education Perspectives, 30*(2), 69.

Chapter 18

Forterra Systems Inc. (n.d.). *Healthcare.* Retrieved from http://www.forterrainc.com/index.php/industries/healthcare

IBM. (2008). *IBM Develops a "Rehearsal Studio" to Let You Practice Your Job in a 3-D World.* Retrieved from http://www-03.ibm.com/press/us/en/pressrelease/23798.wss

Johnson, C., Vorderstrasse, A., & Shaw, R. (2009). Virtual worlds in health care higher education. *Journal of Virtual Worlds Research, 2*(2). Retrieved from http://jvwresearch.org/index.php?_cms=1248968023

Lofgren, E., & Fefferman, N. (2007). The untapped potential of virtual game worlds to shed light on real world epidemics. *The Lancet Infectious Diseases 7*(9), 625–629. Retrieved from http://www.thelancet.com/journals/laninf/article/PIIS1473-3099(07)70212-8/abstract.

Prensky, M. (2009). H. Sapiens Digital: From Digital Immigrants and Digital Natives to Digital Wisdom, *Innovate.* Retrieved from http://www.innovateonline.info/pdf/vol5_issue3/H._Sapiens_Digital-__From_Digital_Immigrants_and_Digital_Natives_to_Digital_Wisdom.pdf

Royse, M., & Newton, S. (2007). How gaming is used as an innovative strategy for nursing education. *Nursing Education Perspectives, 28*(5), 263–267. Retrieved from http://findarticles.com/p/articles/mi_hb3317/is_5_28/ai_n29380070/?tag=content;col1

Second Life Education Wiki. Retrieved from SimTeach, http://www.simteach.com/wiki/index.php?title=Second_Life_Education_Wiki

Serious Games for Healthcare Markets. Retrieved from Breakaway Games Ltd, http://www.breakawaygames.com/serious-games/solutions/healthcare/

Solution Provider Directory. Retrieved from Second Life, http://solutionproviders.secondlife.com/

The New Media Consortium and The Educause Learning Initiative (0029). *2009 Horizon Report.* Retrieved from http://wp.nmc.org/horizon2009/

Vasileiou, V., & Paraskeva, F. (2010) Teaching role-playing instruction in Second Life: An exploratory study. *Journal of Information, Information Technology, and Organizations, 5.* Retrieved from http://www.jiito.org/articles/JIITOv5p025-050Vasileiou431.pdf

Virtual Ability Inc. Retrieved from http://virtualability.org/default.aspx

Virtual Worlds for Training and Education. (2010). Retrieved from Daden Limited, http://www.daden.co.uk/news/25_may_2010_daden_release_whit.html

Wiecha, J., Heyden, R., Sternthal, E., & Merialdi, M.(2010). Learning in a virtual world: Experience with using Second Life for medical education. *Journal of Medical Internet Research, (12)*1. Retrieved from http://www.ncbi.nlm.nih.gov/pmc/articles/PMC2821584/

World of Warcraft. (2010). Retrieved from http://www.worldofwarcraft.com/index.xml

Note: Page numbers followed by *f* indicate figures, page numbers followed by *b* indicate boxes, page numbers followed by *t* indicate tables.